Endovascular Treatment of Arterial Emergencies

Stevo Duvnjak

Endovascular Treatment of Arterial Emergencies

Springer

Stevo Duvnjak
Department of Vascular Surgery
Rigshospitalet
København
Denmark

ISBN 978-3-030-68831-8 ISBN 978-3-030-68832-5 (eBook)
https://doi.org/10.1007/978-3-030-68832-5

This Springer imprint is published by the registered company Springer Nature Switzerland AG
The registered company address is: Gewerbestrasse 11, 6330 Cham, Switzerland

To all my teachers in Interventional Radiology and Vascular Surgery in Serbia and Denmark.

Preface

The endovascular treatment of arterial and venous diseases is unavoidable in daily practice. The development of new devices and improvements in currently available devices ensure the steadily increasing usage of endovascular methods. Emergencies are a part of everyday practice, and mastering endovascular knowledge and techniques provides a good outcome for our patients. This book presents a practical overview of endovascular treatment in an arterial emergency, including the most common clinical scenarios. The cases presented in the book are from my experience during work at the Department of Radiology, Odense University Hospital, Denmark. There are many books available covering endovascular treatment, but few have focused on arterial emergencies alone. Therefore, this book may be valuable for different target groups, including vascular surgery, interventional radiology, cardiology, and emergency surgery. Experienced, resident, and young doctors can use this book for a quick overview and to reference treatment options in acute cases during their clinical work. The book covers the majority of arterial emergencies than can be seen in clinical practice. Many quality images of arterial emergencies and treatments and their descriptions can provide readers with the necessary knowledge on and provide insight into endovascular options.

The book describes the treatment of complex and standard thoracic vascular emergency cases, followed by abdominal emergency and peripheral arterial emergency cases. At the beginning of each case, a few critical remarks that should be considered during the decision-making process are emphasized.

Copenhagen, Denmark — Stevo Duvnjak

Contents

Abbreviations

ABI	Ankle-brachial index
ACT	Activating clotting time
CRP	C reactive protein
CT	Computed tomography
DMSO	Dimethyl sulphoxide
ECG	Electrocardiogram
ECMO	Extracorporeal membrane oxygenation
eGFR	Estimated glomerular filtration rate
EVAR	Endovascular aortic aneurysm repair
FDG-PET	Fluorodeoxyglucose positron emission tomography
FEVAR	Fenestrated endovascular aortic repair
Fr	French
HHT	Haemorrhagic hereditary telangiectasia
IM	Intramural haematoma
IU	International unit
LIMA-LAD	Left internal mammary-left descending artery bypass
mmHg	Millimetre of mercury
MR	Magnetic resonance
MRI	Magnetic resonance imaging
NSCLC	Non-small-cell lung cancer
PAU	Penetrating aortic ulcer
PAVM	Pulmonary arteriovenous malformation
PC	Phase-contrast
PTFE	Polytetrafluorethylene
SMA	Superior mesenteric artery
SSFP	Balanced steady-state free precession
TEVAR	Thoracic endovascular aortic repair
TOF	Time of flight

1 Endovascular Armamentarium in Vascular Emergencies

Contents

1.1 Introduction

Existing endovascular devices are constantly being improved and new devices are continuously being developed, allowing for more effective treatment of arterial emergencies. There are a variety of diagnostic catheters and microcatheters available on the market, both of which are necessary tools for treating these conditions. Stent grafts and embolization materials are often used in the treatment of arterial emergencies, with many different kinds currently available. It is of utmost importance to familiarize oneself with the different types of stent grafts and their indications, and deployment mechanisms. Knowledge and proper use of various embolic materials are absolute prerequisites for the delivery of successful and safe treatments.

1.1.1 Catheters and Microcatheters

There are two types of catheters: flushing with multiple side holes and selective angiographic catheters. Flushing catheters are used for diagnostic angiography, and selective catheters with different shapes enable the selective catheterization of target vessels. Most catheters are made of polyethene, polyurethane, nylon or Teflon and come in different sizes, lengths, and forms [1]. Usually, for diagnostic aortography, a 5 Fr flush catheter such as the Pigtail or Omni Flush is used (Fig. 1.1). Catheters are 0.035- or 0.038-in. guidewire compatible, while the over-the-wire technique is used for catheter advancement and exchange. The catheter length is usually 65 cm or 100 cm, but some are 125 cm or 135 cm long. The French unit (Fr) is used for sizing the catheter outer diameter [2]. Diagnostic catheters usually have a size of 4 or 5 Fr. Catheters with radiopaque marks tend to be used for determining the stent-graft length. Guiding catheters are used to advance different balloons, stents and

S. Duvnjak, *Endovascular Treatment of Arterial Emergencies*,
https://doi.org/10.1007/978-3-030-68832-5_1

stent grafts in the target vessels. They are also used for angiography during the deployment of the different devices. Guiding catheters have a length of 40 or 100 cm. They usually do not have a haemostatic valve, which is the main difference with sheaths [3].

Microcatheters, used for peripheral arterial emergencies, are small catheters with sizes of 2.0 and 2.1 Fr, 2.4 Fr or 2.7 and 2.8 or 2.9 Fr. A microcatheter is used for super-selective angiography and embolization because it is possible to place them distally in small and tortuous vessels. They are made from the same material as catheters and come in different shapes, lengths and sizes (Fig. 1.2). 0.021 in. microcatheters are compatible with micro-coils, while 0.027 in. microcatheters are high-flow microcatheters used for microsphere embolization.

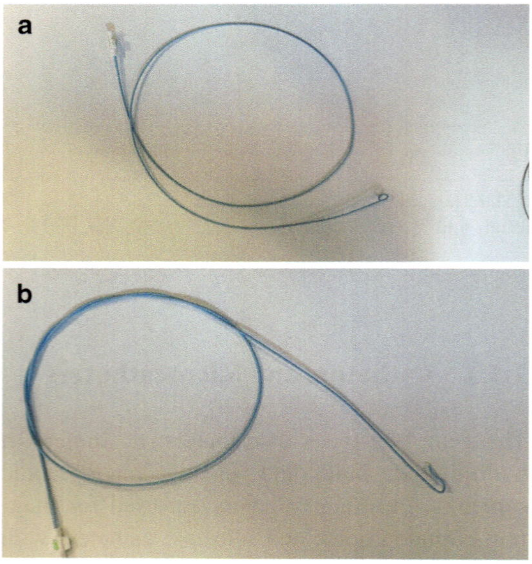

Fig. 1.1 Flushing catheter with multiple side holes for diagnostic angiography (**a**). Selective catheter for selective angiography (**b**)

1.1.2 Stent Grafts

Generally, there are two major types of stent grafts: peripheral stent grafts used for peripheral artery treatment (Fig. 1.3) and aortic stent grafts used for either thoracic or abdominal aortic diseases (Figs. 1.4 and 1.5). Stent grafts

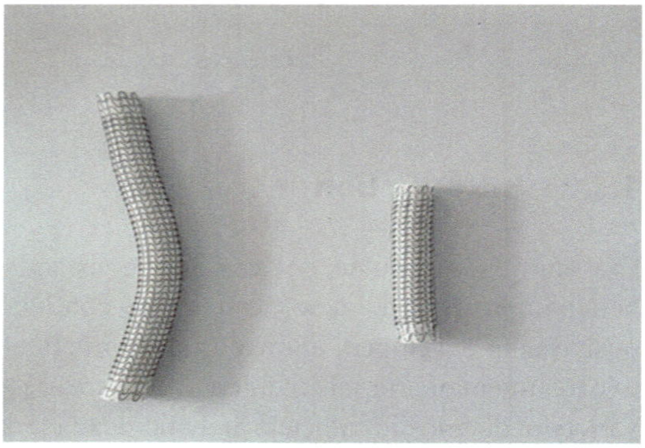

Fig. 1.3 Examples of one kind of peripheral stent graft available in different lengths

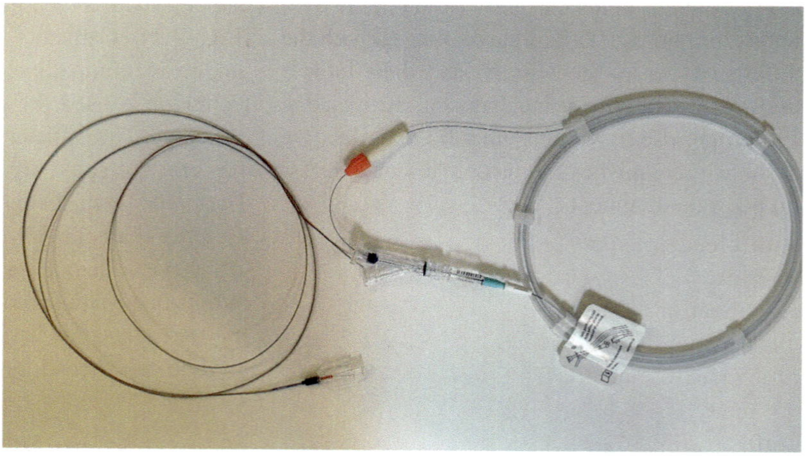

Fig. 1.2 Microcatheter compatible with 0.010, 0.014, 0.016 or 0.018 micro guidewire

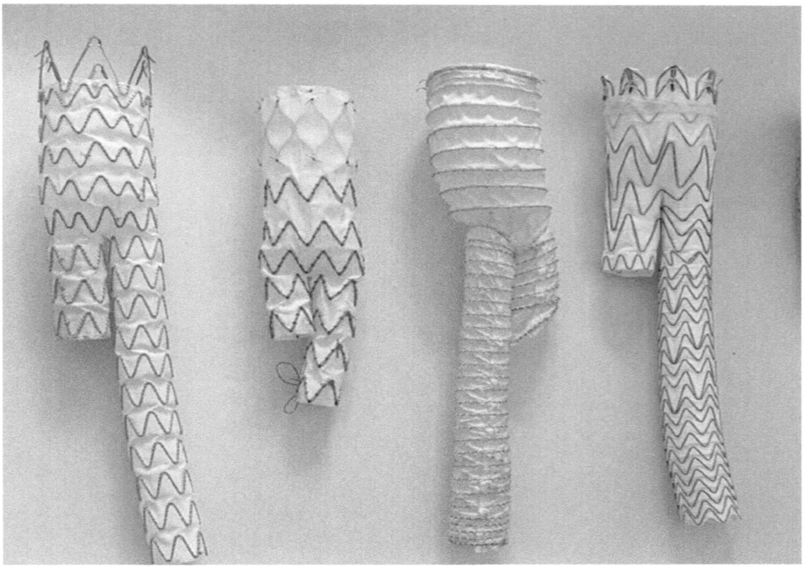

Fig. 1.4 Different types of abdominal aortic endografts for the treatment of infrarenal abdominal aortic aneurysms

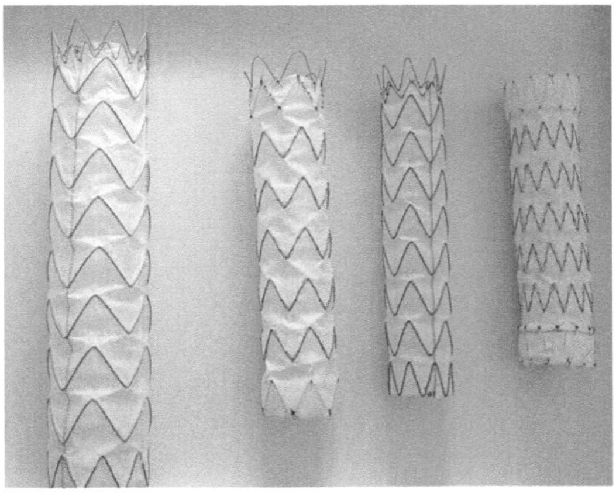

Fig. 1.5 Different types of thoracic endovascular grafts for the treatment of thoracic aorta pathologies

are made of polyester (Dacron) or polytetrafluorethylene (PTFE) and a metallic frame [4]. They are primarily used for treating aortic or peripheral aneurysms and traumatic lesions with bleeding, recovering thrombi or atherosclerotic debris and avoiding further distal embolization. Stent grafts are also used to treat aortic dissections, peripheral atherosclerotic diseases and arteriovenous fistulas. There are many types of aortic and peripheral stent grafts available; however, a detailed overview of their designs, use, and characteristics is beyond the scope of this book.

1.1.3 Mechanical Embolization Materials

Mechanical embolization materials include micro- and macro-coils and vascular plugs made mostly of platinum or alloy (although stainless steel was used previously) (Fig. 1.6) [5]. Micro-coils come in sizes from 2 mm up to 32 mm and in different lengths and be delivered through a microcatheter. Macro-coils can be advanced to the target vessels through a 4 Fr catheter. Vascular plugs are used for large vessel occlusion and can be delivered through a 5 Fr catheter or a 6 to 8 Fr sheath. Micro plugs can also be delivered through a microcatheter. Mechanical embolization materials are very safe and can be used alone or together with other embolization materials. Macro- and micro-coils can be classified as detachable or pushable; detachable coils can be retrieved if the initial position is unsatisfactory. Micro- and macro-coils oversizing should be approximately 15% of the target vessel diameter, while that for vascular plugs is usually between 30 and 50%.

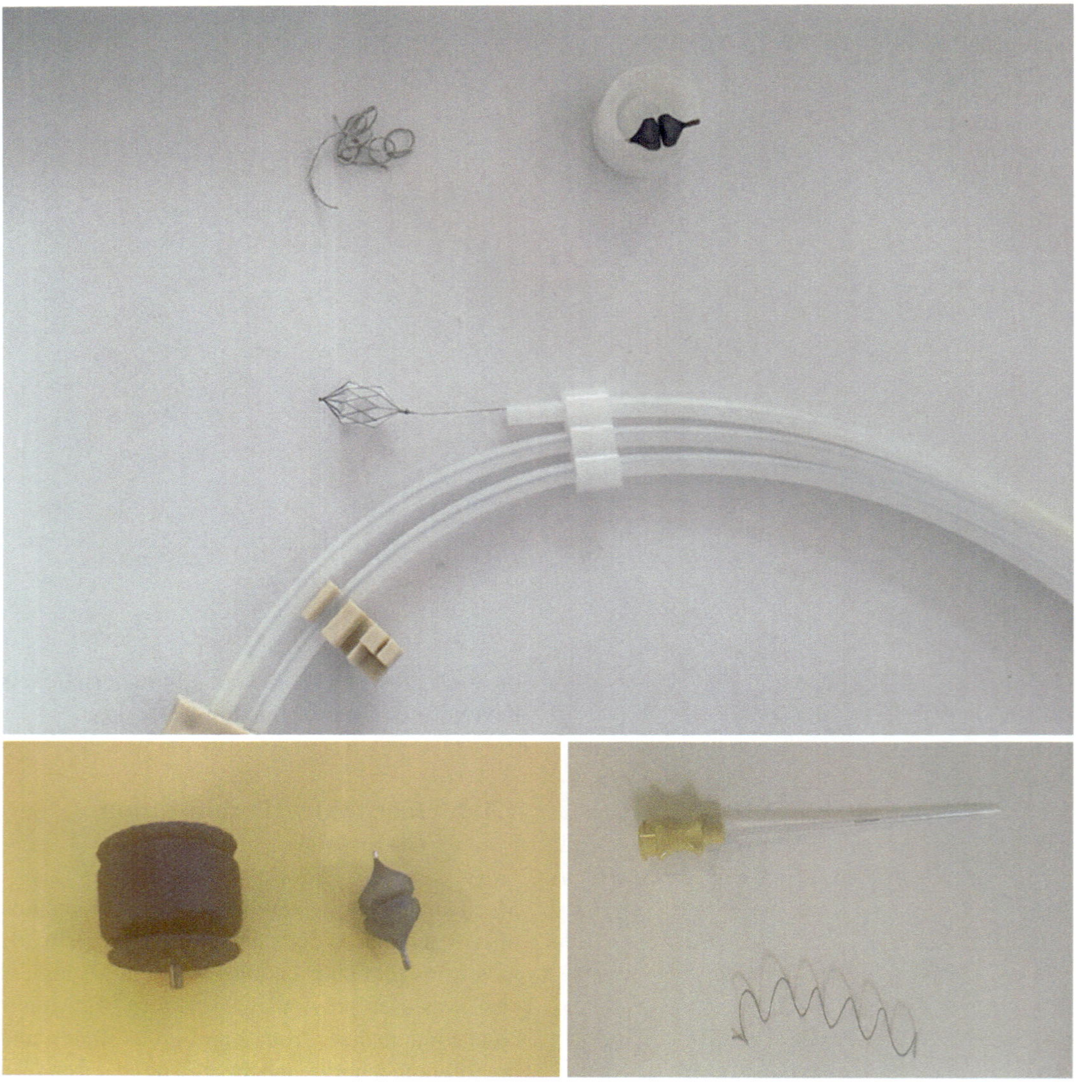

Fig. 1.6 Mechanical embolization devices, micro-coils, micro-plugs and Amplatz vascular plugs

1.1.4 Liquid Embolization Materials and Microspheres

Liquid embolic agents destroy the endothelium of the artery permanently. There are various liquid embolic materials available today. Generally, embolic agents are challenging to control, and experience is essential to avoid non-target embolization. Ethanol is one example of a liquid embolic agent that is very challenging to use, as many complications can occur. Therefore, the use of ethanol today is limited. *N*-butyl-2-cyanoacrylate glue or tissue adhesive is another liquid embolic agent that is challenging to use but very useful, especially in the treatment of bleeding in patients with an abnormal coagulation status. Glue causes an inflammatory endothelial reaction with fibrotic changes [6]. Onyx, an ethylene-vinyl alcohol copolymer, is a non-adhesive biocompatible liquid agent that is frequently used for embolization due to its more comfortable and safer handling than glue or ethanol [7]. Microcatheters compatible with dimethyl sulfoxide (DMSO) need to be flushed with DMSO prior to the use of Onyx.

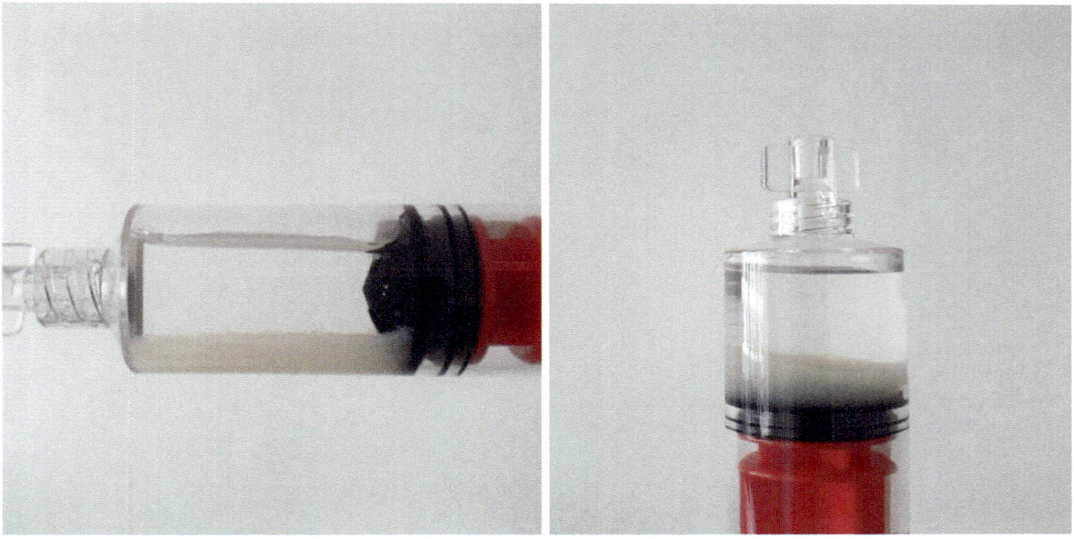

Fig. 1.7 Spherical microparticles of different sizes, ranging from 40 to 1200 μm

Spherical microspheres (Fig. 1.7) and non-spherical polyvinyl alcohol particles (PVA) are primarily used for tumour embolization. Today, microspheres are usually used due to their uniform size, which ranges from 40 to 1200 μm. The microspheres are delivered through a microcatheter and are used for more distal occlusions. In an arterial emergency, microspheres are used in the treatment of bronchial and postpartum bleeding [8]. Postpartum bleeding can be successfully treated with a temporary embolic agent such as spongostan.

References

1. Geschwind J, Dake M. Abrams' angiography: interventional radiology. 3rd ed. Philadelphia: Wolters Kluwer/Lippincott Wiliams & Wilkins; 2014. p. 442–588.
2. Pretorius E, Solomon J. Radiology secrets plus. 3rd ed. Amsterdam: Mosby/Elsevier; 2010. p. 217–22.
3. Morgan RA, Walser E, editors. Handbook of angioplasty and stenting procedures, techniques in interventional radiology. London: Springer-Verlag London Limited; 2010. p. 1–12.
4. Sidawy AP, Perler AB. Rutherford's vascular surgery and endovascular therapy, vol. 2. 9th ed. Amsterdam: Elsevier; 2018. p. 856–67.
5. Golzarian J, editor. Vascular embolotherapy: a comprehensive approach. Berlin: Springer; 2006. p. 15–42.
6. White RI, Standberg JV, Gross GS, Barth KH. Therapeutic embolization with long-term occlusion agents and their effects on embolized tissues. Radiology. 1977;125:677–87.
7. Numan F, Omeroglu A, Kara B, Cantasdemir M, Adaletli I, Kantarci F. Embolization of peripheral vascular malformations with ethylene-vinyl alcohol copolymer (Onyx). J Vasc Interv Radiol. 2004;15:939–46.
8. Golzarian J, editor. Vascular embolotherapy: a comprehensive approach. Berlin: Springer; 2006. p. 263–75.

2 Diagnosis of Vascular Emergencies

Contents

2.1 Diagnosis of Endovascular Emergency

Focused anamnesis and clinical examination are inevitable for every vascular patient and are used to guide further diagnostic and treatment steps. Some vascular emergencies can be diagnosed only with anamnesis and clinical examination or with handheld Doppler and bedside ultrasound; therefore, further treatment delay with advanced diagnostic procedures is unnecessary and can even be harmful. Focused anamneses include the onset, characteristics, and duration of and changes in the symptoms, previous vascular symptoms, and haemodynamic status. Cardiovascular risk factors should be noted, including the presence of diabetes mellitus, renal insufficiency, and cardio-, respiratory, gastrointestinal and brain diseases. The clinical examination begins with inspection and palpation. Pulse status should be noted, as well as sensitive motor function and any pulsatile palpable masses. Simple ankle pressure and ankle-brachial index (ABI) can be measured very easily and quickly, providing information about the status of the lower extremities. Handheld Doppler examinations for the presence of arterial and venous signals are additional quick and straightforward techniques for examining the lower extremities. Differences between measurements of arm pressure can be caused by subclavian or brachiocephalic trunk occlusive diseases. Patients with a previously diagnosed abdominal aortic aneurysm who came to the hospital with sharp acute abdominal pain and hypotension may be suspected of having aortic rupture, which can be

S. Duvnjak, *Endovascular Treatment of Arterial Emergencies*,
https://doi.org/10.1007/978-3-030-68832-5_2

diagnosed with ultrasound. If the patient is haemodynamically unstable, immediate operation is indicated without delay. The colour duplex ultrasound examination is non-invasive, fast, widely available and used in vascular diagnosis, including for the carotid, visceral, and aortic vessels and the vessels of the upper and lower extremities. Detailed descriptions of the ultrasound techniques are beyond the scope of this practical guide.

2.2 Computed Tomography (CT) Diagnosis of Endovascular Emergencies

Diagnosis via CT has almost completely replaced invasive angiographic diagnosis in current practice. Modern CT scanners can rapidly provide imaging of the whole body, and special semiautomated techniques and software programs can quickly reconstruct the arterial system. CT is indispensable in an arterial emergency, capable of diagnosing all emergencies with high sensitivity and specificity. Typically, 100–120 mL of contrast agent is delivered via the cubital vein at a rate of 3–4 mL/s, then flushed with saline. Automated computed tomography programs help to determine when to administer the contrast agent depending on the region of interest. The precise diagnosis of carotid, aortic, visceral and upper and lower extremity vessel diseases can be achieved with CT within a few minutes [1]. The multiplanar reconstruction and high spatial resolution of CT provide images with great detail and allow the making of confident diagnoses and further treatment (Fig. 2.1). The CT diagnosis of aortic aneurysms and dissections is necessary for planning endovascular treatments and ordering proper stent grafts. Thoraco-abdominal aneurysms that require complex stent-graft fenestration and branch technology cannot be treated without useful, quality CT imaging and specialized reconstruction (Fig. 2.2). Peripheral arterial diseases can be diagnosed with CT very effectively and provide all necessary information for further treatment. The presence of extensive calcifications in the lower limbs can cause problems in CT imaging due to the beam hardening effect [2]. Patients with renal impairment are at risk of worsening renal insufficiency after contrast administration, but in a vascular emergency, every patient's risk and need for CT are analysed.

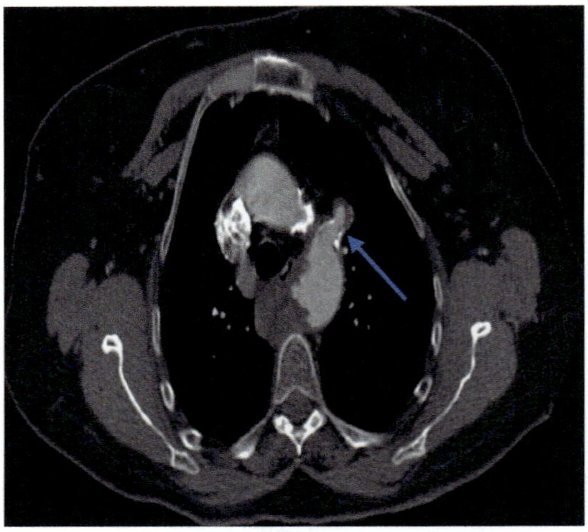

Fig. 2.1 Contrast-enhanced CT-axial image of a penetrating ulcer in the aortic arch (arrow)

2.3 Magnetic Resonance Imaging (MRI) Diagnosis of Endovascular Emergencies

MRI offers an advanced form of radiological examination, and for vascular diagnosis, it can be formed either in non–contrast- and contrast-enhanced modes. MRI is generally time consuming and, and there are a few contraindications for the technique; therefore, in an acute situation, MRI is of limited use. MRI is radiation-free, and different types of contrast can typically be used during follow-up after treatment and for elective patients with vascular diseases. Non–contrast-enhanced MRI techniques primarily include time

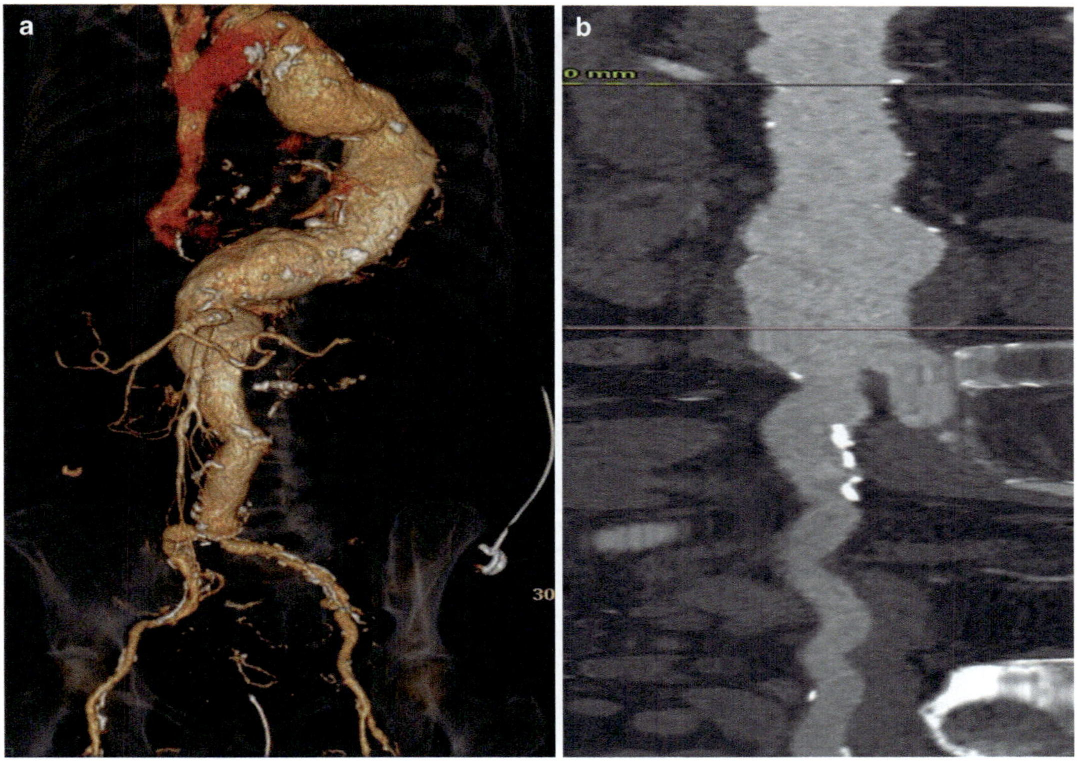

Fig. 2.2 3-D reconstruction of a thoracoabdominal aorta aneurysm (**a**). (**b**) Example of the centreline measurement of an infrarenal aortic aneurysm for EVAR planning

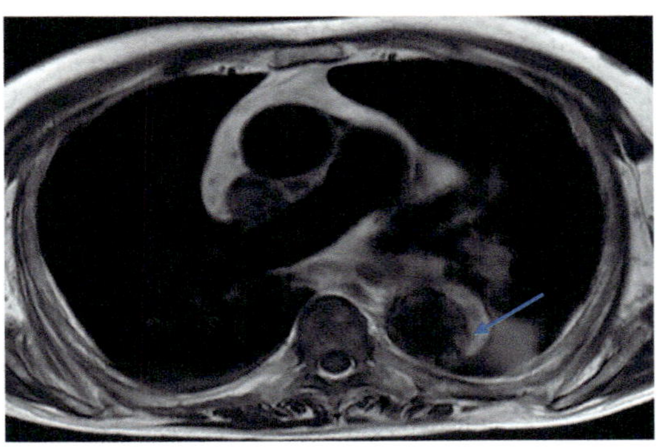

Fig. 2.3 Non–contrast-enhanced T2-weighted MRI of the thoracic aorta with intramural haematoma (arrow)

of flight (TOF), followed by others such as phase-contrast (PC) MRI and balanced steady-state free precession (SSFP) (Fig. 2.3). SSFP is useful in diagnosing large vessel, primarily aortic, diseases [1–3] (Fig. 2.4) [3]. Nevertheless, longer examination times and motion artefacts are problems with non–contrast techniques [4]. TOF techniques for small vessels are inaccurate and overestimate stenosis/occlusion, usually requiring us to perform contrast-enhanced MRI in such cases. The MRI contrast agent in use today, gadolinium, is safer than those used in previously, but some patients with advanced renal diseases can develop systemic fibrosis following its use [5]. Precisely timed contrast administration is essential to obtain high-quality images. Long segments can pose challenges, such as lower limb angiograms, requiring sequential scanning (Fig. 2.5). The development and introduction of the 3 T MR scanner shortened the examination time and provided much better images, so in the future, MRI can expect to see greater utilization in vascular emergencies [6].

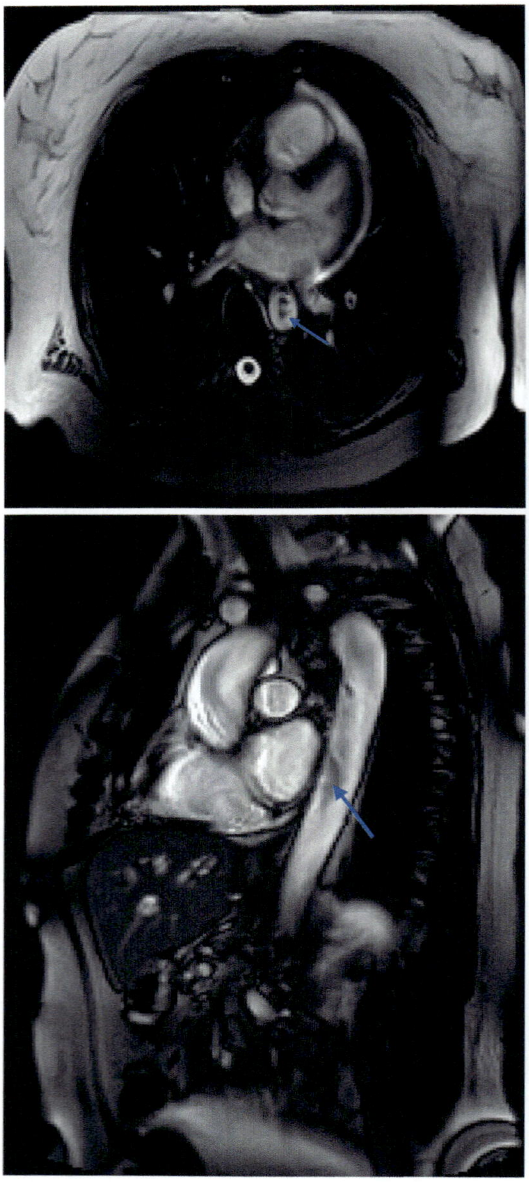

Fig. 2.4 TOF and SSFP non–contrast-enhanced MRI of the thoracic aorta with a mobile thrombus inside the descending portion (arrows)

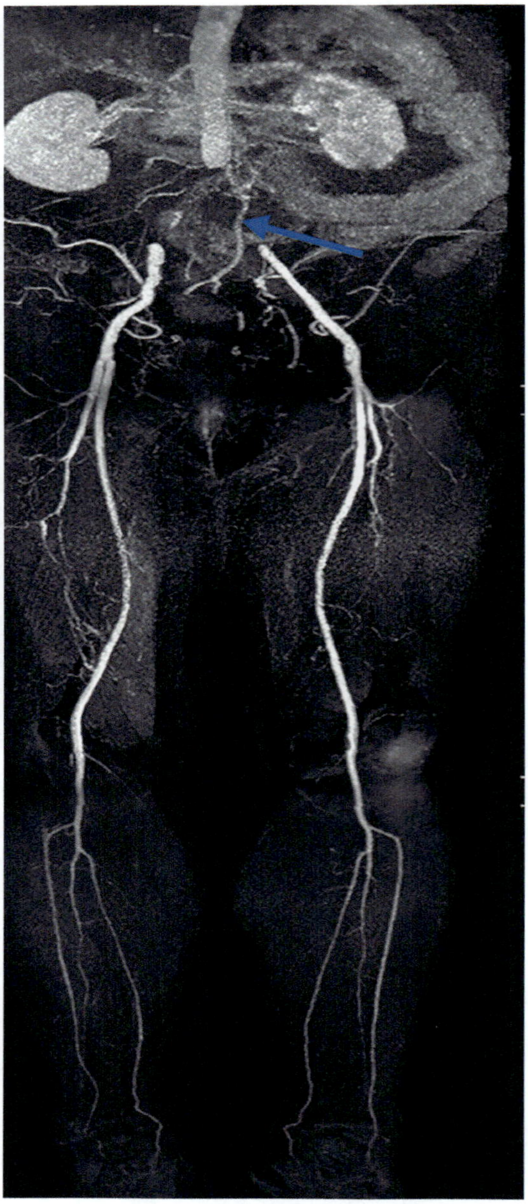

Fig. 2.5 Contrast-enhanced MRI of the lower limb extremities with infrarenal aortic occlusion (arrow)

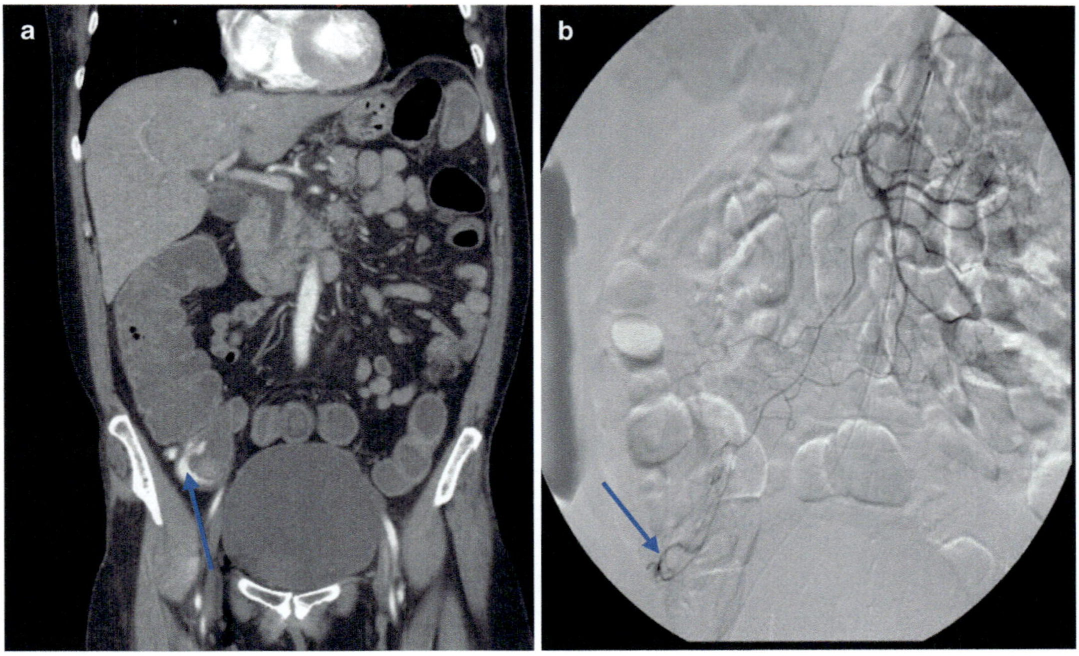

Fig. 2.6 Lower gastrointestinal bleeding (**a**). CT showing contrast extravasation into caecum-(arrow). (**b**) Selective angiography of the superior mesenteric artery prior to embolization of the bleeding in the caecal artery (arrow)

2.4 Invasive Angiographic Diagnosis of Endovascular Emergencies

Today, invasive angiography is used as one step during endovascular treatment. Advances in CT and MRI imaging have almost entirely led to the replacement of invasive diagnostic angiography. There are some situations where additional invasive angiography is needed, however, such as in critical lower limb ischaemia with extensive calcification and stenosis and, in certain situations, gastrointestinal bleeding. The risk for local complications during invasive angiography is low, with haematoma that requires treatment and pseudoaneurysm occurring for approximately 1% of patients [7]. Bleeding and dissection are other local complications and have also been recorded in approximately 1% of patients. In gastrointestinal bleeding, CT can detect a bleeding rate of 0.3–0.5 mL/min [8] and is usually followed by angiography and embolization (Fig. 2.6). Patients diagnosed with gastrointestinal bleeding and clinical signs of re-bleeding can be sent directly to undergo angiography for a new embolization (Fig. 2.7) instead of a new CT imaging scan. Furthermore, invasive angiography is used after the completion of endovascular interventions to confirm that the result is satisfactory (Fig. 2.8).

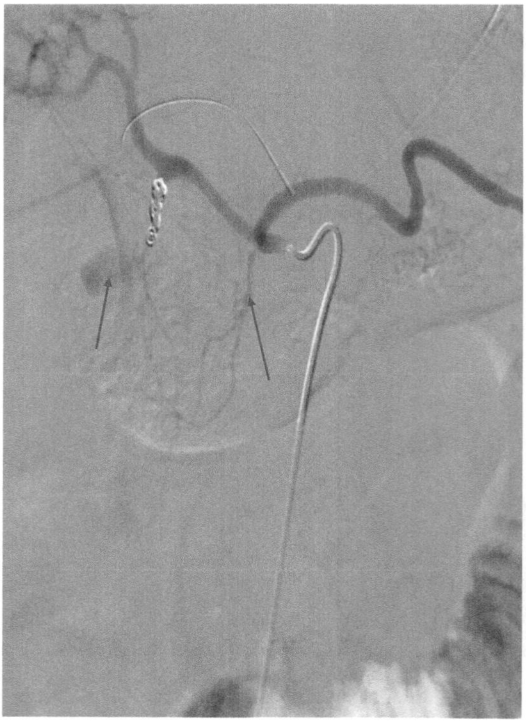

Fig. 2.7 Patient with upper gastrointestinal bleeding who had previously undergone embolization of the gastroduodenal artery. A new angiogram was obtained due to re-bleeding from the dorsal pancreatic artery (arrows)

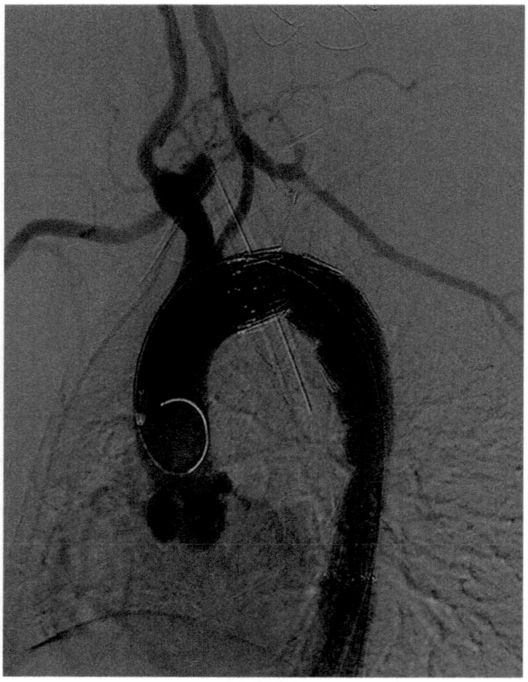

Fig. 2.8 Control angiography after TEVAR stent-graft deployment and left carotid-subclavian bypass (arrow)

References

1. Sidawy AP, Perler AB. Rutherford's vascular surgery and endovascular therapy, vol. 2. 9th ed. Amsterdam: Elsevier; 2018. p. 265–390.
2. Barrett JF, Keat N. Artifacts in CT: recognition and avoidance. Radiographics. 2004;24:1679–91.
3. Kuo AH, Nagpal P, Ghoshhajra BB, Hedgire SS. Vascular magnetic resonance angiography techniques. Cardiovasc Diagn Ther. 2019;9:S28–36.
4. Hartung MP, Grist TM, François CJ. Magnetic resonance angiography: current status and future directions. J Cardiovasc Magn Reson. 2011;13:19.
5. Perazella MA. Advanced kidney disease, gadolinium and nephrogenic systemic fibrosis: the perfect storm. Curr Opin Nephrol Hypertens. 2009;18:519–25.
6. Tomasian A, Salamon N, Lohan DG, Jalili M, Villablanca JP, Finn JP. Supraaortic arteries: contrast material dose reduction at 3.0-T high-spatial-resolution MR angiography-feasibility study. Radiology. 2008;249:980–90.
7. Bhatty S, Cooke R, Shetty R, Jovin SI. Femoral vascular access-site complications in the cardiac catheterization laboratory: diagnosis and management. Interv Cardiol. 2011;3:503–14.
8. Wells ML, Hansel SL, Bruining DH, Fletcher JG, Froemming AT, Barlow JM, et al. CT for evaluation of acute gastrointestinal bleeding. Radiographics. 2018;38:1089–107.

3 Thoracic Vascular Emergencies

Contents

S. Duvnjak, *Endovascular Treatment of Arterial Emergencies*,
https://doi.org/10.1007/978-3-030-68832-5_3

Thoracic aortic dissection is defined classically using the Stanford classification system either as type A, involving the ascending aorta, or type B involving the descending aorta distally from the left subclavian artery. Type A aortic dissections are the most common, constituting approximately 60% of all dissections; this kind of vascular emergency is still primarily treated with open surgery (Fig. 3.1).

3.1 Thoracic Aortic Dissections

3.1.1 Acute Complicated Aortic Dissection Type B

Key Points

- It is sometimes difficult to estimate renal ischaemia and the potential for renal function recovery. Patients with renal malperfusion should not be excluded from treatment too quickly.
- The best initial treatment if possible is TEVAR followed by eventually additional visceral artery stenting and covering of the primary entry instead of primary visceral artery stenting alone.
- The stent graft should be advanced under fluoroscopic guidance at all times.

3.1.1.1 Aetiology and Clinical Presentation

A 65-year-old patient was admitted to another hospital with a sudden onset of sharp retrosternal pain radiating into the back and primary right lower limb. The patient was known to have hypertension treated with two drugs. Renal function rapidly deteriorated, and the patient was in anuria on the first day. Previously, the patient had normal renal function.

3.1.1.2 Pre-interventional Diagnosis

In the admitting hospital, non–contrast-enhanced CT was performed the day after symptom onset (Fig. 3.2). The patient's status deteriorated over the next few days, and dialysis was required due to increasing creatinine and hyperkaliaemia. Furthermore, the patient developed severe hypertension and back pain and was transferred to our hospital 3 days after symptom onset. The patient's renal function severely deteriorated, and a non–contrast-enhanced MR scan was performed to establish the diagnosis (Fig. 3.3). The scan confirmed a diagnosis of aortic dissection type B distally from the left subclavian artery complicated with renal malperfusion. The true lumen was compressed by the false lumen, but no mesenteric ischaemia or symptoms were present. The true lumen of the right common iliac artery was compressed as well but without clinical manifestations of limb ischaemia.

3.1.1.3 Endovascular Treatment

The duration of renal ischaemia was at least 4 days, and the function of the renal parenchyma was not known. Endovascular treatment of aortic dissections consists of TEVAR, including covering the primary entry and opening of the true lumen, which leads to better perfusion of the renal arteries. The present case was potentially complicated by a fragile aorta and the risk for retrograde dissection if a TEVAR stent graft was to be deployed in the acute phase and with unknown results on the renal function. Other problems included the status of the left subclavian artery and the decision to cover the artery or to perform first carotid-subclavian bypass. We decided first to place stents into the renal arteries in order to prolong our decision time and to see if the renal function would improve as well as to deploy a 16 mm self-expandable stent in the infrarenal aorta to open the true lumen. The stents were inserted percutaneously via the left brachial artery and left femoral artery. First, the self-expandable stent (Fig. 3.4) was placed into the infrarenal abdominal aorta to open the true lumen, but during its manipulation, the stent was placed into the false lumen, preventing satisfactory opening of the true lumen and flow through the renal arteries.

Three renal stents measuring 6 mm × 39 mm and one measuring 7 mm × 39 mm were deployed in the right kidney, and two balloon-expandable stents measuring 7 mm × 39 mm were deployed in the left renal artery. Control angiography still showed a severely compressed true lumen (Fig. 3.5).

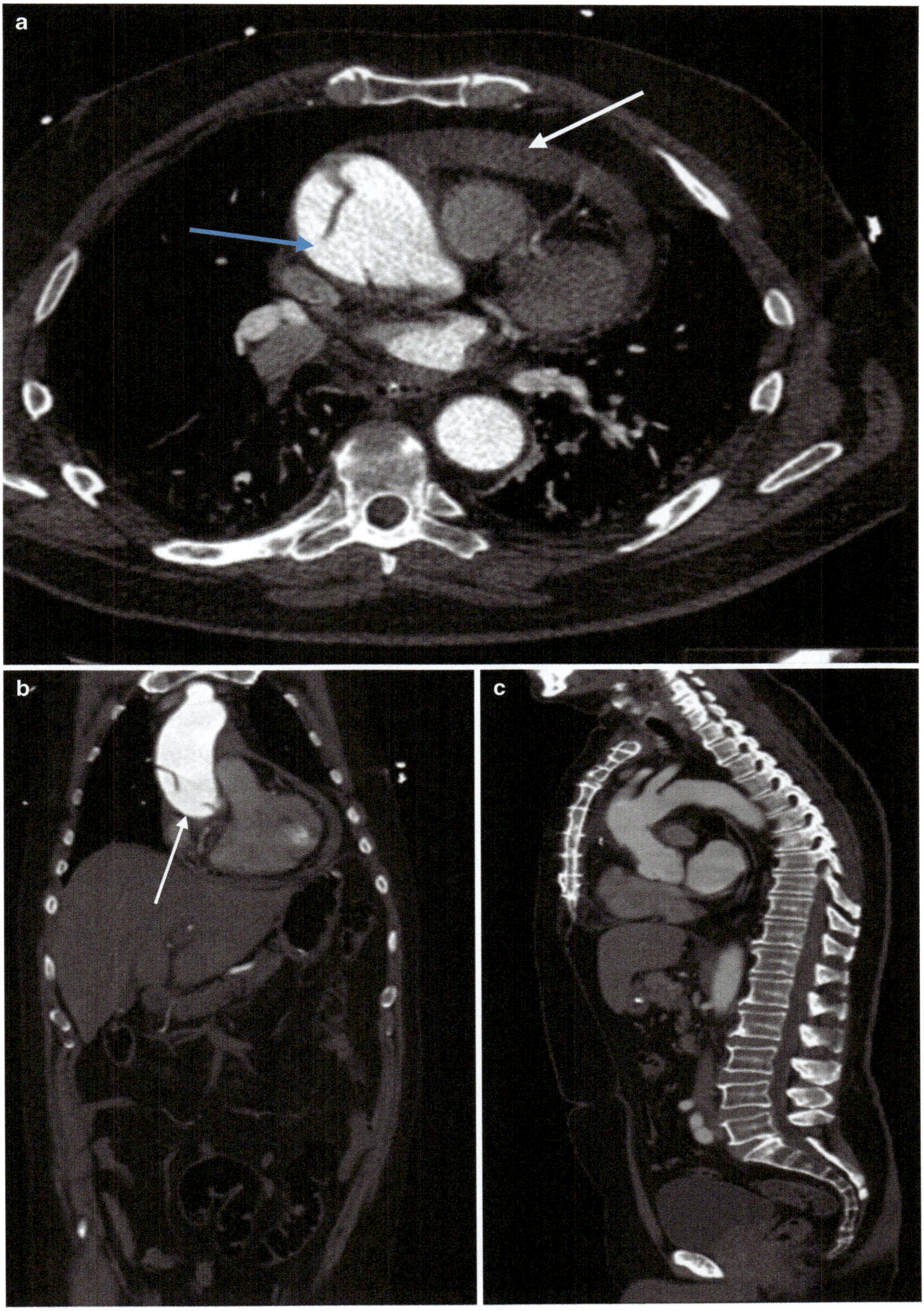

Fig. 3.1 (**a**) Acute aortic dissection type A (blue arrow). White arrow indicates haemopericardium. (**b**) White arrow indicates the primary entry and origin of the dissection. (**c**) Control CT images after ascending aorta replacement by open surgery

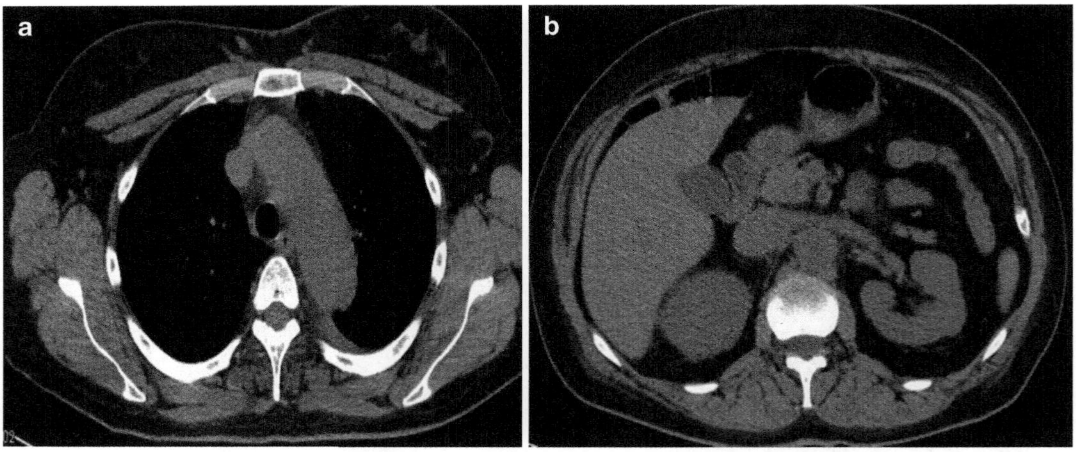

Fig. 3.2 Non–contrast-enhanced CT scan showing no pathological changes at the level of either the aortic arch/descending aorta (**a**) or the renal artery (**b**)

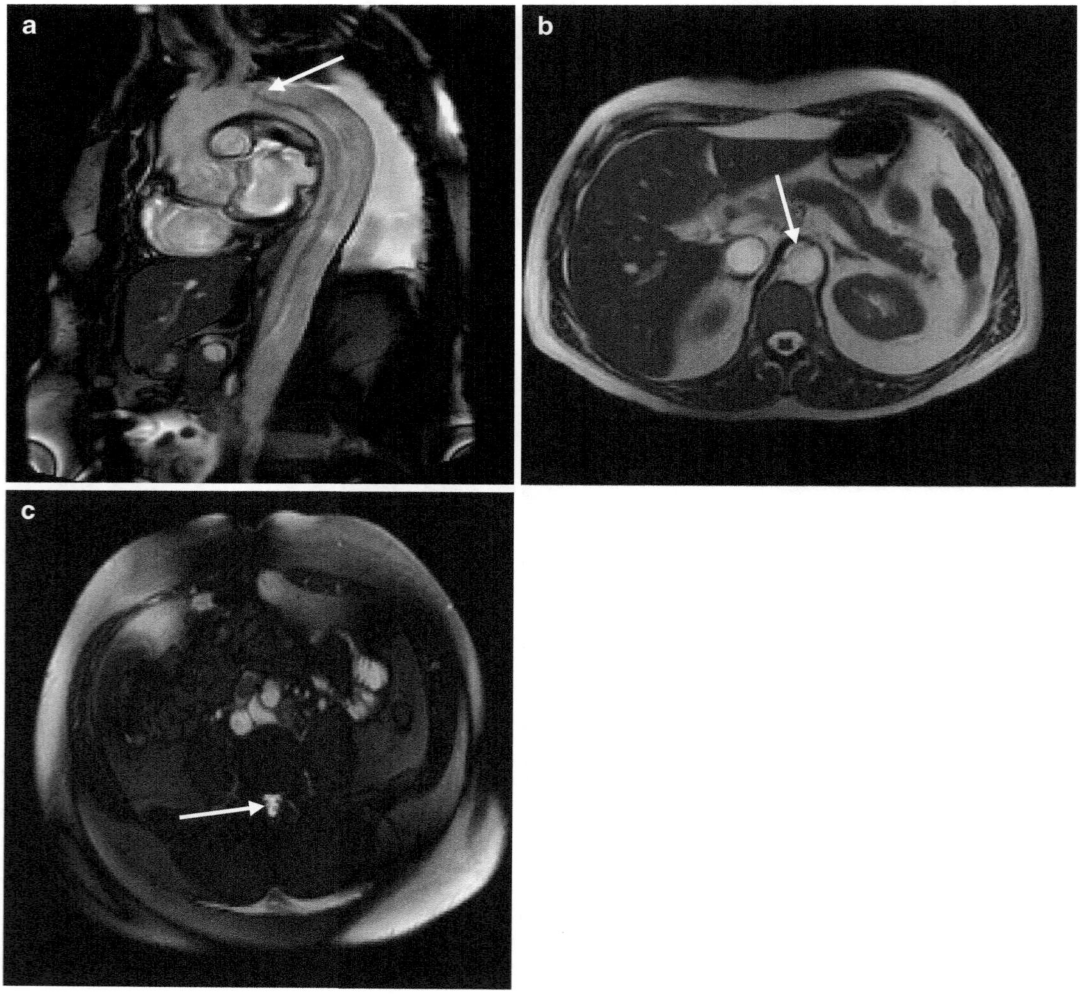

Fig. 3.3 Non–contrast-enhanced MR scan depicts an aortic dissection type B with the primary entry distal from the left subclavian artery (white arrow) (**a**). Severely compressed true lumen and ostium of all visceral arteries are indicated by arrows (**b**). Compression of the true lumen in the right common iliac artery is indicated by the (white arrow) (**c**)

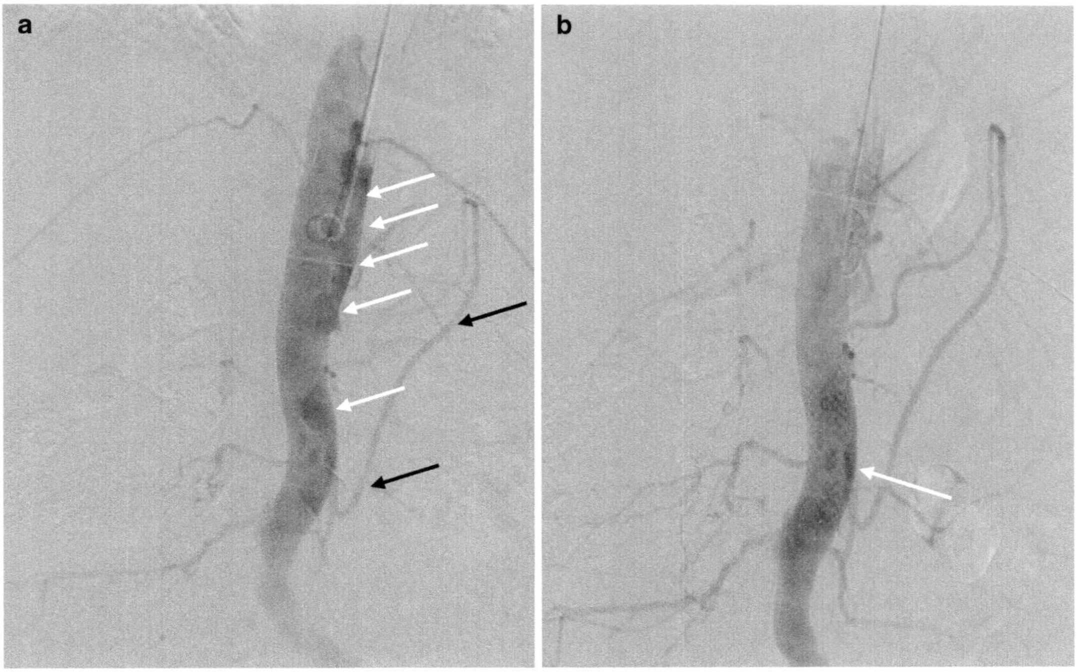

Fig. 3.4 Angiography through the catheter advanced into the false lumen, with the compressed true lumen shown with arrows (**a**) and no flow in the renal arteries. The inferior mesenteric artery has a fast flow, and the superior mesenteric artery shows sufficient flow passing retrograde through the inferior mesenteric artery (black arrow). (**b**) The self-expandable stent is incorrectly deployed into the false lumen (arrow)

The following day, renal ultrasound confirmed renal perfusion and an open stent. The patient was still on dialysis, but the hypertension was under control, and the patient started experiencing diuresis. Renography 1 week after renal stenting showed bilateral renal perfusion without side differences but significantly decreased flow in both kidneys (Fig. 3.6). Two weeks after renal stenting, we decided to perform TEVAR and occlude the primary entry in order to improve the flow through all the visceral arteries. The aortic wall was not as fragile after 2–3 weeks, and the risk for retrograde dissection had decreased. Under general anaesthesia, the true lumen was negotiated through the surgically exposed left femoral artery. The index contrast-enhanced CT showed the primary entry close to the left subclavian artery and the open renal stent (Fig. 3.7). It was challenging to cannulate the true lumen, after confirmation of the cannulation, a catheter with a super-stiff guidewire was advanced through the ascending aorta with some difficulties. We maintained attention on the tip of the super-stiff guidewire, and during the advancement of the TEVAR stent graft, the right renal artery stent was pushed out from the artery unnoticed and became attached to the stent graft.

During the manipulation, the renal stent followed the movement of the stent graft, and we realized that the guidewire had been placed through the renal stent struts (Fig. 3.8).

We advanced the TEVAR stent graft distally from the left subclavian artery and withdrew the guidewire. The renal stent was now free. Furthermore, after advancing the guidewire through the TEVAR stent graft, the graft was intentionally deployed to cover approximately one-third of the left subclavian artery. The distal part of the stent graft insufficiently secured the loosened renal stent. Therefore, a new, short stent graft was advanced and deployed distally, covering and ultimately securing the loosed renal stent. Control angiography showed the excellent opening of the true lumen and much better anterograde flow through the superior mesenteric artery and both renal arteries (Fig. 3.9). The right renal

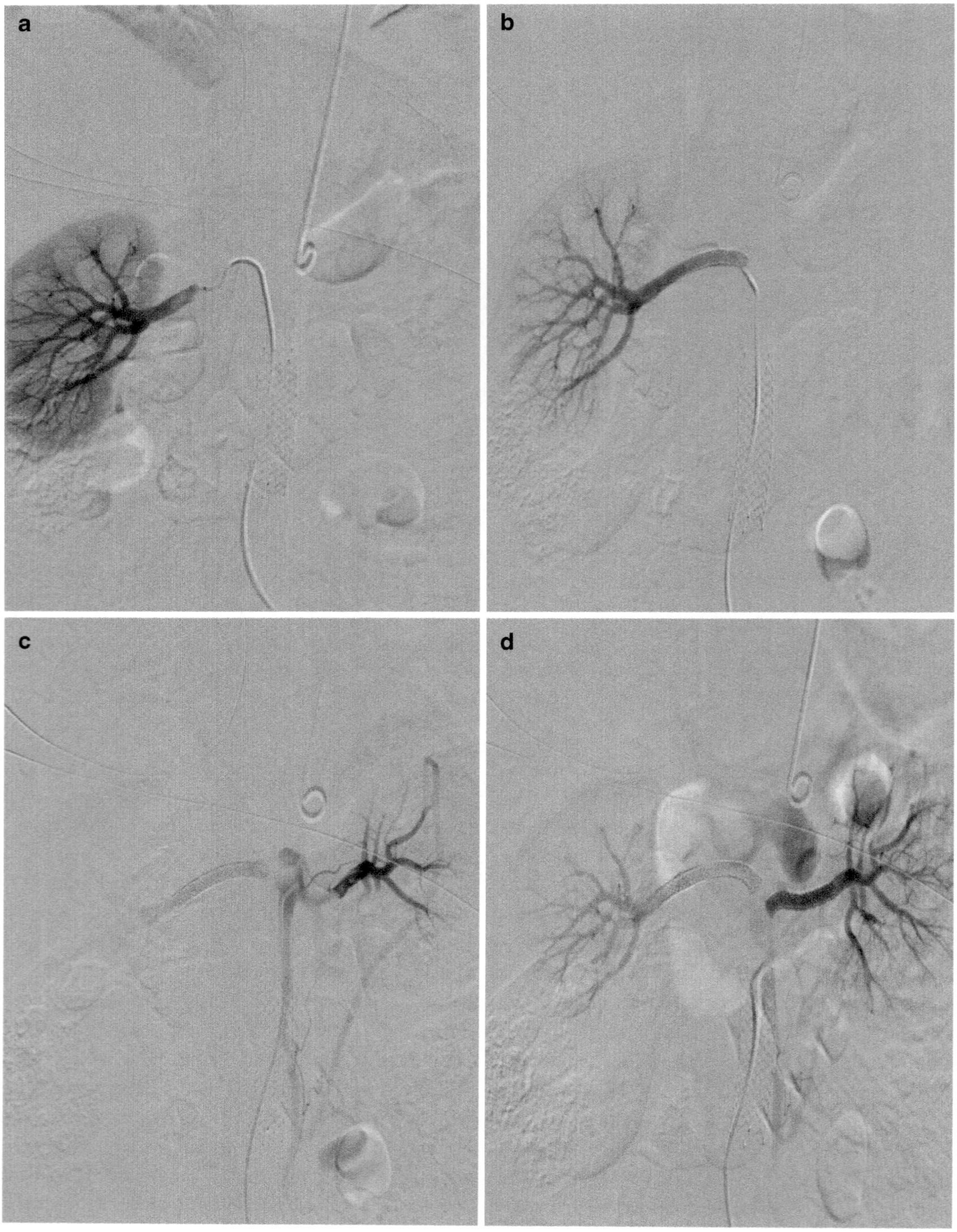

Fig. 3.5 Control angiography after bilateral renal stenting still showing compression of the true lumen. (**a**, **b**) showed the deployed stent in the right renal artery. (**c**, **d**) showed the deployed stent in the left renal artery

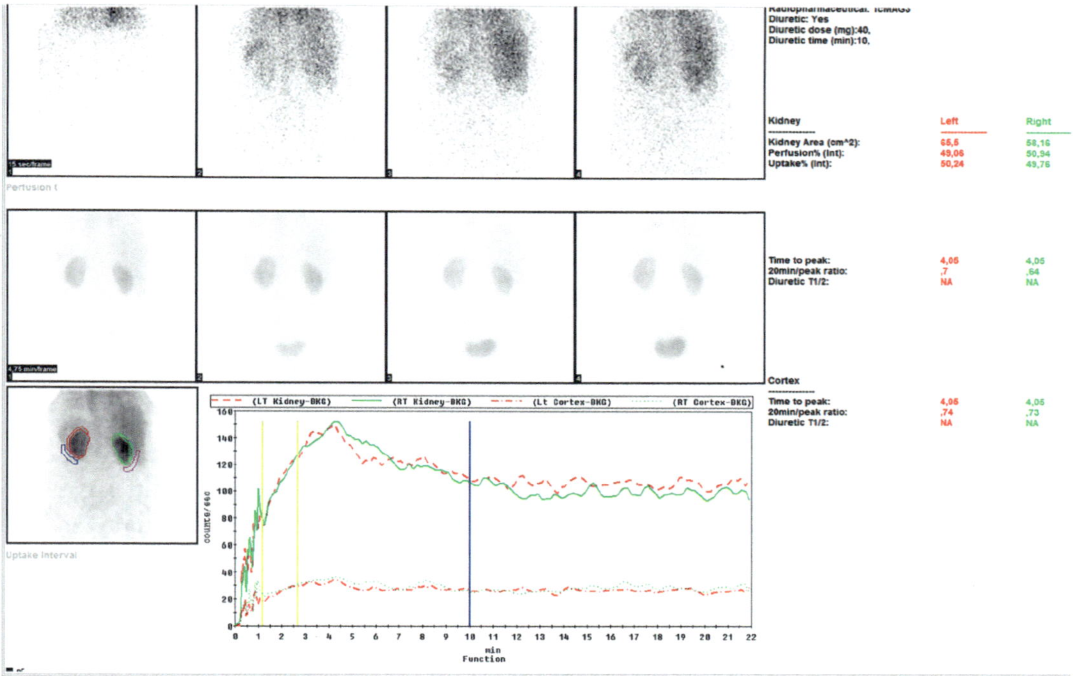

Fig. 3.6 Functional renography showing no side differences and significant flow decrease in both kidneys

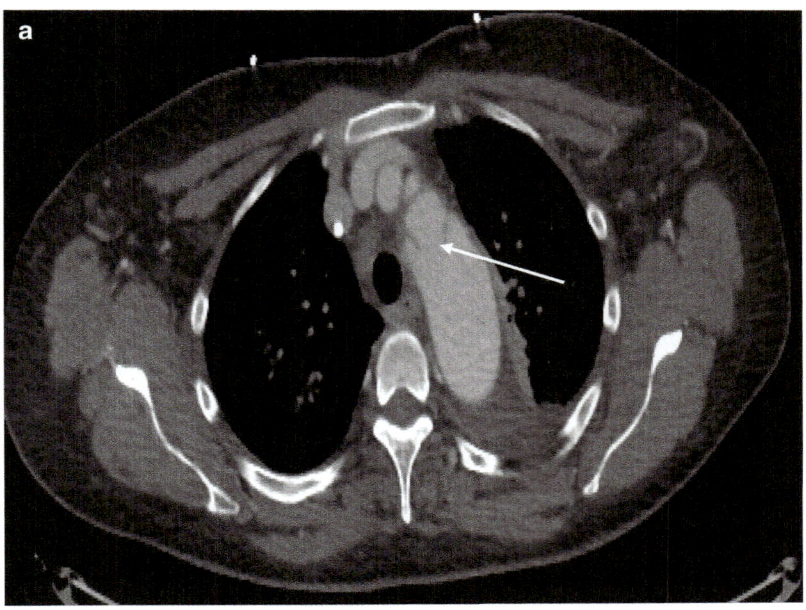

Fig. 3.7 Pre-TEVAR CT showing the type B dissection. The primary entry was 10 mm wide and close to the left subclavian artery (arrow) (**a**). The bilateral renal stents were patent (**b**)

Fig. 3.7 (continued)

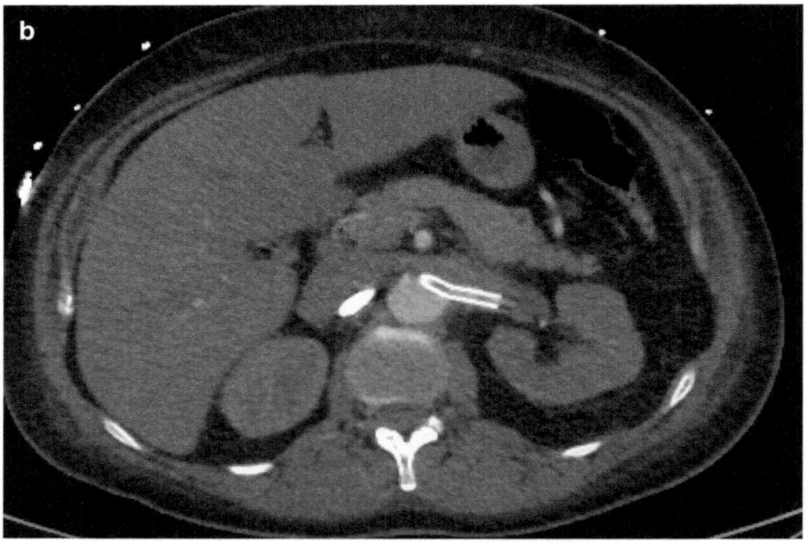

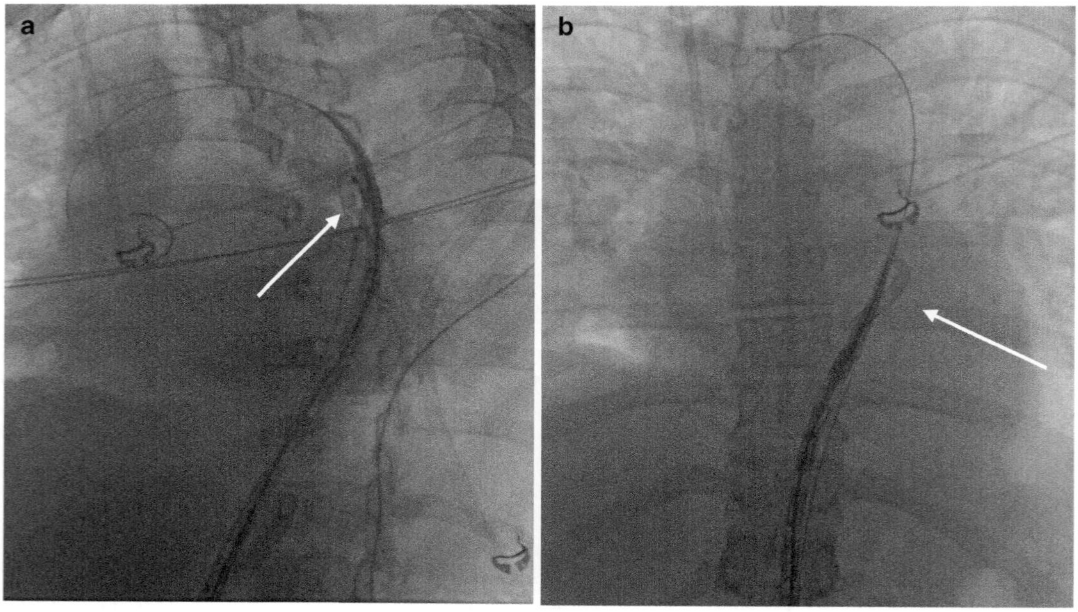

Fig. 3.8 Advancement of the TEVAR stent graft and "attached" renal stent (white arrow) (**a**). Withdrawal of the super-stiff guidewire inside the TEVAR stent graft, leaving the renal stent in the descending aorta (arrow) (**b**). Advancement of the TEVAR stent graft into the aortic arch (**c**). Securement of the loosed renal stent with additional short stent-graft placement (arrow) (**d**)

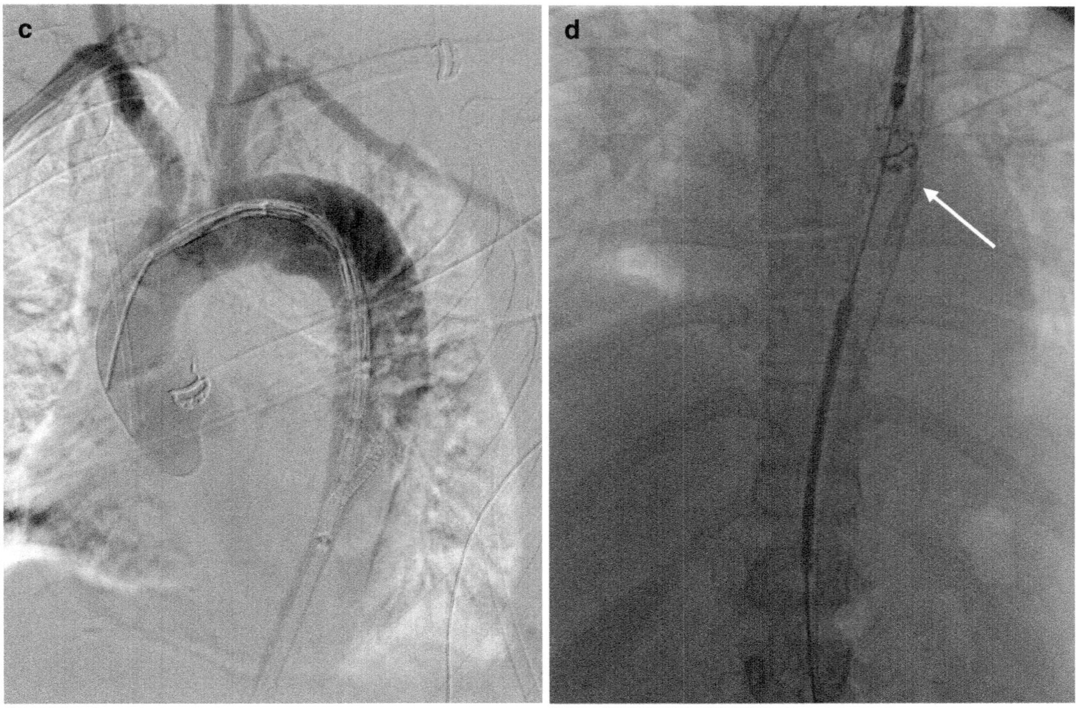

Fig. 3.8 (continued)

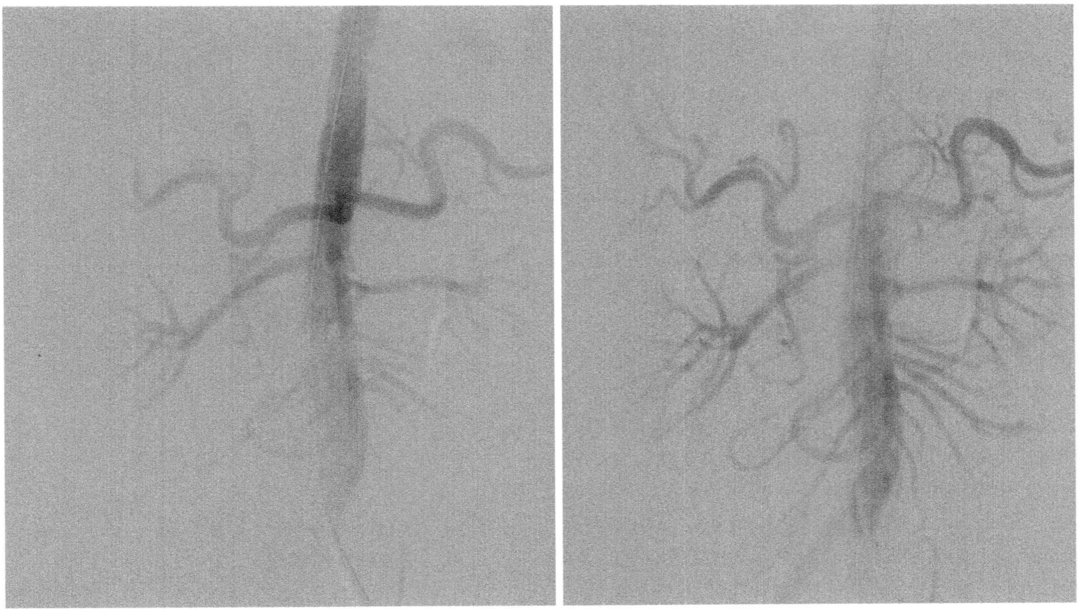

Fig. 3.9 Control angiography showing much better flow through all visceral arteries

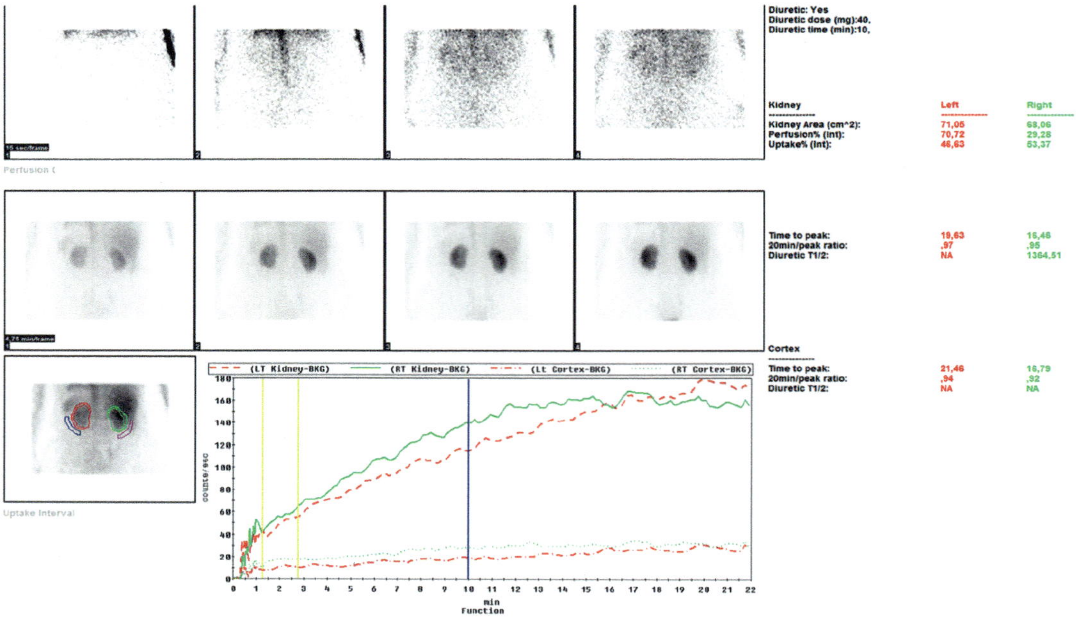

Fig. 3.10 Control renography 1 week after TEVAR showing remarkable improvement in renal function

artery was not dissected after the renal stent was removed from the artery. The left renal artery stent was open, and the right common iliac artery was stented as well. Renal function recovery was remarkable as confirmed on control renography, and the patient was removed from dialysis (Fig. 3.10). Hypertension was well controlled with the two drugs, and no other symptoms were observed. The patient was discharged from the hospital 2 months later with almost normal renal function, an eGFR of 54 and a slightly increased creatinine level.

3.1.1.4 Outcome

One-month control images showed aortic remodelling and a thrombosed false lumen proximally. Both renal arteries were patent. The superior mesenteric artery and the coeliac trunk were patent. The self-expandable stent placed in the infrarenal aorta demonstrated a small thrombus and fracture (Fig. 3.11). We decided to perform open surgery to remove the stent. The surgery was performed without complications, and control CT showed good results (Fig. 3.12). The patient showed no symptoms and well-controlled hypertension during the three-year follow-up.

3.1.2 Subacute Complicated Aortic Dissection Type B

Key Points

- Close surveillance is very important in cases of acute dissection to promptly diagnose complications and provide treatment.
- MRI scanning can be used for control, avoiding the use of radiation and contrast agents.
- If possible, TEVAR should planned in the subacute phase for at least >14 days and up to 3 months.

3.1.2.1 Aetiology and Clinical Presentation

A 75-year patient with previously diagnosed hypertension treated with a combination of three drugs was admitted after an acute onset of retrosternal pain. Acute myocardial infarction was excluded. After admission, emergency CT was performed, and aortic dissection type B was

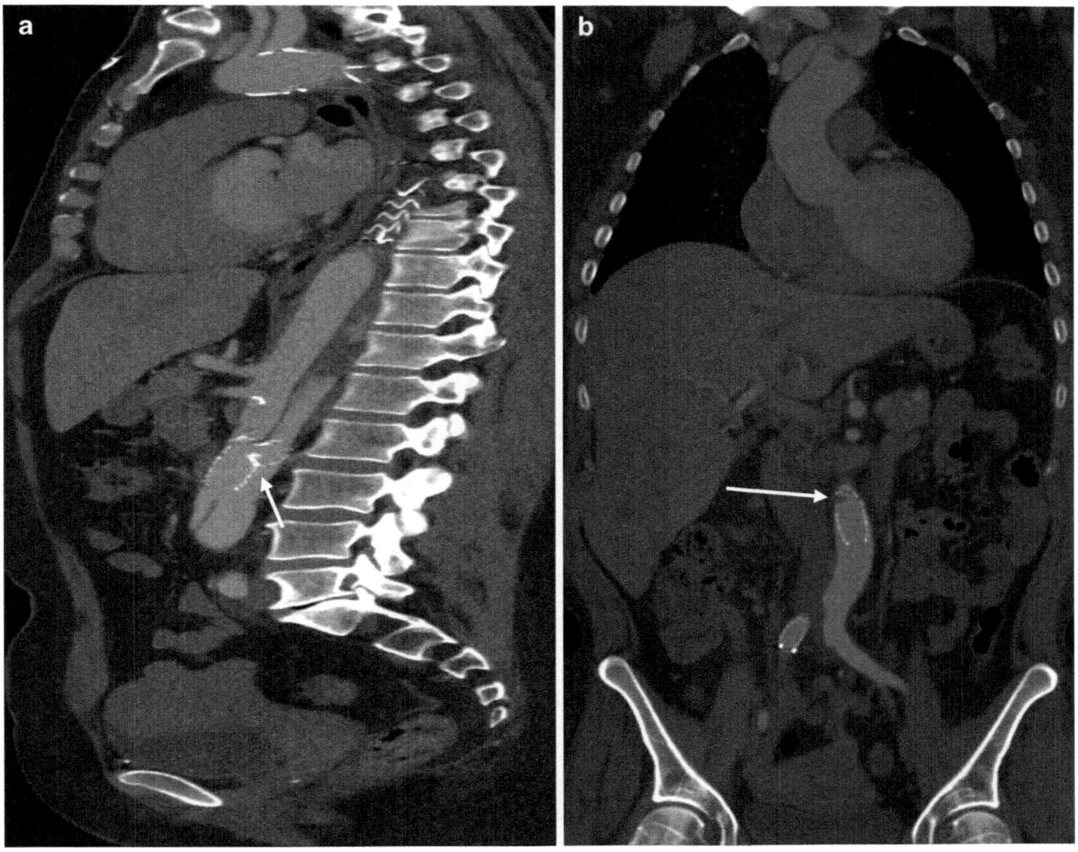

Fig. 3.11 The fractured self-expandable stent is partly deployed in the false lumen and partly in the true lumen in the infrarenal aorta (white arrow) (**a**). (**b**) Arrow indicates thrombus

diagnosed with primary entry just distal from the left subclavian artery and localized only to the descending aorta (Fig. 3.13). The patient responded well to conservative medical treatment, including nitroprusside, beta-blockers and pain control. The patient was kept in the hospital for 4 days and remained asymptomatic. On the fifth day, the patient was discharged, and a one-month control MR scan was scheduled.

3.1.2.2 Pre-interventional Diagnosis

One-month control ambulant non–contrast-enhanced MRI (SSFP sequence) showed that the aortic dissection had progressed and that the false lumen had become enlarged. The diameter of the false lumen was almost double that at the initial CT scan, and the dissection had propagated distally (Fig. 3.14). The patient remained asymptomatic, but due to the rapid enlargement of the false lumen despite a well-controlled blood pressure, we decided to perform subacute TEVAR, which was scheduled for the following week.

3.1.2.3 Endovascular Treatment

A 37 mm diameter, 100 mm long thoracic stent graft (COOK, IN, USA) was advanced through the surgically exposed right common femoral artery in order to cover the primary entry. The aorta diameter was 34–35 mm. Control angiography via a diagnostic catheter introduced via the left femoral artery was performed, showing even more enlargement of the false lumen (Fig. 3.15).

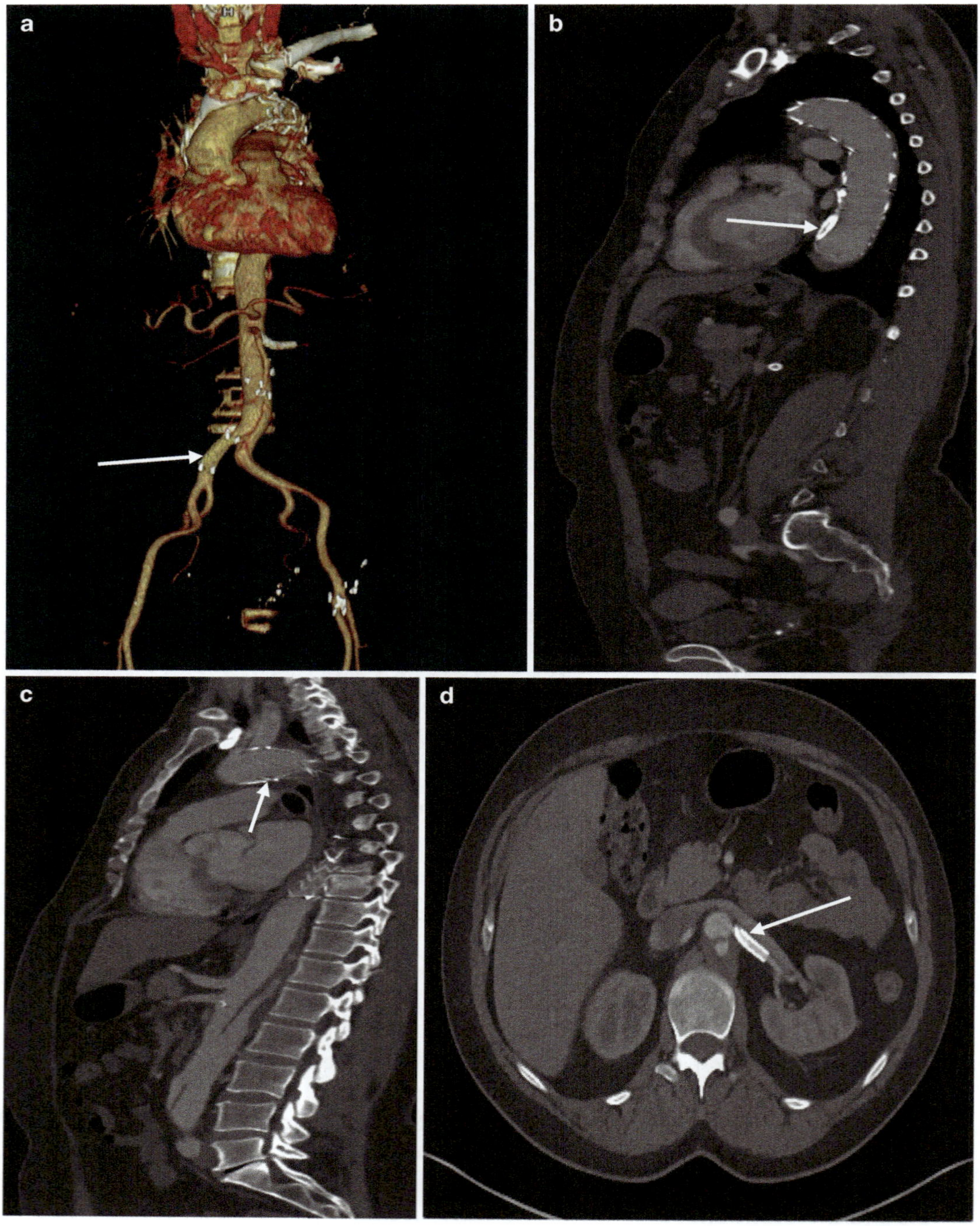

Fig. 3.12 Control CT after removal of the self-expandable stent in the infrarenal aorta. Patent stent in the right common femoral artery (white arrow) (**a**). (**b**) nice descending aorta remodelling. The arrow indicates the renal stent trapped between the stent graft and aorta. (**c**) partially covered ostium of the left subclavian artery, asymptomatic. (**d**) patent left renal stent

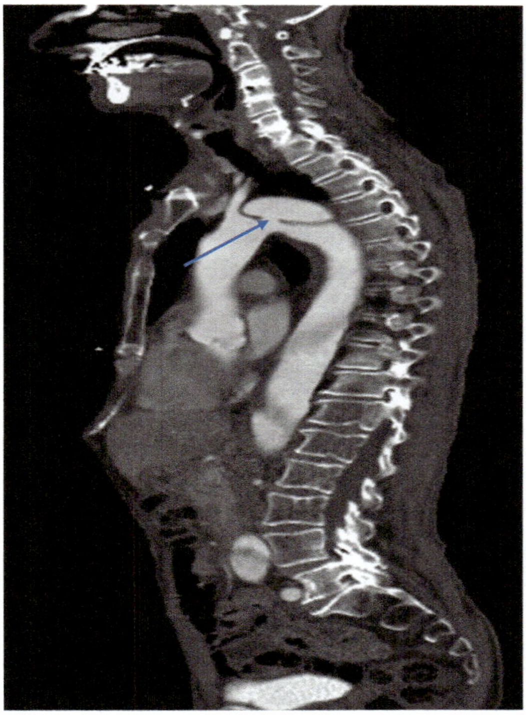

Fig. 3.13 Initial CT scan with type B aortic dissection localized to the proximal descending aorta. Arrow indicates the primary, 7 mm wide entry

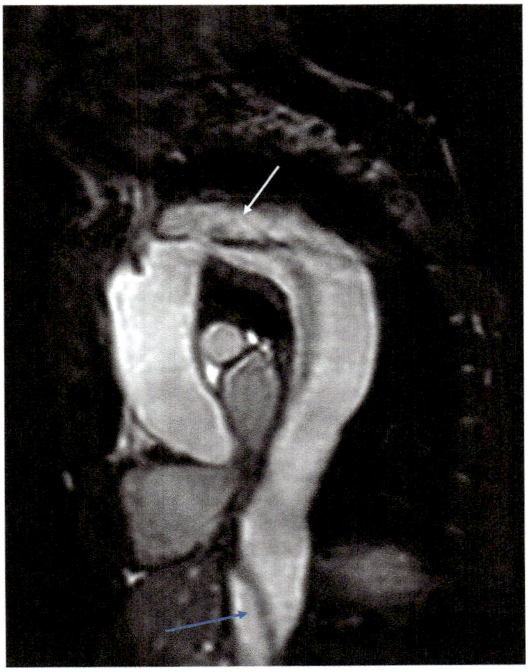

Fig. 3.14 One-month control MR with rapid enlargement of the false lumen (white arrow). Blue arrow indicates the distal progression of the dissection

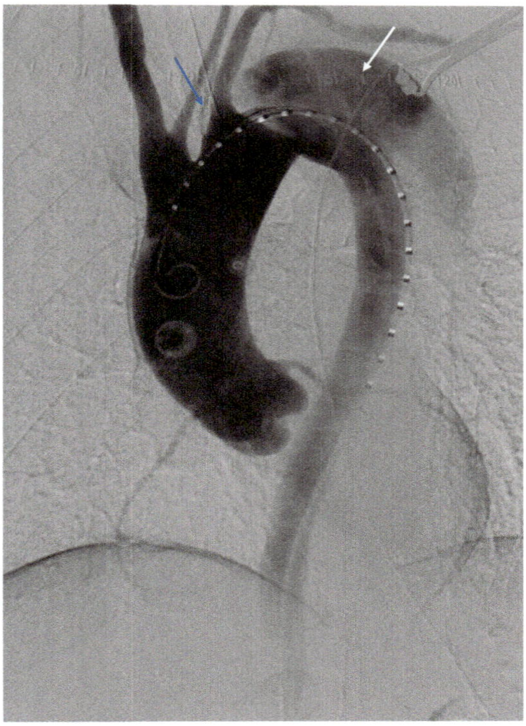

Fig. 3.15 Diagnostic angiography with continuous false lumen enlargement relative to that of the control MR scan (arrow). Note the common stem of the left carotid artery and brachiocephalic trunk. The blue arrow indicates the small left vertebral artery branching directly from the aortic arch

The stent graft was intentionally placed to cover the left subclavian artery aiming to create a proximal landing zone of at least 20 mm, and the result was satisfactory. No post-dilatation was observed. The intimal membrane remained elastic, and complete opening of the true lumen was achieved (Fig. 3.16). The left vertebral artery was small and arose directly from the aortic arch. Therefore, we did not perform carotid-subclavian bypass first before TEVAR. The right vertebral artery was dominant. However, the patient developed left arm ischaemia and underwent carotid-subclavian bypass later.

3.1.2.4 Outcome

The patient recovered without any complications and was discharged 5 days after the intervention. Over the 4 year follow-up, the patient had no complaints, and complete aortic remodelling was achieved.

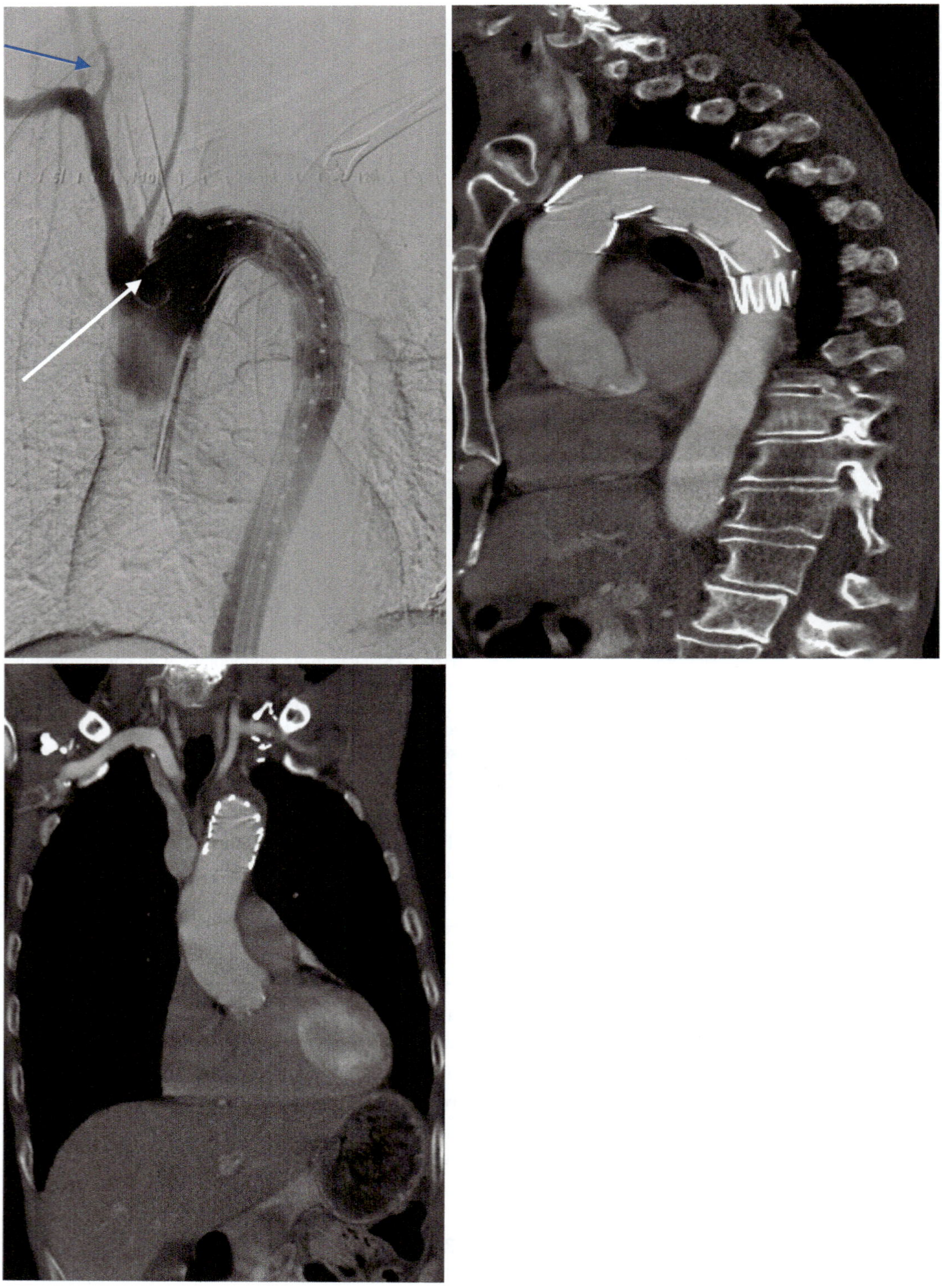

Fig. 3.16 Control angiography after TEVAR stent-graft deployment with intentional covering of the left subclavian artery. The arrow indicates the proximal stent graft, placed close to the carotid arteries. The blue arrow indicates the dominant right vertebral artery

3.1.3 Acute Aortic Dissection Type B Presented with Rupture

Key Points

- In certain acute cases, suboptimal treatment can provide additional time for a second, more permanent option, as in the present case.
- Typically, there is reactive pleura effusion in the aortic dissection, which should not be described as blood.
- In some cases, it is not necessary to retrograde occlude the left subclavian artery; if needed, however, it can be done easily via left brachial access.

3.1.3.1 Aetiology and Clinical Presentation

A 68-year-old patient with a previous aortic surgery due to aortic valve insufficiency and previously diagnosed arterial hypertension was admitted with low blood pressure (80/60 mmHg) and chest pain. The patient indicated that the sharp chest pain started shortly after becoming hypotensive. ECG was normal with no signs of myocardial ischaemia.

3.1.3.2 Pre-interventional Diagnosis

Emergency CT revealed a ruptured aortic dissection type B with retrograde dissection propagation slightly above the left subclavian artery (Fig. 3.17). Left haemothorax and mediastinal haematoma were present. Because of the rupture,

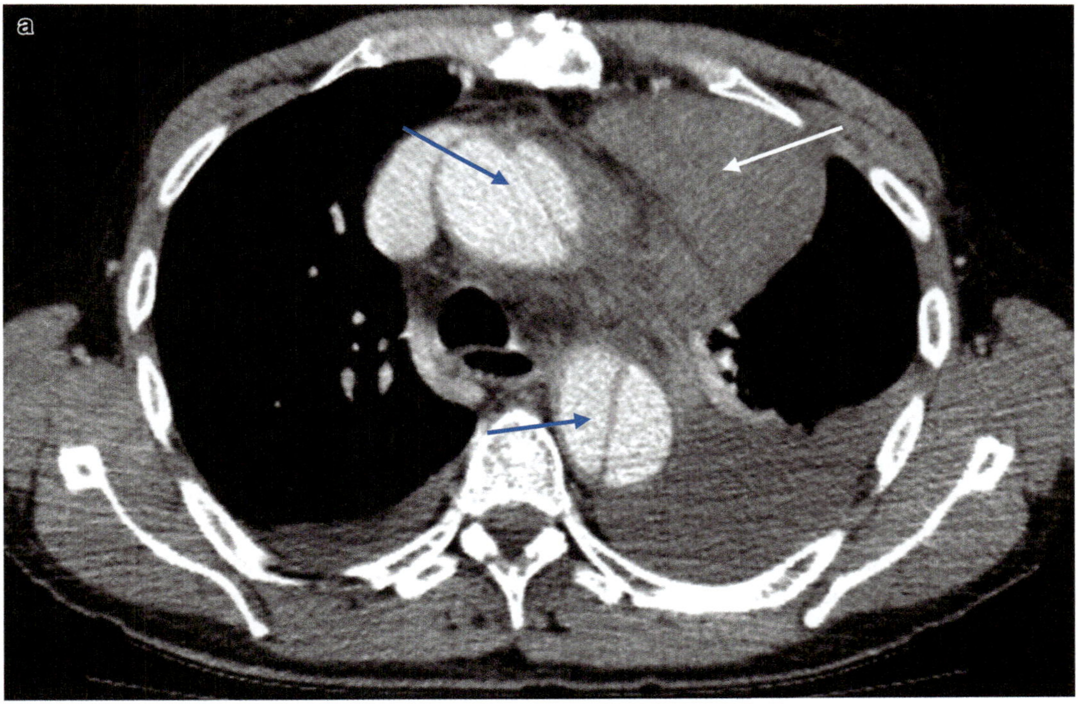

Fig. 3.17 Ruptured complicated aortic dissection type B. (**a**) blue arrows indicate the dissection membrane. White arrow indicates haemothorax. (**b**) white arrow indicates a reactive pleural effusion. Blue arrows point to the dissection membrane. (**c**) gull arrow points to the left common carotid artery. Blue arrow indicates retrograde propagation of the dissection. White arrow pointed haemothorax

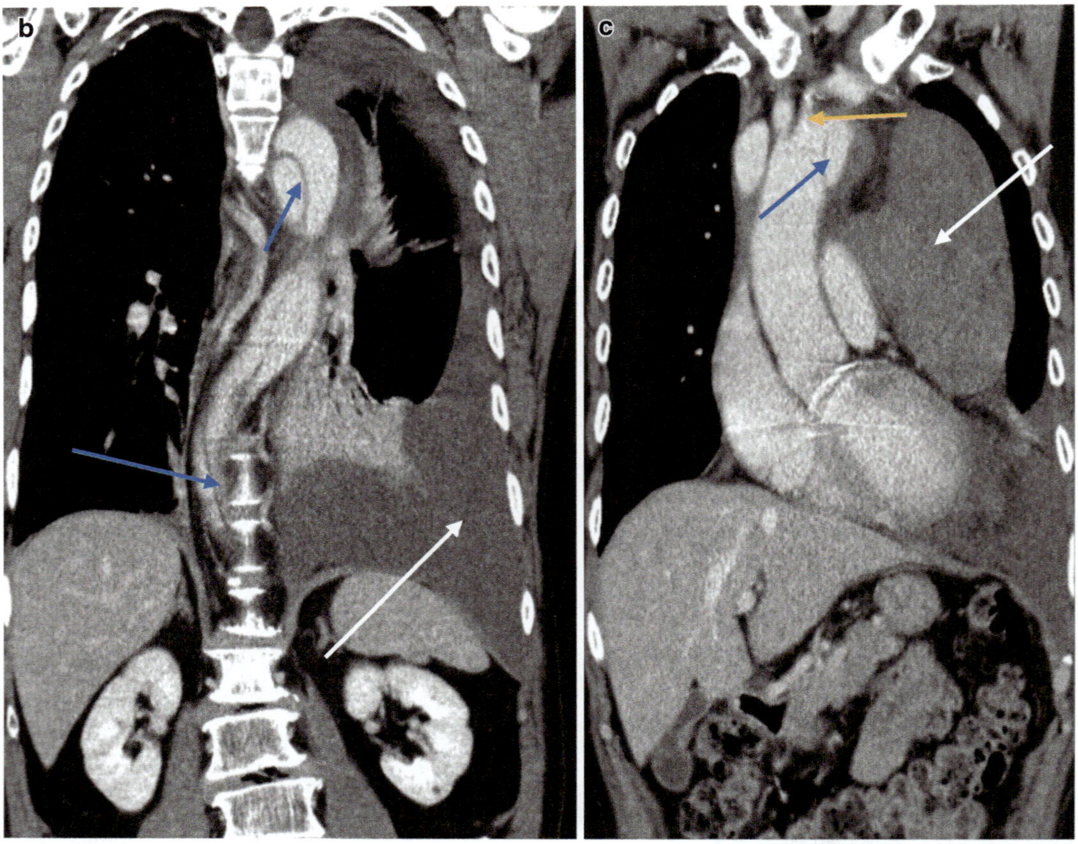

Fig. 3.17 (continued)

emergency TEVAR was scheduled. The patient responded to blood transfusion.

3.1.3.3 Endovascular Treatment

The aortic wall in an acute dissection is fragile, and the risk for retrograde dissection following stent graft implantation is higher than that for subacute dissection. In rupture cases, we must act immediately and need to accept the risks for complications. In this case, another issue was the need to eventually perform carotid-carotid-subclavian bypass to create at least a 20 mm long proximal landing zone. The patient's status deteriorated, however, and we had no time for bypass surgery. Therefore, we proceeded with a direct TEVAR stent-graft operation with the goal of covering the left subclavian artery and deploying a stent graft close to the left common carotid artery. The right common femoral artery was surgically exposed, and a TEVAR stent graft with a diameter of 42 mm (aorta diameter 37 mm) was deployed close to the left common carotid artery, intentionally covering the left subclavian artery (Fig. 3.18). The arterial pressure was kept below 90 mmHg during stent graft deployment to avoid stent graft migration and to precisely deploy the stent. The diagnostic catheter used for control angiography during stent graft deployment was advanced through the left femoral artery. The patient's status improved, and no clinical signs of bleeding were detected after TEVAR. The control CT performed the day after TEVAR showed an expected endoleak due to an insufficient proximal landing zone and unchanged haemothorax (Fig. 3.19). Three days after the first TEVAR, the patient was in a much better clinical status, and we proceeded with total supra-aortic transposition, creating an anastomosis in the ascending aorta distal to both carotid arteries.

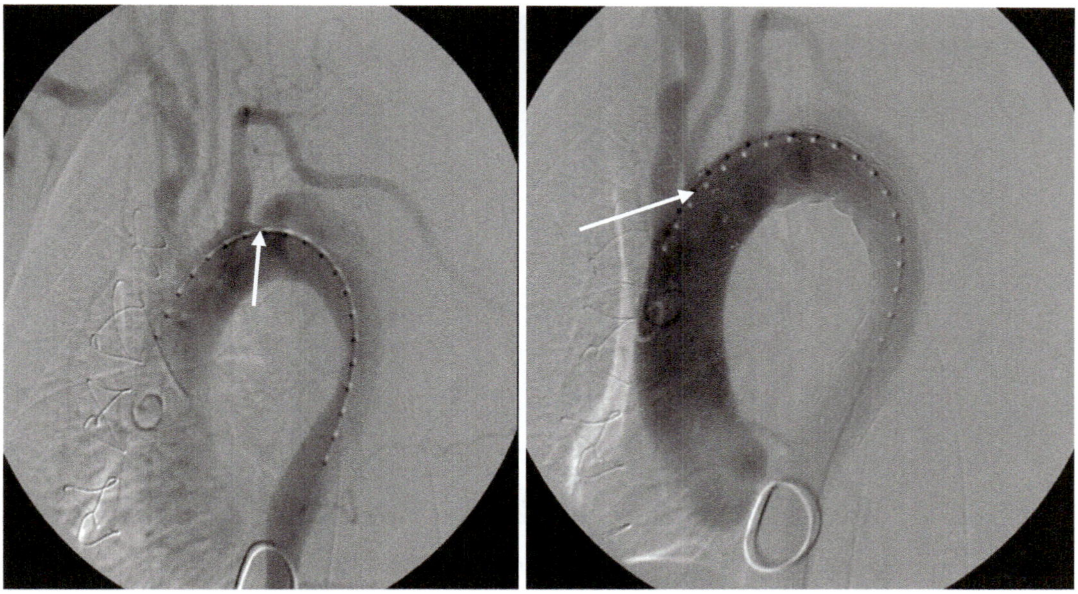

Fig. 3.18 Details of the TEVAR intervention. (**a**) angiograph of the thoracic aorta. Arrow indicates primary entry. (**b**) control angiograph after deployment of the stent graft close to the left common carotid artery (arrow)

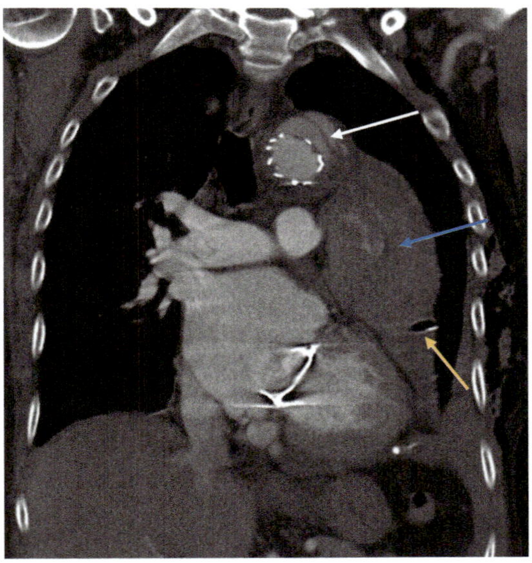

Fig. 3.19 Control CT 1 day after TEVAR. Endoleak type 1 resulting from an insufficient proximal landing zone, and an expected and retrograde endoleak via a non-occluded left subclavian artery (white arrow). Gull arrow points to the chest tube. Blue arrow indicates haemothorax

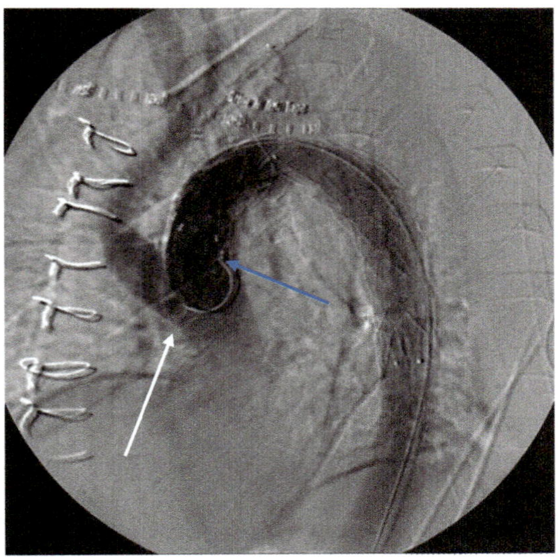

Fig. 3.20 Details from the second TEVAR intervention and supra-aortic bypass. The white arrow indicates the supra-aortic bypass and anastomosis in the ascending aorta. The blue arrow indicates the proximal part of the stent graft. No endoleak was observed

Furthermore, left carotid-subclavian bypass was performed, including ligation of the left subclavian artery. After that, a new TEVAR stent graft was advanced proximally and deployed in the ascending aorta, overlapping with the first stent graft (Fig. 3.20). The stent graft had a diameter of 44 mm. The patient recovered from the surgery very well, and to date no complications have occurred.

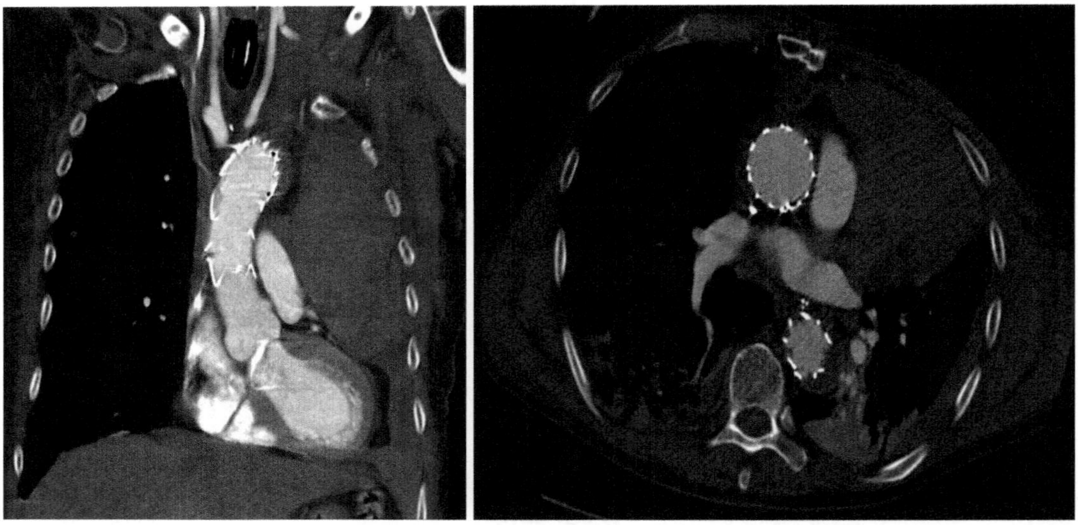

Fig. 3.21 One-month control CT showing a patent bypass and well-deployed stent-graft without endoleak

3.1.3.4 Outcome

The patient was discharged from the hospital after 14 days without any complications. Control CT was performed 1 month later, showing a well-deployed stent graft and open supra-aortic bypass (Fig. 3.21). Nevertheless, haemothorax was still present, but the saturation was 100%.

3.1.4 Subacute Aortic Dissection Type B Presented with Rupture

Key Points

- It is difficult to predict rupture; however, some anatomical characteristics, such as a false lumen diameter over 20 mm, a primary entry over 10 mm, and a total aorta diameter over 40 mm are some proposed features for early TEVAR.
- All effort should be made to treat acute B dissections in the subacute phase to avoid possible retrograde dissection.
- Minimal stent graft oversizing and no post-dilatation are recommend.

3.1.4.1 Aetiology and Clinical Presentation

A 56-year-old patient was sent to the emergency department after complaints of chest pain radiating into the back. The patient was haemodynamically stable with constant chest and back pain. Systolic pressure was 180/110 mmHg. No ECG changes were observed, and no myocardial infarction was suspected.

3.1.4.2 Pre-interventional Diagnosis

Acute contrast-enhanced CT showed an acute aortic dissection type B (Fig. 3.22). Proximal intramural haematoma was present in the descending aorta, and the primary entry was in the middle part of the descending aorta. No signs of malperfusions were present. The patient responded to conservative medical therapy for blood pressure control, including intravenous nitroprusside and beta-blockers, and pain control. After a few hours, the patient was without pain, normotensive and in good shape. The patient was kept in the department for 3 days and discharged in stable clinical condition without pain. A control CT or MRI was scheduled for 1 month later. Twenty-two days later, the patient was admitted again, haemodynamically unstable with blood pressure

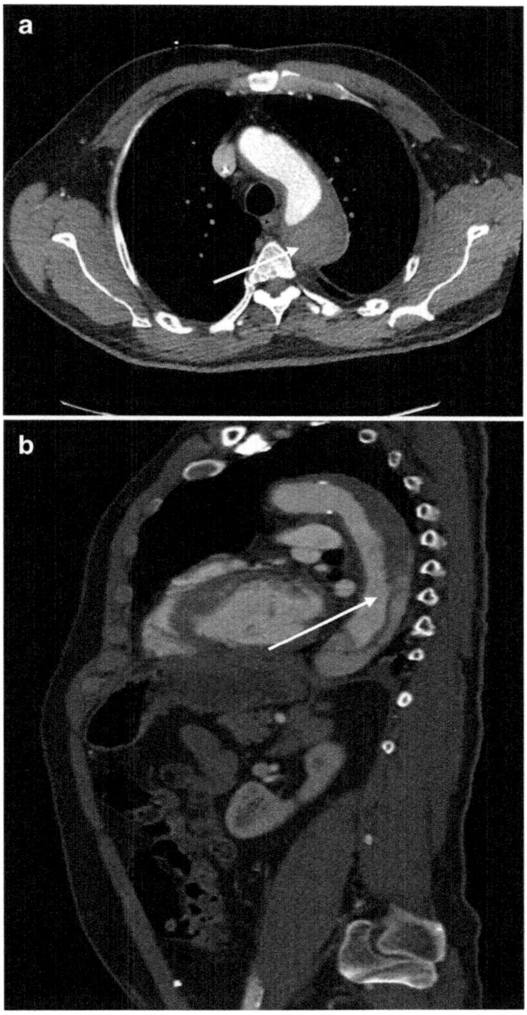

Fig. 3.22 Primary CT showing type B aortic dissection. (**a**) arrow indicates intramural haematoma in the proximal descending aorta. (**b**) arrow indicates primary entry in the middle part of the descending aorta

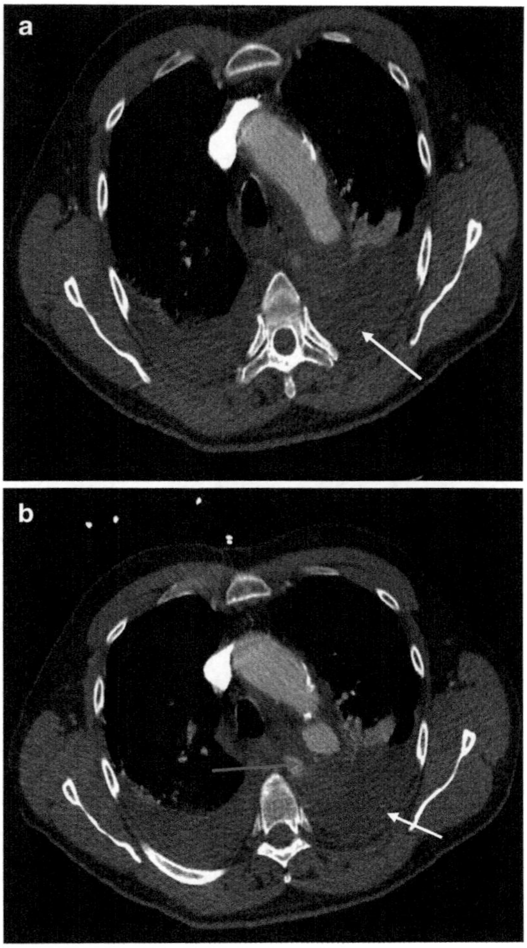

Fig. 3.23 Twenty-two days after the primary CT, the patient developed an aortic rupture and left haemothorax (arrow) (**a**). (**b**) blue arrow indicates rapid enlargement of the false lumen, and white arrow indicates haemothorax

70/40 mmHg and severe pain. Emergency CT showed rapid enlargement of the false lumen and ruptured false lumen with mediastinal haematoma and haemothorax (Fig. 3.23).

3.1.4.3 Endovascular Treatment

Acute TEVAR was conducted. The aorta had different proximal and distal diameters. The proximal aorta had a diameter of 30 mm, and the distal aorta had a diameter of 34 mm. The first stent graft, diameter 34 mm and length 150 mm, was advanced through the exposed right common femoral artery. A diagnostic catheter was advanced via the left femoral artery and used for control angiography. During deployment, blood pressure was kept <90 mmHg. The first stent graft was placed just distal from the left subclavian artery. The second TEVAR stent graft, diameter 38 mm, was then advanced and deployed approximately 5 cm proximal from the coeliac trunk, covering the primary entry and rupture (Fig. 3.24).

3.1.4.4 Outcome

The patient recovered very well and was discharged from the hospital without any complications. One month control CT showed a persistent intramural haematoma in the proximal part of the descending aorta and a shrinking haemothorax

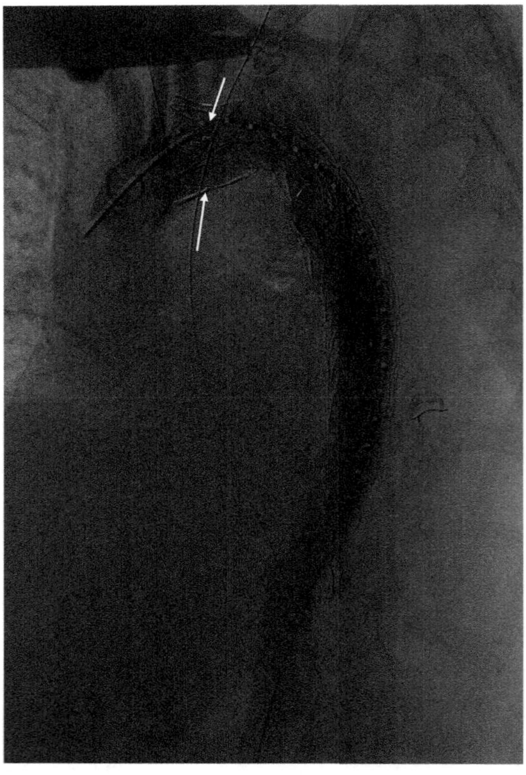

Fig. 3.24 Details from the emergency TEVAR with 34 × 34 × 150 and 38 × 38 × 150 stent grafts, showing satisfactory results. Arrows indicate the proximal covered part of the stent graft deployed just distally from the left subclavian artery

(Fig. 3.25a). Three month control CT showed complete resorption of the intramural haematoma and complete remodelling of the aorta with complete thrombosis of the false lumen and no retrograde dissection (Fig. 3.25b).

3.1.5 Chronic Aortic Dissection with Enlarging Aneurysm-I

Key Points

- Life-long surveillance is necessary for patients with aortic dissection
- Spinal ischaemia should be considered in cases requiring long coverage of the aorta
- Embolization of the false lumen can help in some cases

3.1.5.1 Aetiology and Clinical Presentation

A 67-year-old patient with arterial hypertension underwent urgent surgery because of aortic dissection type A 1 year prior with ascending aortic tube graft replacement. The patient recovered very well, and the dissection in the aortic arch and descending aorta was conservatively treated. The right kidney was hypoperfused on CT imaging; however, the creatinine level was normal (Fig. 3.26). The diameter of the aortic arch and descending aorta was unchanged. Control CT 1 year later revealed rapid enlargement of the false lumen in the descending aorta at a diameter of 55 mm (Fig. 3.27). The patient did not have any other significant comorbidities, and frozen elephant trunk surgery was planned.

3.1.5.2 Pre-interventional Diagnosis

The surgery was performed without permanent complications, and the patient recovered gradually and discharged home. Two years after the second surgery, control CT revealed rapid enlargement of the false lumen in the aortic arch and descending aorta. The aortic diameter was 70 mm versus the previous 52 mm, and the perfusion of the false lumen from the distally uncovered descending aorta persisted (Fig. 3.28).

3.1.5.3 Endovascular Treatment

TEVAR stent graft extension and embolization of the false lumen were performed. First, the TEVAR stent graft was advanced, and after that, a diagnostic catheter was advanced into the false lumen. Through a microcatheter advanced into the diagnostic catheter, a number of 0.018 in. detachable micro-coils were deployed in the false lumen, ranging from 20 to 30 mm in diameter and from 20 to 50 cm in length. After that, the TEVAR stent graft was deployed with at least 3–4 cm overlapping with the frozen trunk graft (Fig. 3.29). Final control angiography showed a satisfactory result and no endoleak or opacifications of the false lumen. All visceral arteries were patent. The patient was discharged from the hospital 2 days later without any complications. The potential risk for spinal ischaemia was a concern. However, the internal iliac, lumbar and subclavian arteries were open,

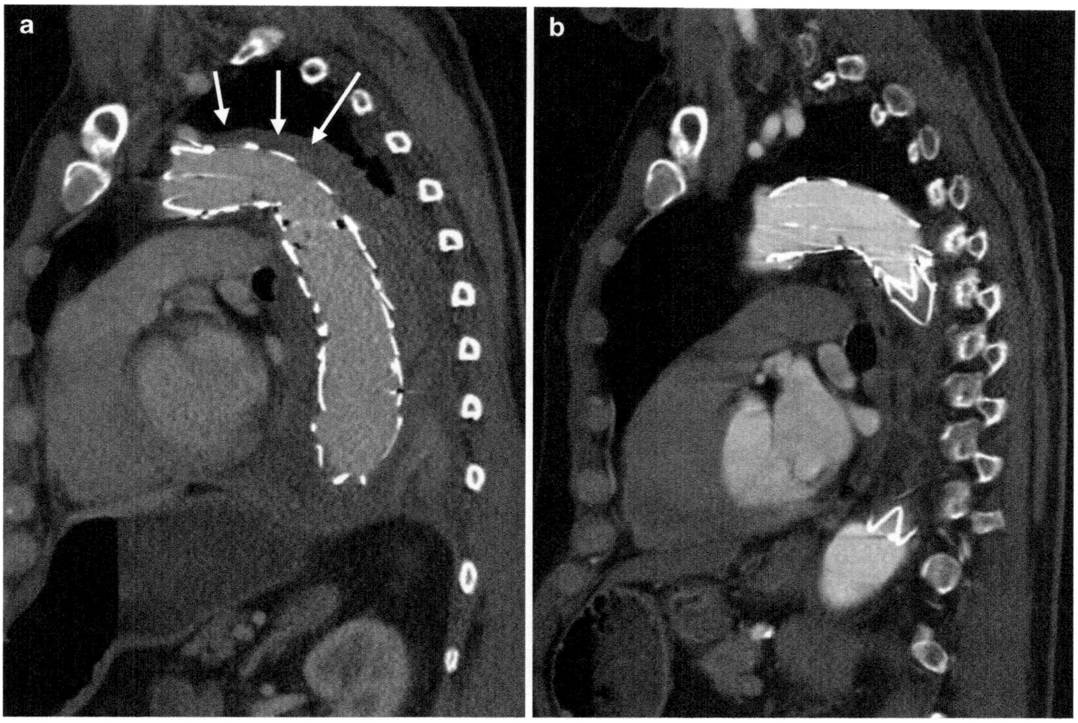

Fig. 3.25 (**a**) One month control CT control showing intramural haematoma (arrows). (**b**) Three month control CT control showing complete intramural haematoma resorption. The left haemothorax and mediastinal haematoma regressed as well

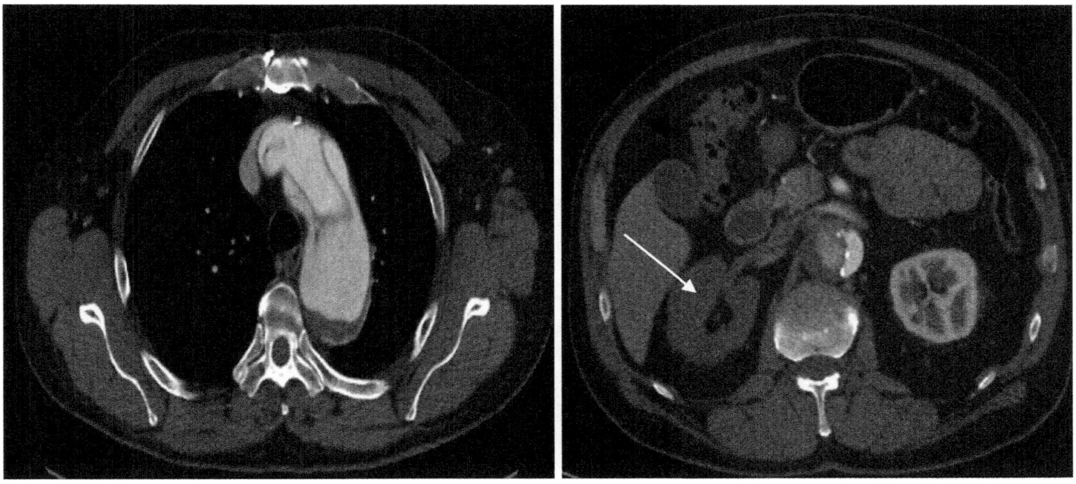

Fig. 3.26 Contrast-enhanced CT after ascending acute aorta surgery. Dissections in the aortic arch and descending aorta were conservatively treated, and the patient was asymptomatic. Note the right kidney showing no contrast despite a normal creatinine level (white arrow)

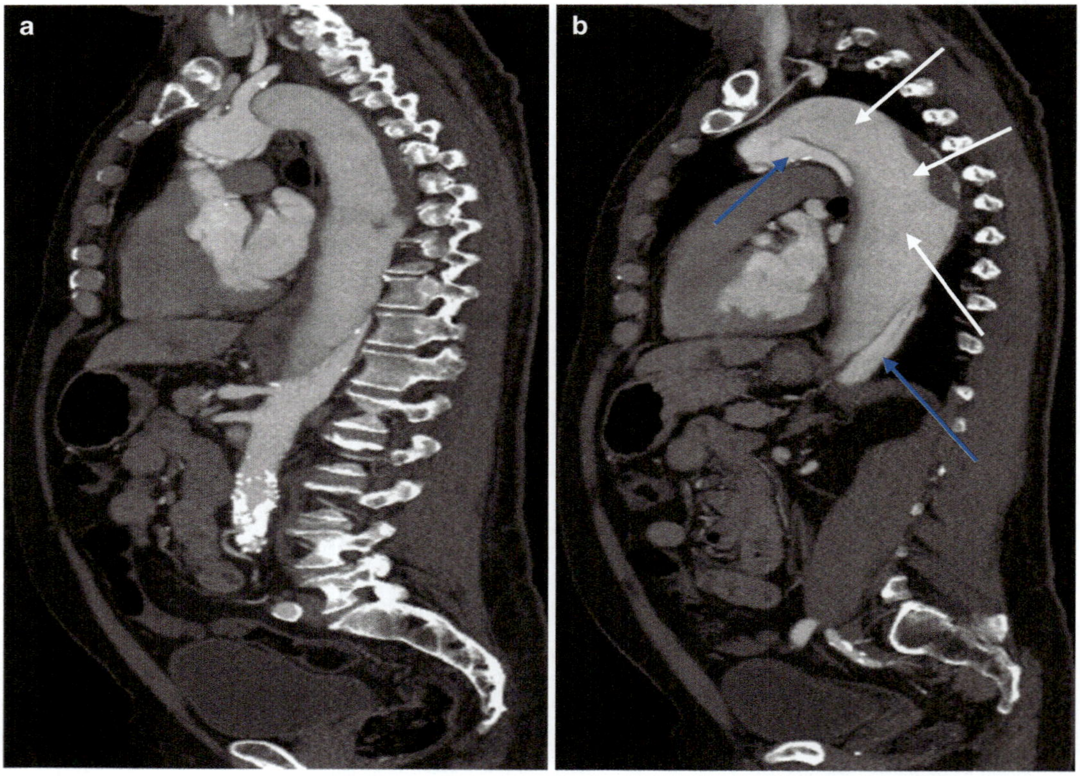

Fig. 3.27 Contrast-enhanced control CT. (**a**) three month control image after ascending aorta surgery. (**b**) one year later, control CT shows rapid enlargement of the false lumen (white arrows). Blue arrows indicate the true lumen

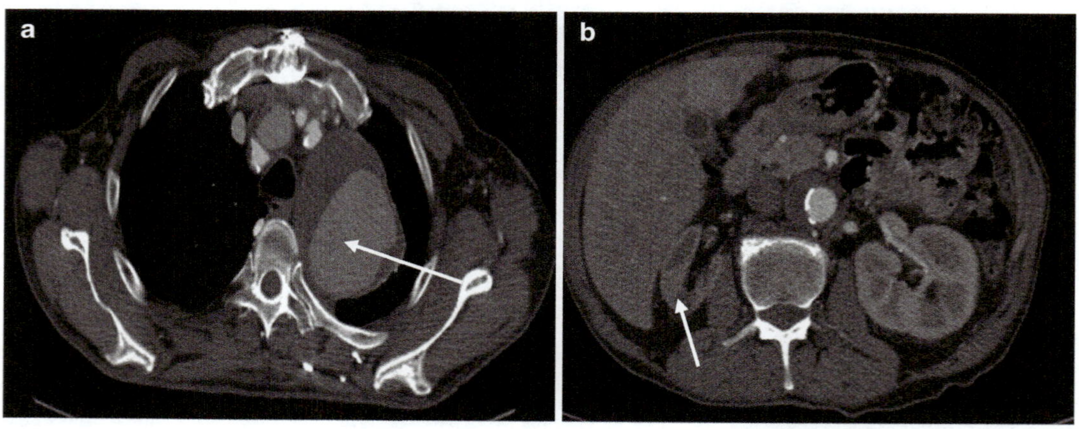

Fig. 3.28 Contrast-enhanced control CT images 2 years after frozen elephant trunk surgery with rapid enlargement of the false lumen. White arrows in panels **a**, **c** and **d** indicate endoleak and contrast in the false lumen. Panel **b** shows better right kidney perfusion (white arrow). The blue arrow in panel C indicates the frozen elephant trunk stent

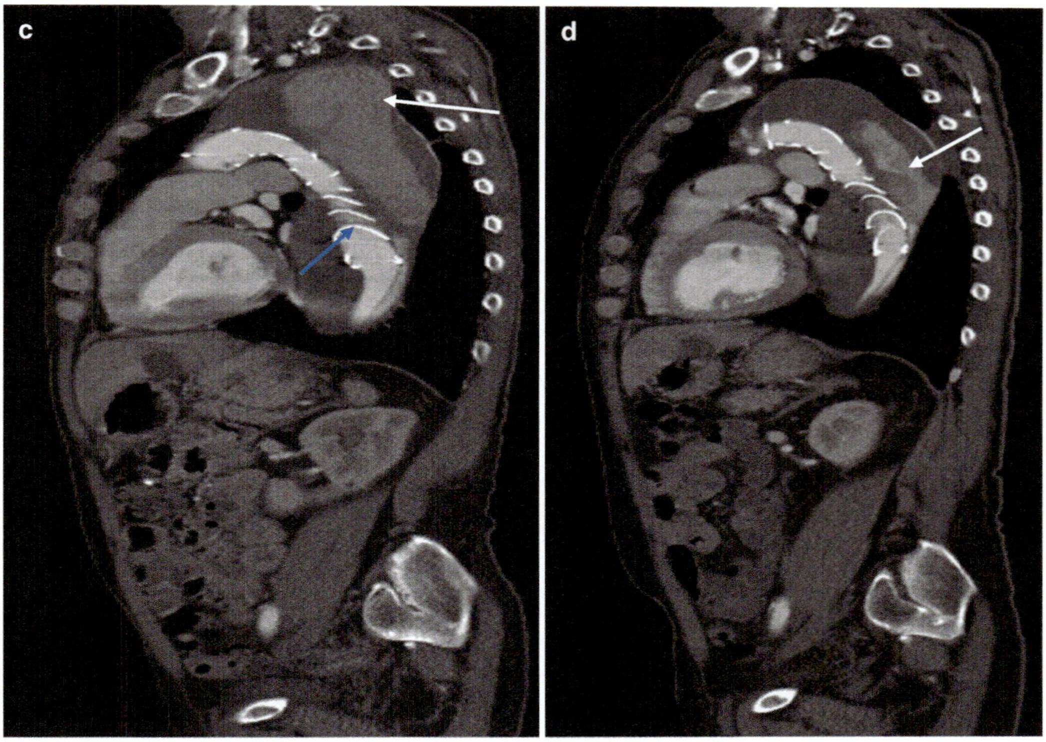

Fig. 3.28 (continued)

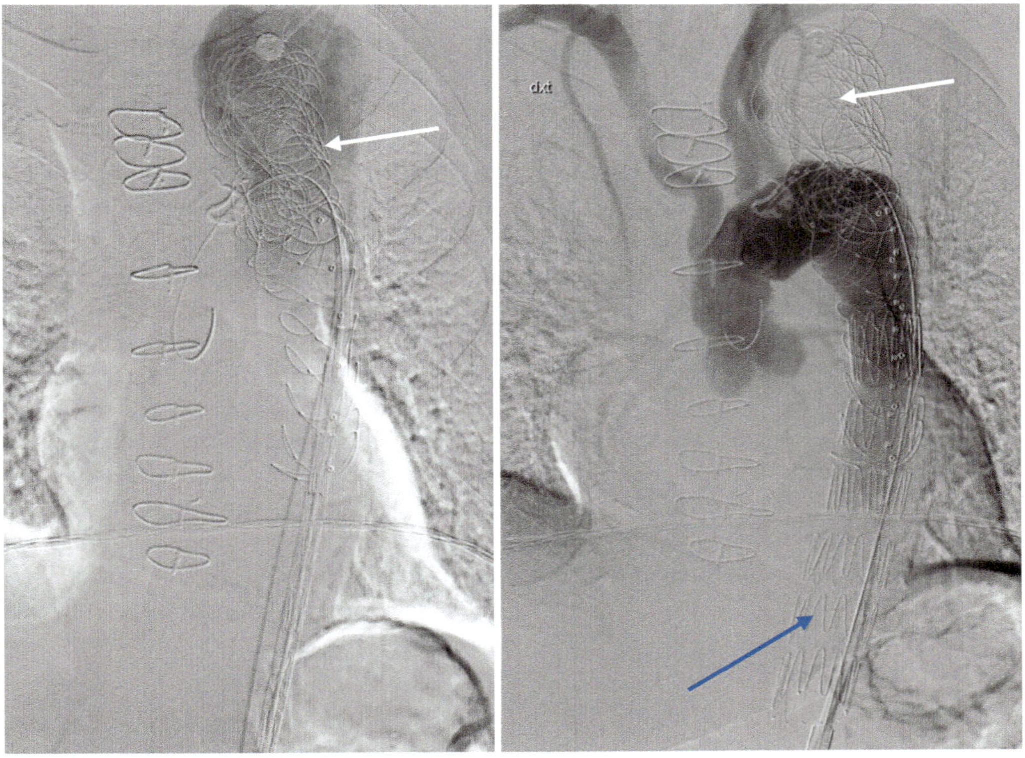

Fig. 3.29 Details from the TEVAR stent graft deployment and embolization of the false lumen with micro-coils, indicated with white arrows. Blue arrows indicate the TEVAR stent graft

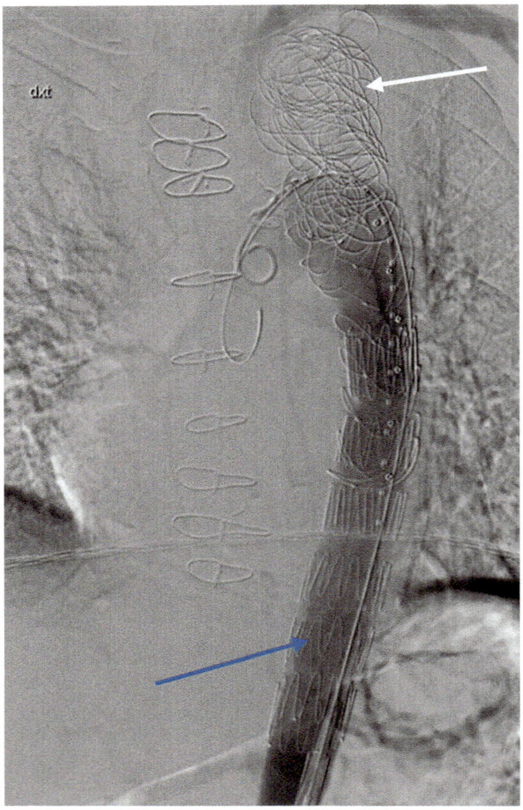

Fig. 3.29 (continued)

and staged covering of the descending aorta minimized the risk for spinal ischaemia. False lumen embolization, a relatively simple technique that can promote thrombosis, was performed. Most likely, only TEVAR stent graft extension can achieve the same result, but embolization can be used in some complex situations as well.

3.1.5.4 Outcome

The patient is asymptomatic and doing well. Contrast-enhanced control CT showed no new events, and the false lumen diameter remains stable (Fig. 3.30). Strict blood pressure control is mandatory and being performed with two drugs.

3.1.6 Chronic Aortic Dissection with Enlarging Aneurysm-II

Key Points

- Frequent control scans is advisable for some patients with aortic dissection.
- In non-ruptured cases and if the duration of the complex fenestrated aortic stent graft operation is prolonged, it would be better to stop the intervention and complete it at a later date.
- The guidewire should be controlled to avoid forcible advancing of the branch stent graft and thus rupture. Alternative access should be used instead.

3.1.6.1 Aetiology and Clinical Presentation

A 67-year-old patient with an advanced-stage chronic obstructive lung disease and arterial hypertension was admitted to the emergency centre because of severe back abdominal pain. The patient was haemodynamically stable, and the arterial pressure was 180/120 mmHg. The pain was constant. There were no signs of coronary ischaemia.

3.1.6.2 Pre-interventional Diagnosis

Contrast-enhanced CT showed aortic dissection with primary entry in the distal descending aorta and intramural haematoma in the proximal part of the descending aorta (Fig. 3.31). There was no dissection or haematoma in the ascending aorta or aortic arch. The patient was admitted to the hospital and treated conservatively with intravenous nitroprusside, beta-blockers and pain control, showing good results. The patient was discharged from the hospital 5 days later without pain or any other complaints. Control CT 1 month later showed false lumen expansion and aneurysm growth,

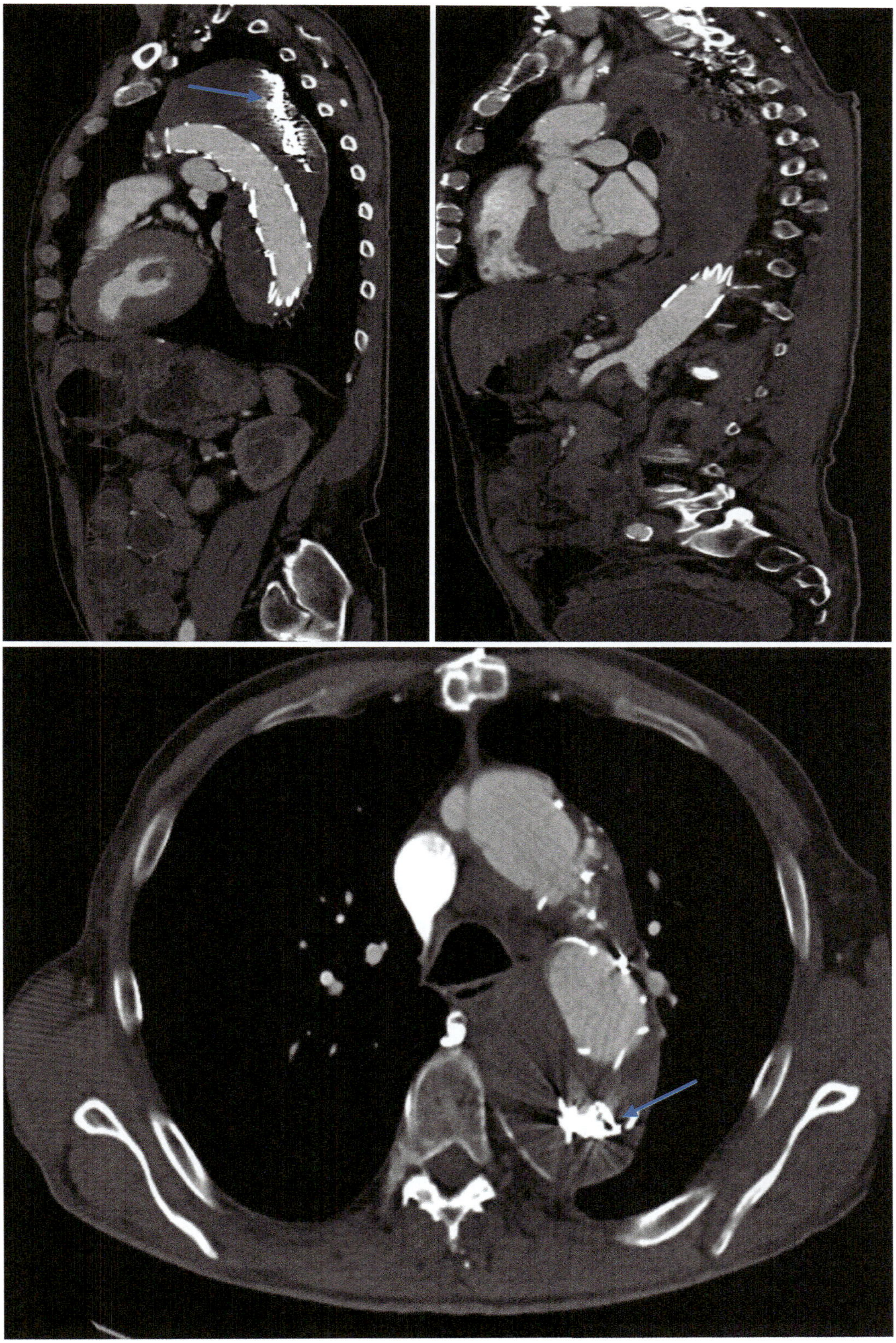

Fig. 3.30 Contrast-enhanced control CT showing satisfactory results. No endoleak is observed. Better opening of the true lumen was achieved. Blue arrows indicate the micro-coils

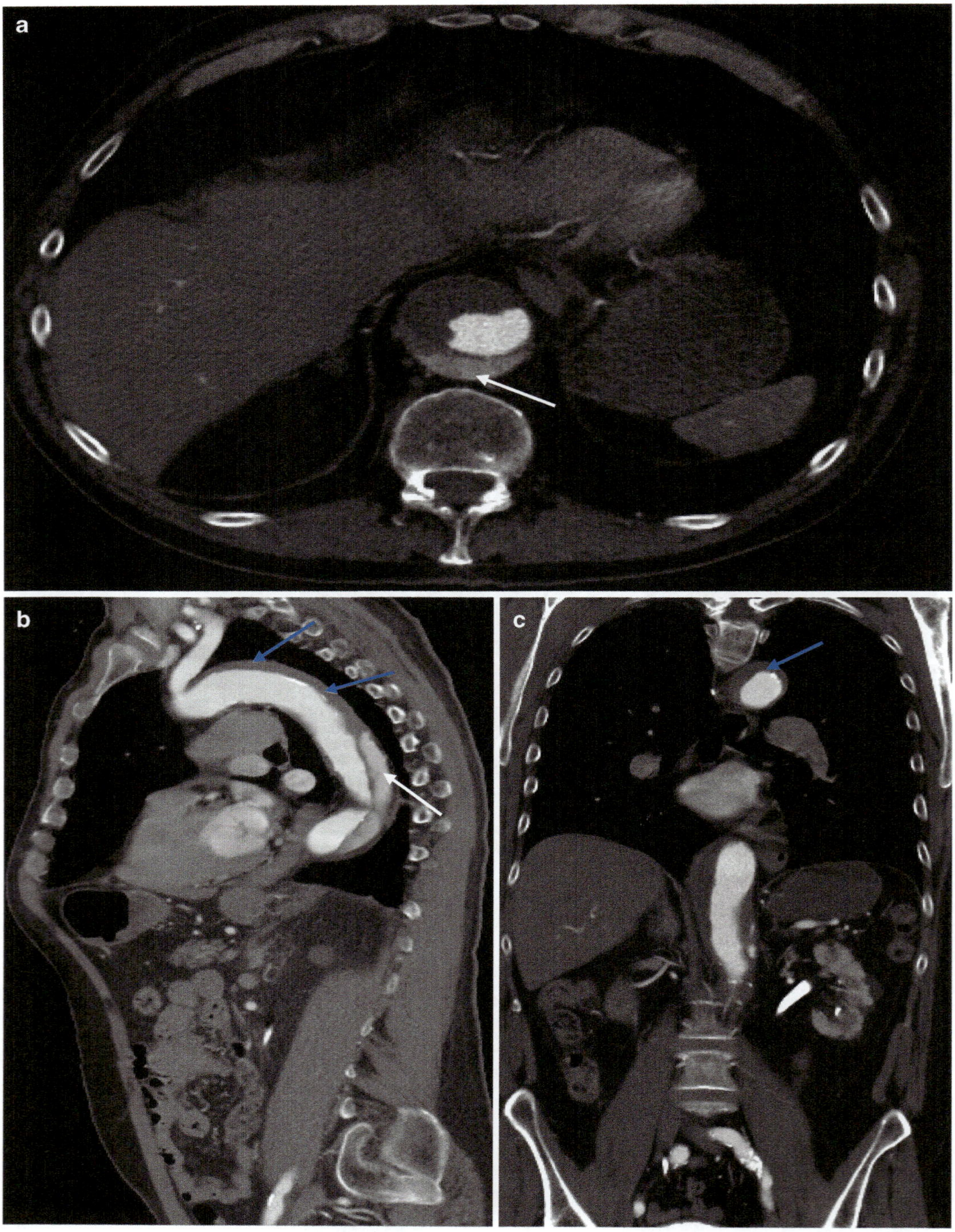

Fig. 3.31 Aortic dissection type B with primary entry in the distal descending aorta. (**a**) white arrow indicates the false lumen. (**b** and **c**) blue arrows indicate intramural haematoma in the proximal descending aorta. White arrow indicates the false lumen

but the patient remained asymptomatic. The diameter of the aorta, including both lumens in the descending aorta, was 57 mm, approximately 1 cm growth beyond that on the initial scan, indicating the need for endovascular treatment (Fig. 3.32). The dissection extended slightly distally from the renal vessels. The intramural haematoma in the proximal part of the descending aorta had regressed.

3.1.6.3 Endovascular Treatment

Two-stage endovascular treatment was planned. First, a TEVAR stent graft was deployed distally from the left subclavian artery approximately 5 cm proximally from the coeliac trunk. The second stage was planned for a few weeks later after ordering a custom-made fenestrated stent graft with four fenestrations. The first TEVAR stent graft was easily deployed distally from the left subclavian artery (Fig. 3.33), and the patient was discharged from the hospital. A few weeks later, the patient was readmitted for second-stage intervention, and the patient remained asymptomatic. The fenestrated stent- graft was advanced and deployed according to the instructions. First, the superior mesenteric artery was cannulated and secured. After that, the left renal artery was cannulated without difficulties (Fig. 3.34). However, it was challenging to cannulate and advance a 6 Fr sheathe into the right renal artery. During the manipulation, one segmental renal branch ruptured, and the patient became haemodynamically unstable. The 0.035 in. guidewire was kept safely in the renal artery, and very carefully, the 5 Fr glide catheter was advanced over the wire into the renal artery.

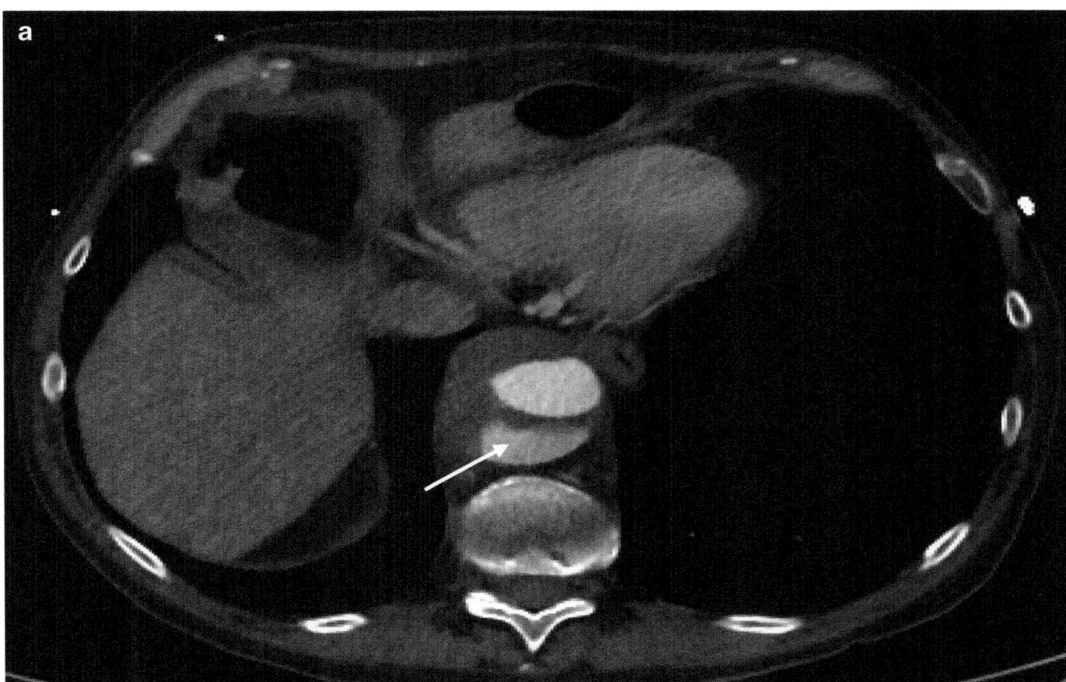

Fig. 3.32 Contrast-enhanced control CT images 1 month later with fast enlargement of the false lumen (white arrows), (**a–c**) Compared with the initial CT findings, **a** and **b** show regression of the intramural haematoma and a healthier aortic wall (blue arrows)

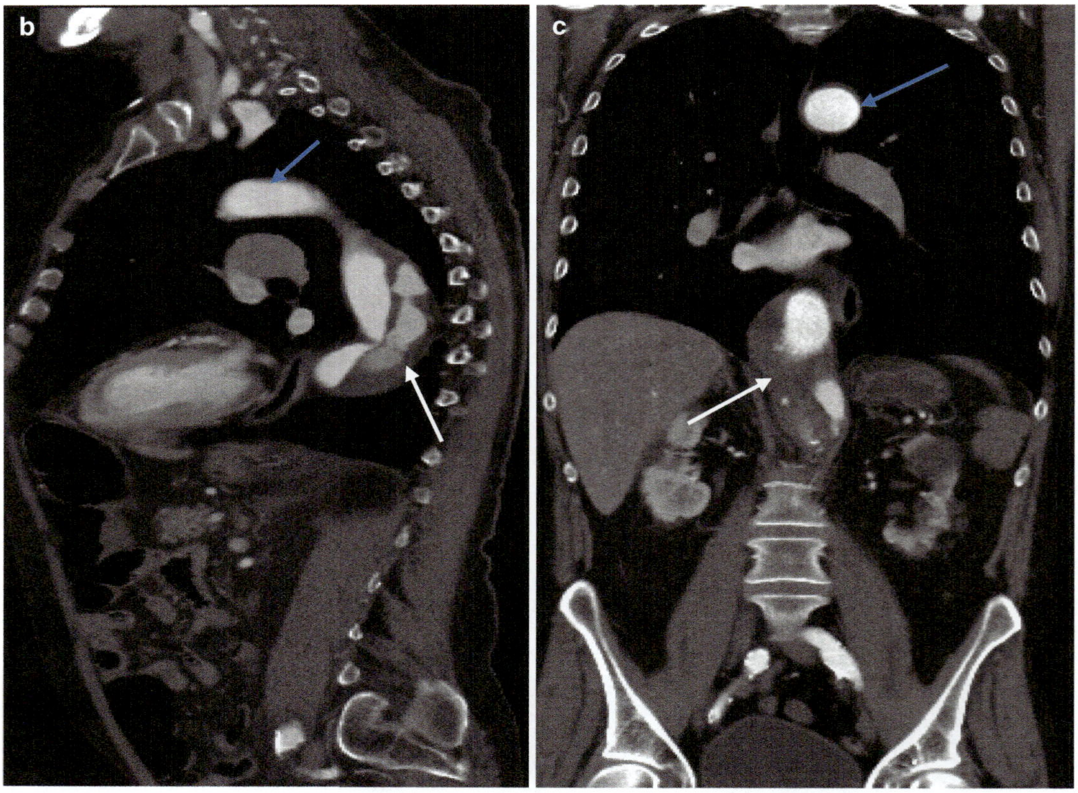

Fig. 3.32 (continued)

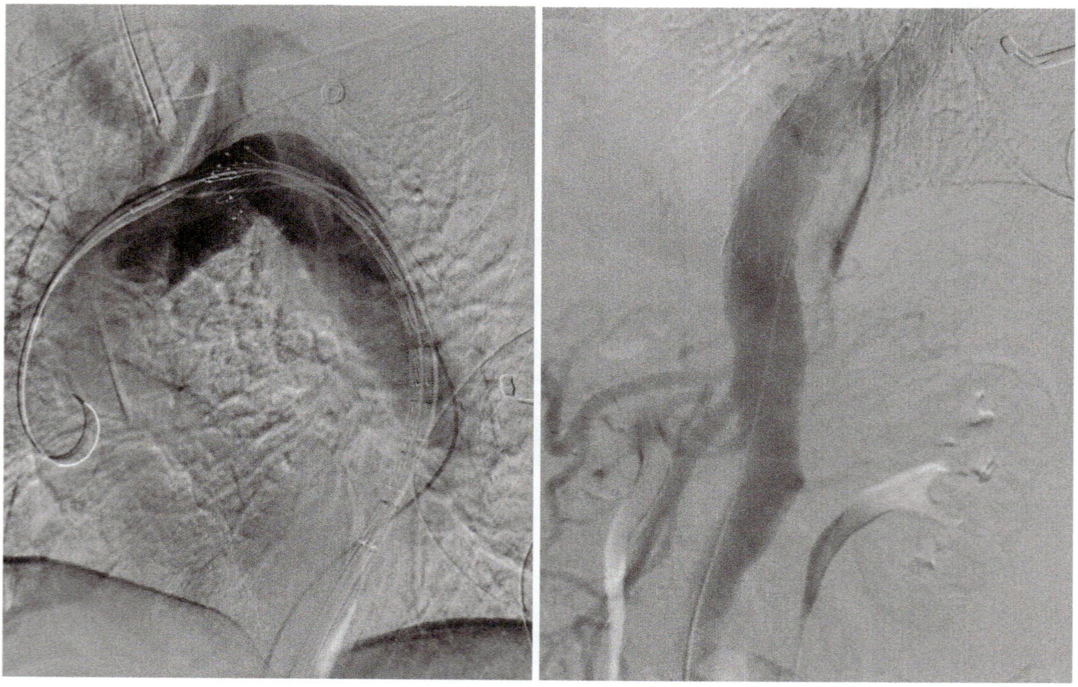

Fig. 3.33 First stage of the intervention showing TEVAR stent graft deployment distal to the left subclavian artery

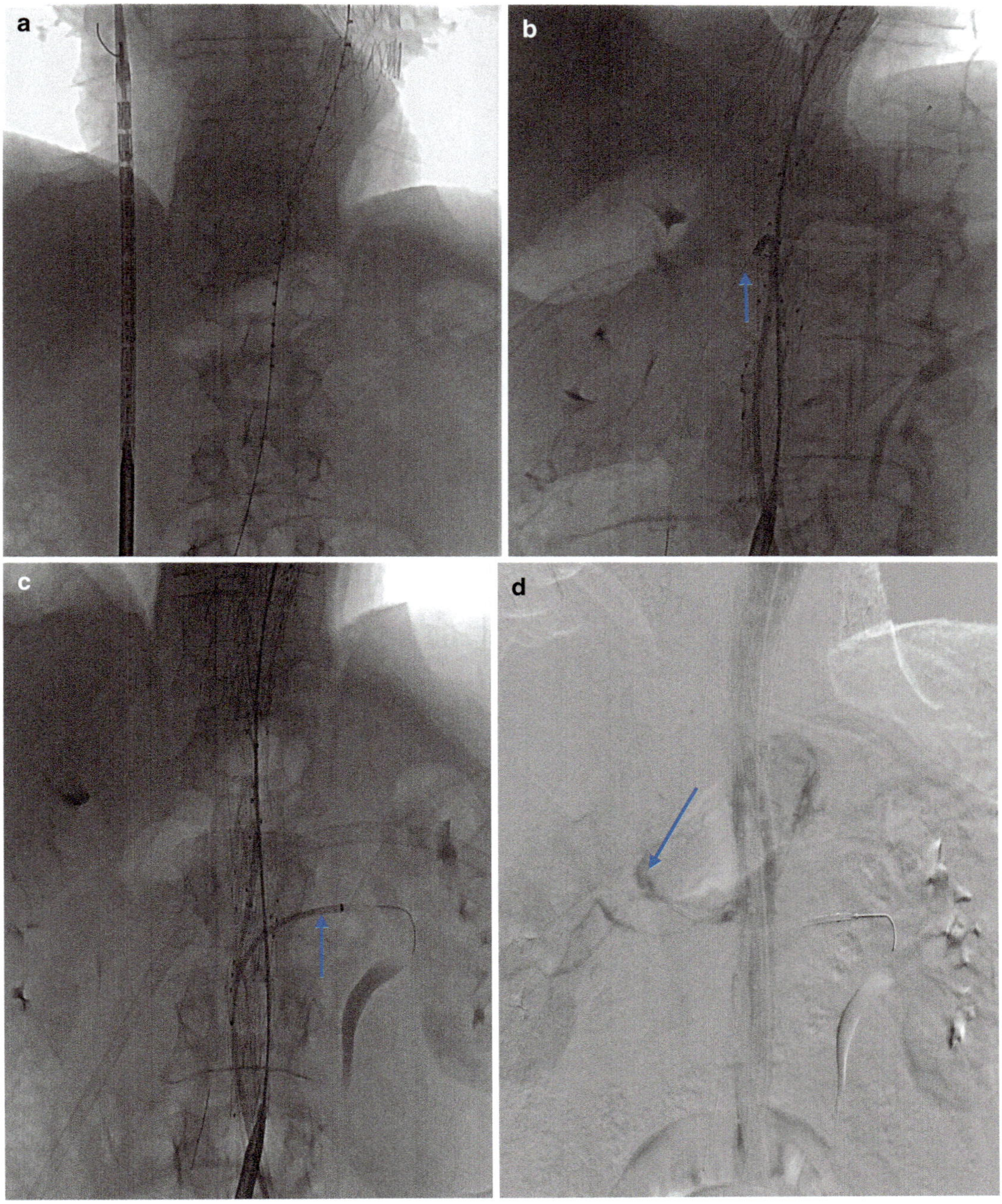

Fig. 3.34 Details form the fenestrated stent graft deployment. (**a**) orientation of the stent graft. (**b**) secured superior mesenteric artery (arrow). (**c**) secured left renal artery (arrow). (**d**) bleeding from the segmental branch of the right renal artery (arrow)

Next, a 0.021 in. microcatheter was advanced coaxially through the glide catheter into the renal artery, the bleeding segmental branch was occluded with a few micro-coils, and bleeding was arrested. The right renal stent was advanced via the left brachial artery. Difficulties were encountered in canulated and advancing a stent through the coeliac trunk; therefore, we decided to stop the intervention and perform coeliac trunk stent deployment later (Fig. 3.35).

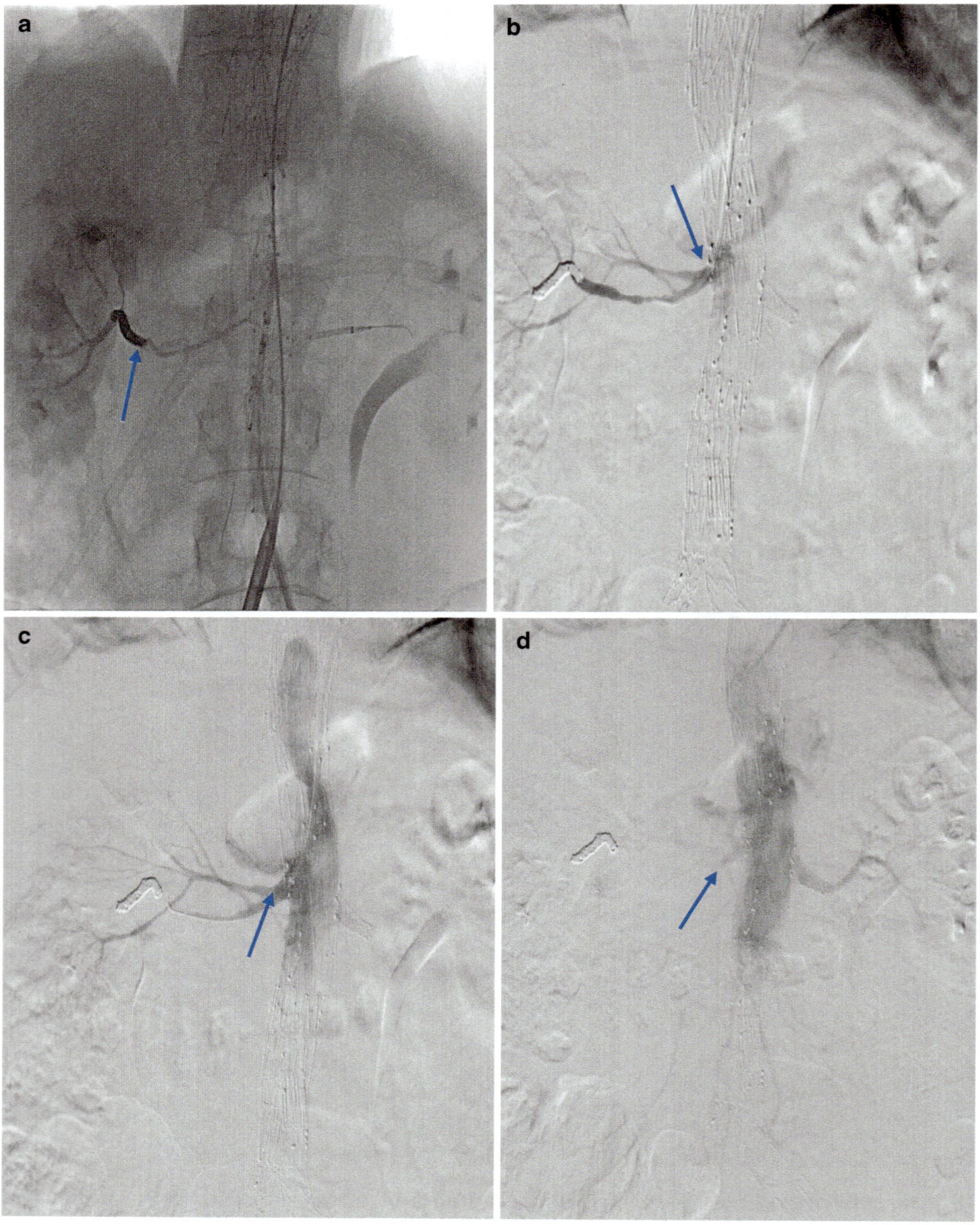

Fig. 3.35 Embolization of the bleeding segmental right renal artery (arrow) (**a**). Advancement and deployment of the stent into the right renal artery via left brachial access (arrow) (**b**, **c**). Control angiography showing persistent spasm of the right renal artery (arrow) (**d**)

3.1.6.4 Outcome

The patient was discharged from the hospital 4 days after the intervention. The coeliac trunk fenestration was still open, and secondary intervention was planned for a few weeks later. Two weeks after the intervention, the patient was admitted to the emergency department with dyspnoea and 88% oxygen saturation. Acute CT

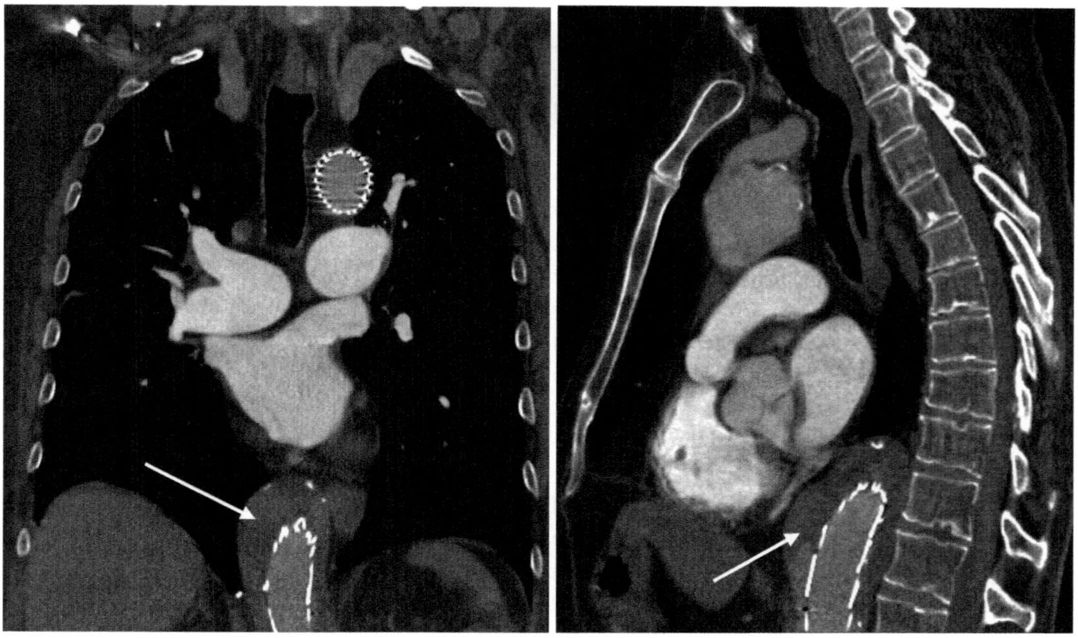

Fig. 3.36 Acute contrast-enhanced CT scan due to clinical suspicion of pulmonary embolism. No pulmonary embolus was detected. An endoleak emerged due to an open fenestration to the coeliac trunk (arrows). Unfortunately, the distal aorta segment was not scanned during this examination

scanning was performed, and the initial clinical suspicion was lung emboli. None were observed, however, and exacerbation of the chronic obstructive diseases was diagnosed. Unfortunately, only chest CT scanning was performed, and none of the stent grafts in the entire length were scanned (Fig. 3.36). The patient is still awaiting secondary intervention and remains asymptomatic.

3.2 Thoracic Aortic Aneurysms

3.2.1 Ruptured Thoracic Descending Aortic Aneurysm

Key Points

- It is difficult to predict rupture; however, some anatomical characteristics, such as a false lumen diameter over 20 mm, a primary entry over 10 mm in length, and a total aorta diameter over 40 mm are some features that may suggest the need for early TEVAR.
- It is very important to lower blood pressure below 90 mmHg during TEVAR stent graft deployment. Constant communication with the anaesthesiologist is imperative.

3.2.1.1 Aetiology and Clinical Presentation

A 66-year-old asymptomatic patient with a chronic type B aortic dissection was conservatively treated. The patient had been controlled twice previously for a stable aortic dissection, and blood pressure was well controlled with two drugs. The patient had a 51 mm abdominal aortic aneurysm. Approximately one and a half years after the dissection was diagnosed, the patient was brought to the emergency department hypotensive and in shock. Retrosternal pain radiating into the back was intense in the beginning, but on admission, the pain was moderate. The patient responded well to resuscitation therapy. There were no signs of coronary ischaemia.

3.2.1.2 Pre-interventional Diagnosis

Emergency contrast-enhanced CT revealed a ruptured aortic type B dissection with mediastinal haematoma. The false lumen had rapidly enlarged compared with the finding on the previous CT scanning, leading to rupture in the proximal part of the descending aorta (Fig. 3.37). The primary entry was just below the left subclavian artery. After stabilization, emergency partial supra-aortic vessel debranching and TEVAR were planned to produce a proximal landing zone of at least a 20 mm proximal landing zone. The dissection extended distally to the level of the coeliac artery.

3.2.1.3 Endovascular Treatment

Carotid-carotid bypass was performed, followed by left carotid-subclavian artery bypass. The right common femoral artery was exposed, and a TEVAR stent graft was advanced and deployed close to the brachiocephalic trunk (Fig. 3.38). The blood pressure was below 90 mmHg during stent graft deployment, allowing us control over graft insertion and avoidance of stent graft migration or coverage of the brachiocephalic trunk. The second stent graft was extended distally. Control angiography showed a satisfactory result and complete rupture coverage.

3.2.1.4 Outcome

The patient recovered well. There were no neurologic complications or spinal ischaemia. The patient remained haemodynamically stable, and no new bleeding complications had occurred. Control CT control 1 month after surgery showed a good result and no endoleaks. The mediastinal haematoma showed evidence of regression. Carotid and subclavian bypass were opened. Bilateral pleural effusion, hiatus hernia and atelectasis were diagnosed on the control CT (Fig. 3.39). Three month control CT showed additional mediastinal haematoma regression and satisfactory results. The bilateral pleural effusion showed evidence of regression. There was no sign of distal progression of the dissection (Fig. 3.40).

3.2.2 Aortic Arch Aneurysm I

Key Points

- Aortic arch aneurysms require partial or total supra-aortic debranching. Usually, a first open surgery is performed, and after a few weeks, the second stage procedure and TEVAR stent raft deployment are conducted.
- It is important to manipulate the superstiff guidewire carefully to avoid dissecting the ascending aorta.
- Systolic pressure during the deployment should be ≤90 mmHg. Other options, such as a temporary pacemaker, are also available.

3.2.2.1 Aetiology and Clinical Presentation

A 67-year-old patient complained of unspecific mild retrosternal discomfort and was caught during the last few weeks. There were no signs of infection, and all laboratory examination results were within standard limits. The patient was afebrile. Chest X-ray indicated possible widening of the mediastinum.

3.2.2.2 Pre-interventional Diagnosis

Contrast-enhanced CT showed a 50 mm aortic arch saccular aneurysm (Fig. 3.41). The left common carotid artery and brachiocephalic trunk shared a common stem-bovine arch. There were no other abnormalities in the thoracoabdominal aorta.

3.2.2.3 Endovascular Treatment

Left carotid-subclavian bypass surgery was performed first. One week later, under general anaesthesia, a TEVAR stent graft 34 mm in diameter and 200 mm in length was advanced through the exposed right femoral artery. Before stent-graft deployment, the left subclavian artery was occluded in the pre-vertebral

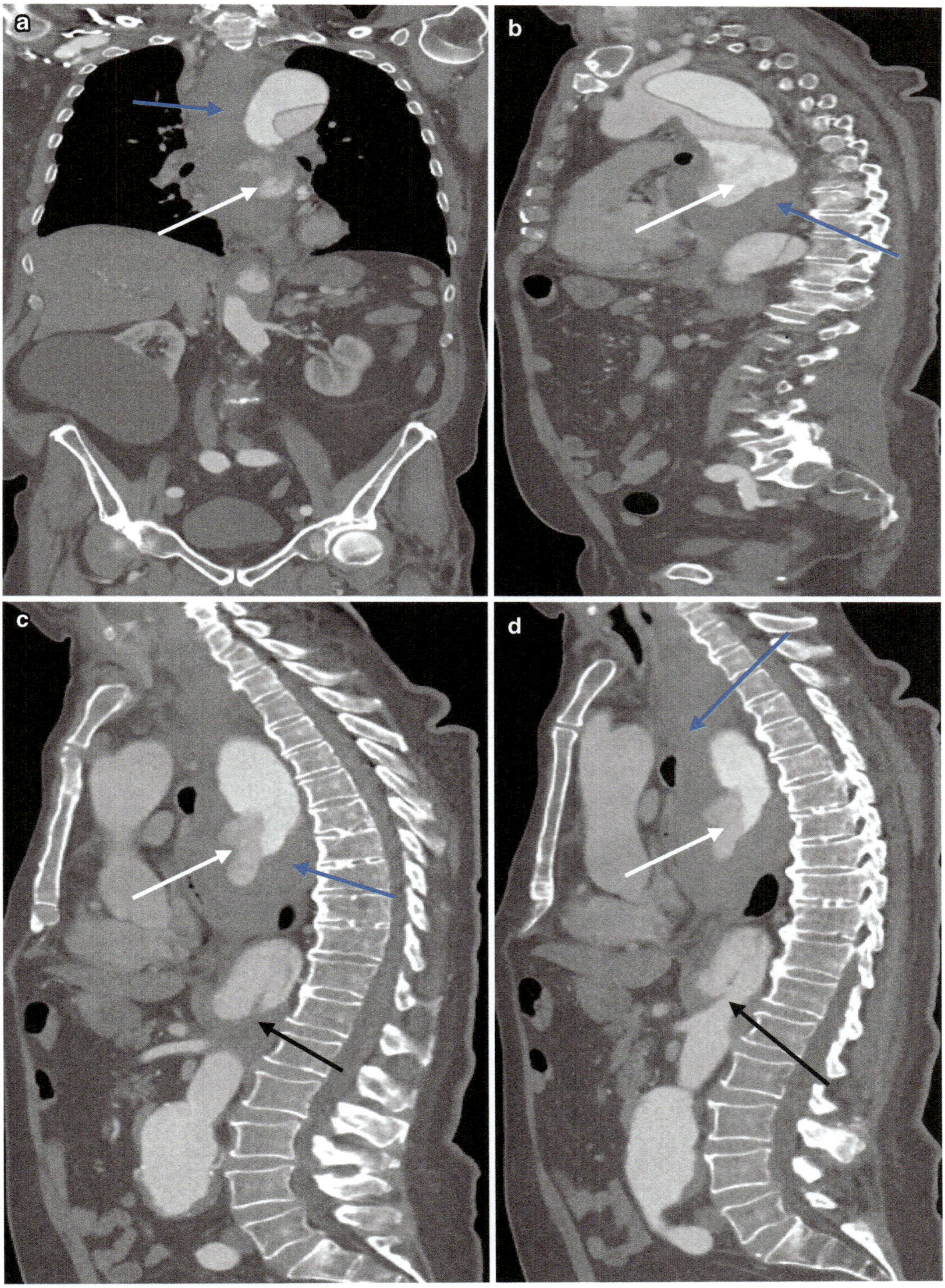

Fig. 3.37 Emergency contrast-enhanced CT showing a ruptured type B aortic dissection. White arrows indicate enlarged and ruptured false lumens. Blue arrows indicate mediastinal haematoma (**a** and **b**). (**c** and **d**) Black arrows indicate distal extension of the dissection up to the level of the coeliac trunk

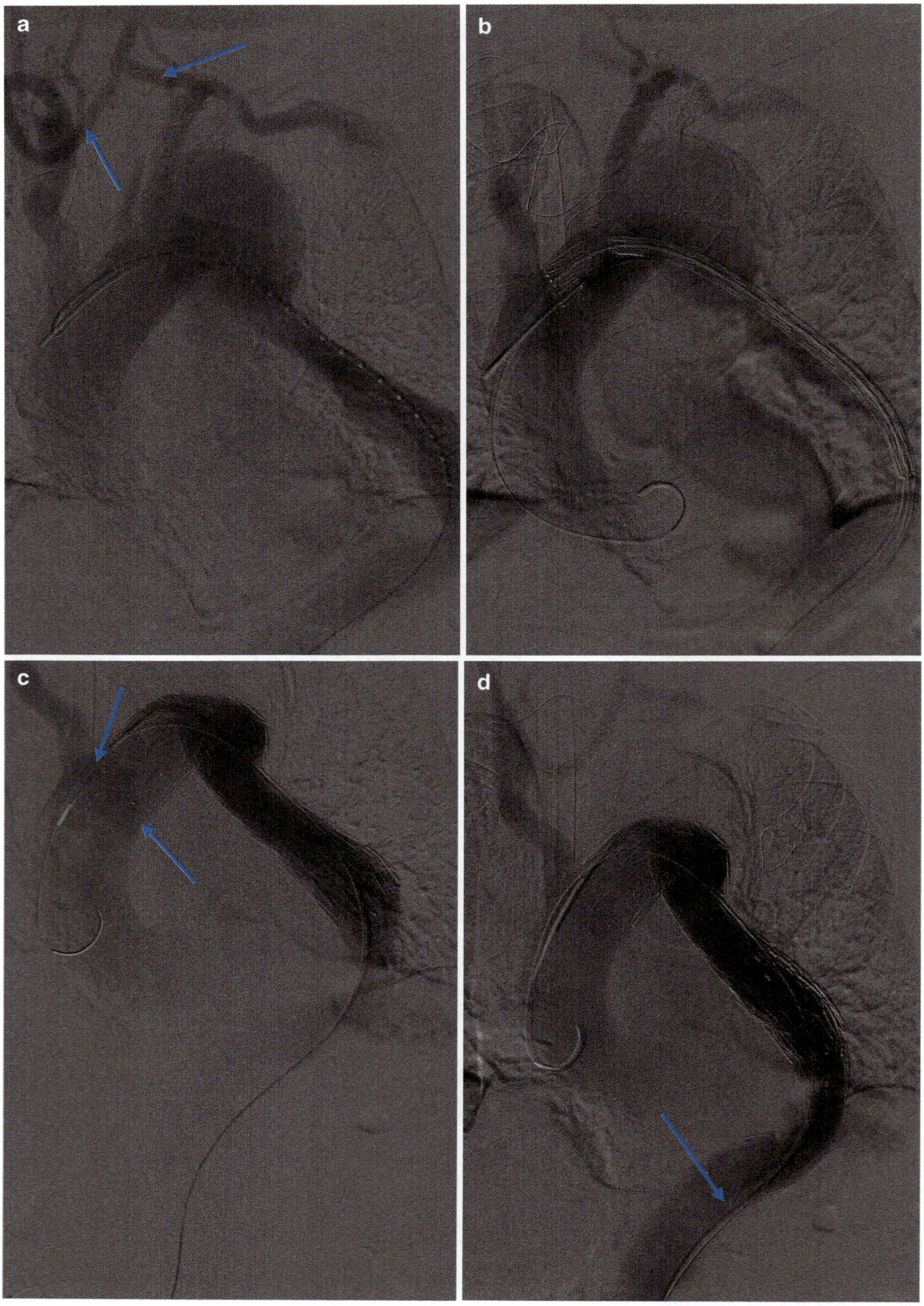

Fig. 3.38 After carotid-carotid bypass and left carotid-subclavian bypass, TEVAR stent-grafts were deployed. (**a**) pre-TEVAR angiography shows patent carotid and subclavian bypass (arrows). (**b**) advancement of the stent graft. (**c**) first TEVAR stent graft deployed close to the brachiocephalic trunk (arrow). (**d**), distally extended TEVAR stent graft with compete coverage of the rupture (arrow)

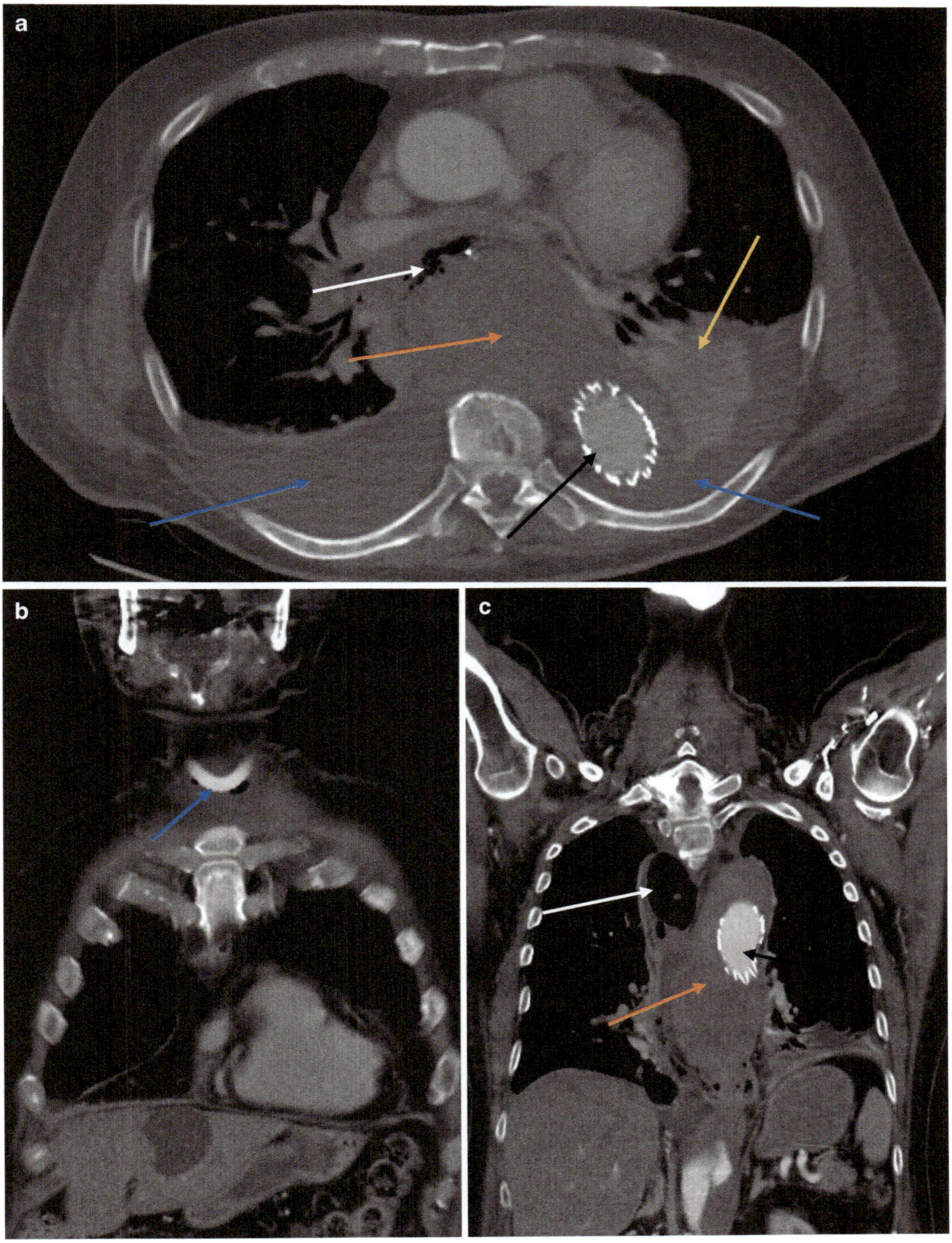

Fig. 3.39 Control images 1 month after surgery. (**a**) Black arrow indicates a well-deployed stent graft and no endoleak. Blue arrows indicate bilateral pleural effusion. Yellow arrow indicates left lung atelectasis. Orange arrow indicates mediastinal haematoma, and white arrow indicates hiatus hernia. (**b**) blue arrow indicates carotid-carotid bypass. (**c**) white arrow indicates a hiatus hernia, and orange arrow indicates a mediastinal haematoma

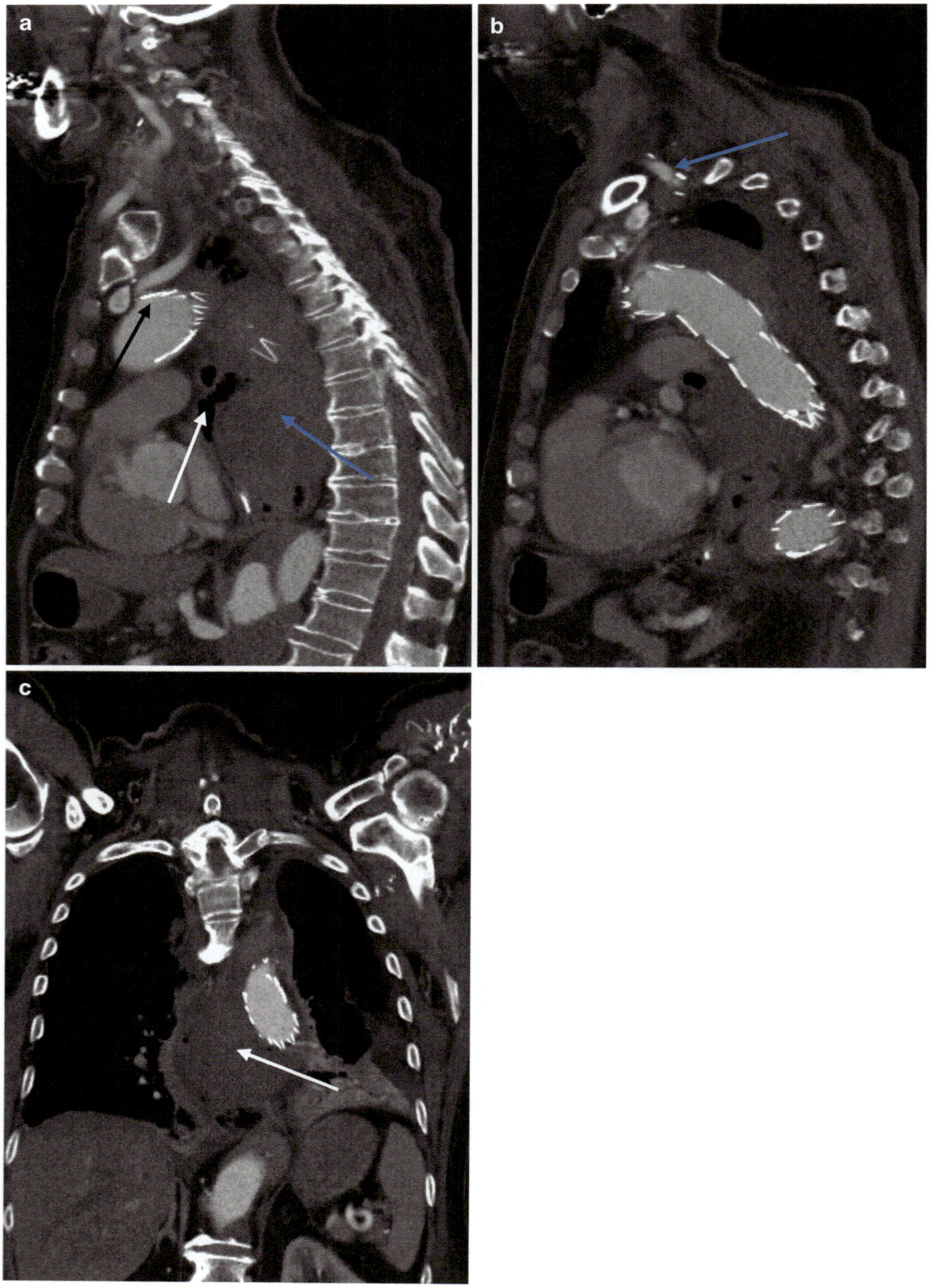

Fig. 3.40 Three months after surgery, control images show a satisfactory outcome. (**a**) black arrow indicates a well-deployed stent close to the brachiocephalic trunk. White arrow indicates hiatus hernia. Blue arrow indicates mediastinal haematoma. (**b**) blue arrow indicates carotid-subclavian bypass. (**c**) white arrow indicates mediastinal haematoma

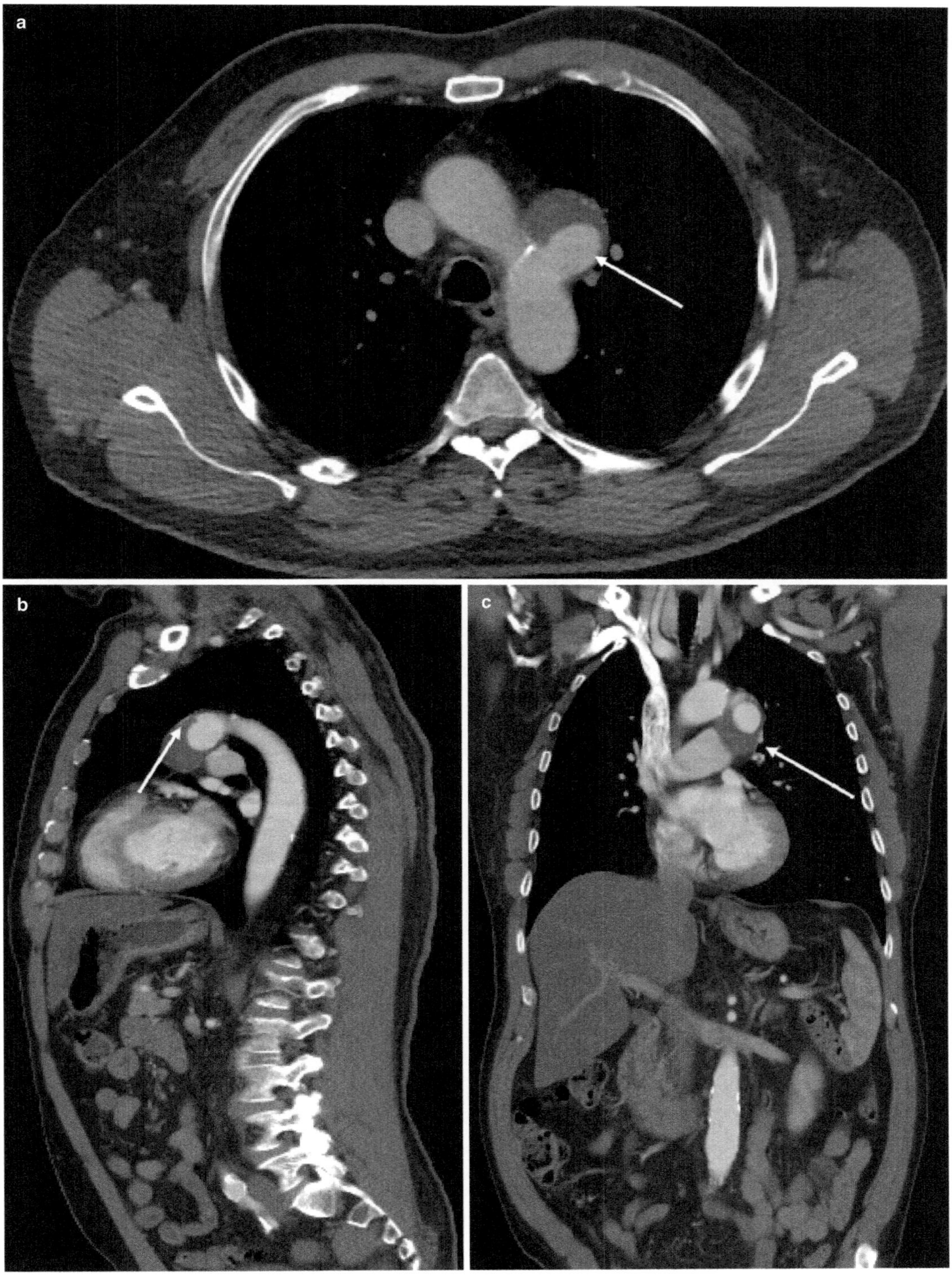

Fig. 3.41 Contrast-enhanced CT showing a 50 mm saccular aortic arch aneurysm (white arrows). (**a**) axial reconstruction. (**b**) sagital reconstruction. (**c**) coronal reconstruction

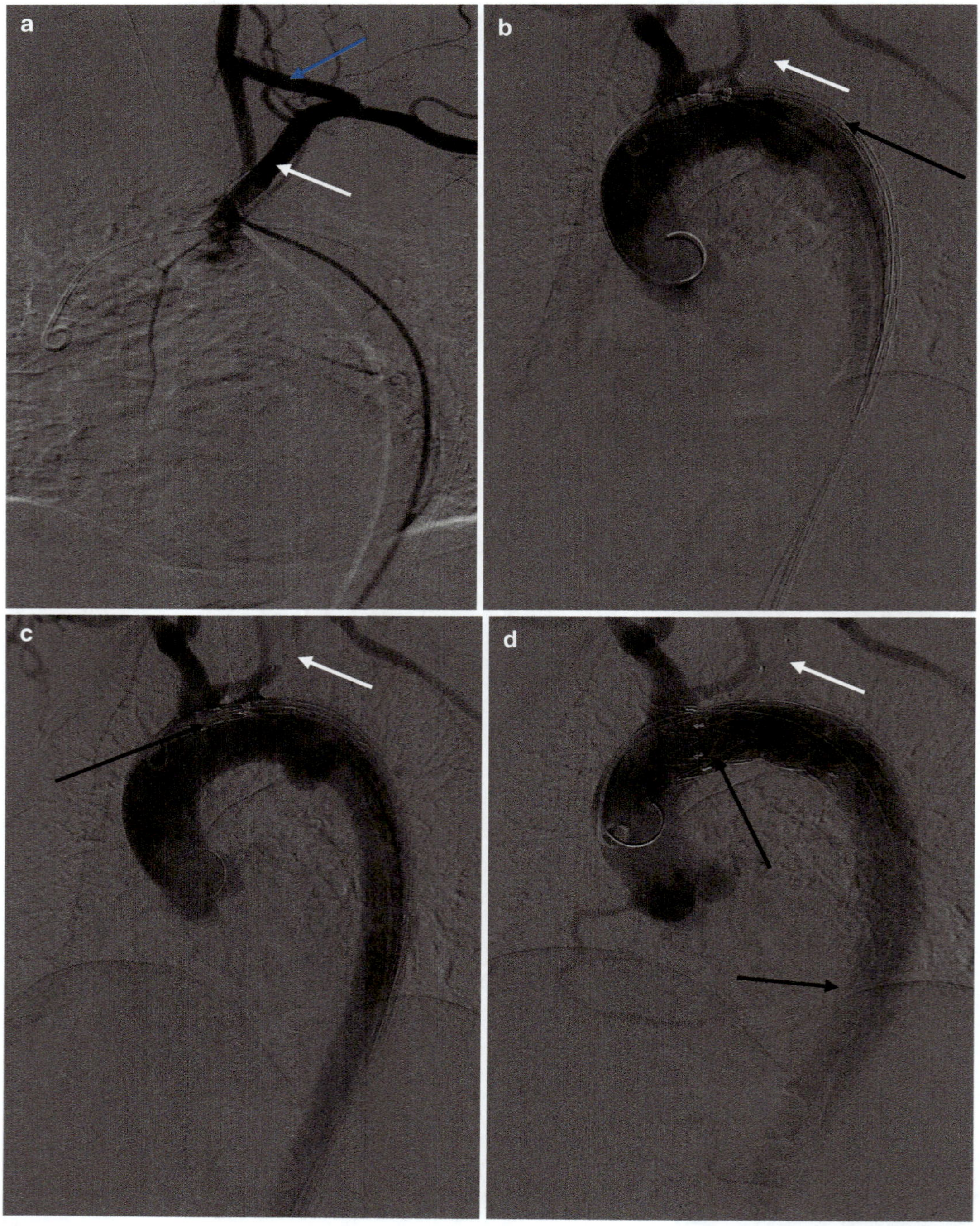

Fig. 3.42 First, the left subclavian artery was occluded with an Amplatz plug placed 16 mm into the pre-vertebral segment (white arrows). Blue arrow indicates the carotid-subclavian bypass. Advancement and deployment of the TEVAR stent graft (black arrows)

segment with an Amplatz plug advanced percutaneously through the left femoral artery. The stent graft was precisely inserted close to the carotid artery, and during deployment, systolic pressure was kept below 90 mmHg (Fig. 3.42).

3.2.2.4 Outcome

The patient was discharged from the hospital without pain, and no complications occurred during the surgery and beyond. Three month control CT (Fig. 3.43) and 1 year post-surgery control MRI (Fig. 3.44) showed satisfactory results and shrinkage of the aneurysm.

3.2.3 Aortic Arch Aneurysm II

> **Key Points**
> - Angiography should always be performed and carotid-subclavian bypass

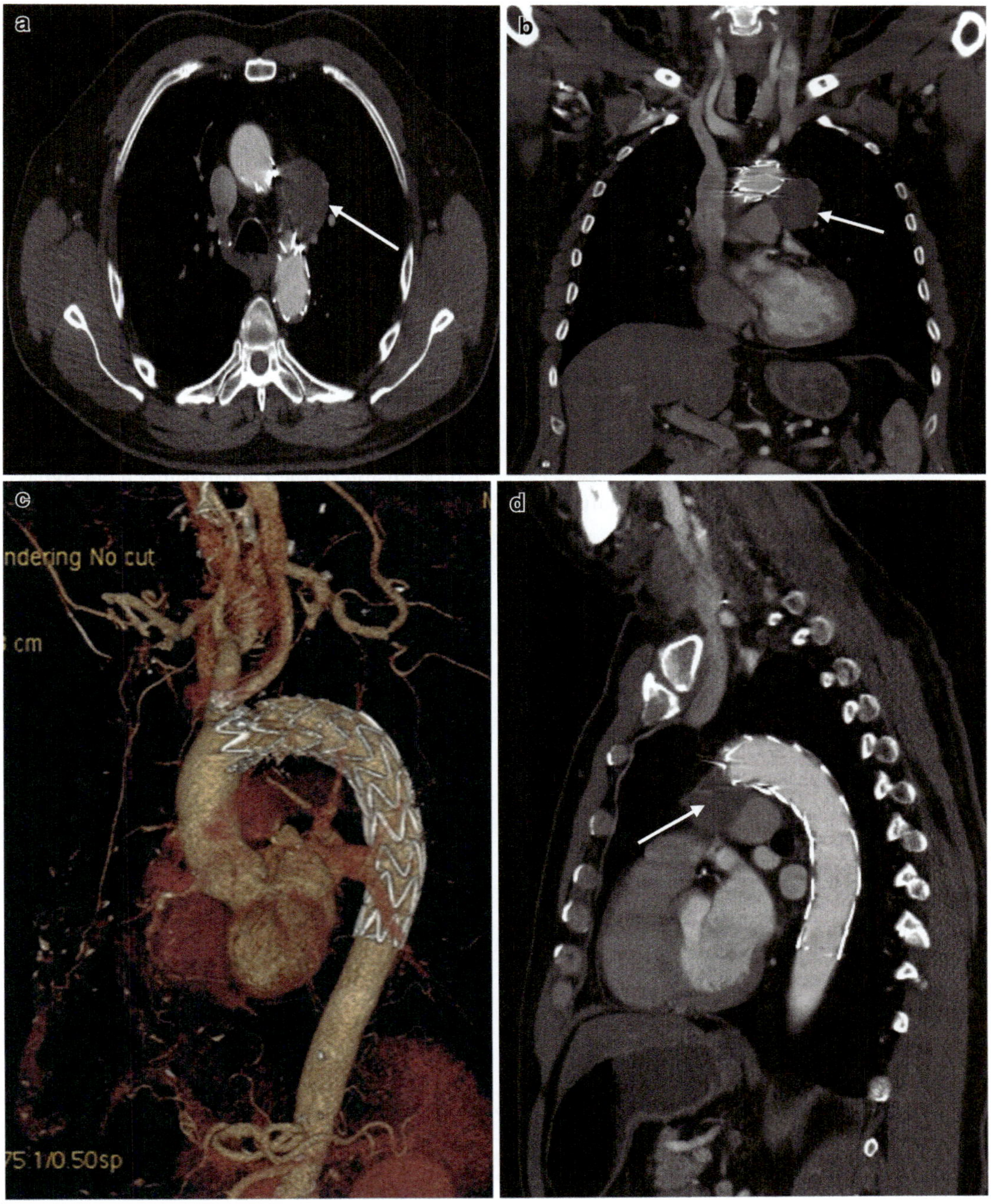

Fig. 3.43 Three month control CT showing complete exclusion of the aneurysm and no endoleak (white arrows)

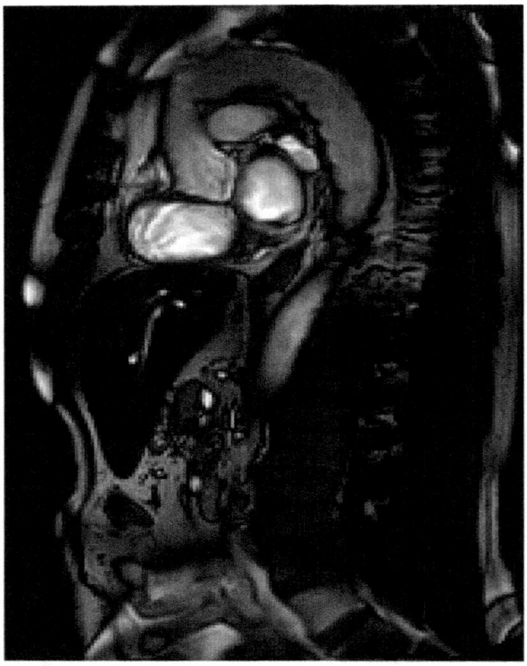

Fig. 3.44 One-year control MR showing a satisfactory result and saccular aneurysm shrinkage

checked before occlusion of the left subclavian artery.
- Concurrent flow thought the bypass and subclavian artery could cause thrombosis of the bypass.
- A tapered stent graft should be used if the proximal and distal diameters are different.

3.2.3.1 Aetiology and Clinical Presentation

A 73-year-old patient had previously undergone open abdominal aortic repair with an aortic tube graft and coronary bypass, including LIMA-LAD bypass. The patient was asymptomatic and had controlled arterial hypertension. An aortic arch aneurysm was incidentally discovered and controlled.

3.2.3.2 Pre-interventional Diagnosis

The previous contrast-enhanced control CT showed a 60 mm aortic arch aneurysm. The entire aortic arch showed a proximal aneurysm with a diameter of 40 mm (Fig. 3.45).

3.2.3.3 Endovascular Treatment

After being informed about the treatment options and risks, the patient chose to undergo treatment. First, left carotid-subclavian bypass was performed uneventfully. Three weeks later, the left subclavian artery was occluded with an Amplatz plug first in the pre-vertebral segment and distally from the LIMA-LAD bypass. The left subclavian artery was occluded directly before confirmation that the bypass was patent. Then, a TEVAR stent graft (Relay NBS, Bolton Medical; a stent graft with a varying diameter) was deployed. The first tapered stent graft (42–38 mm) was deployed distally in the descending aorta (Fig. 3.46). After that, a stent graft with a diameter of 46–24 mm was deployed in the aortic arch, and due to a discrete type 1 endoleak, a few micro-coils were placed through a micro-catheter advanced between the stent graft and aortic wall (Fig. 3.47).

In the intensive care unit, the patient developed signs of myocardial ischaemia and clinical occlusion of the carotid-subclavian bypass. Reviewing the angiographic images, we observed that the bypass was indeed occluded, which we missed during TEVAR. Emergency surgery was performed, creating a new carotid-subclavian bypass with good clinical outcomes. However, a prolonged stay in the hospital due to left phrenic nerve palsy and left diaphragm elevation was required.

3.2.3.4 Outcome

Patient recovery gradually remained a problem with left partial diaphragm paralysis. There were no neurological or spinal ischaemia complications. The first control was performed 3 months after the surgery with a satisfactory result and no endoleak (Fig. 3.48). Two years after surgery, the patient complained of retrosternal pain, and CT revealed new aortic dissection type A and increasing dilatation of the ascending aorta (Fig. 3.49). There was no endoleak, and carotid-subclavian bypass was patent. There was no option for surgical treatment, and the patient was treated conservatively.

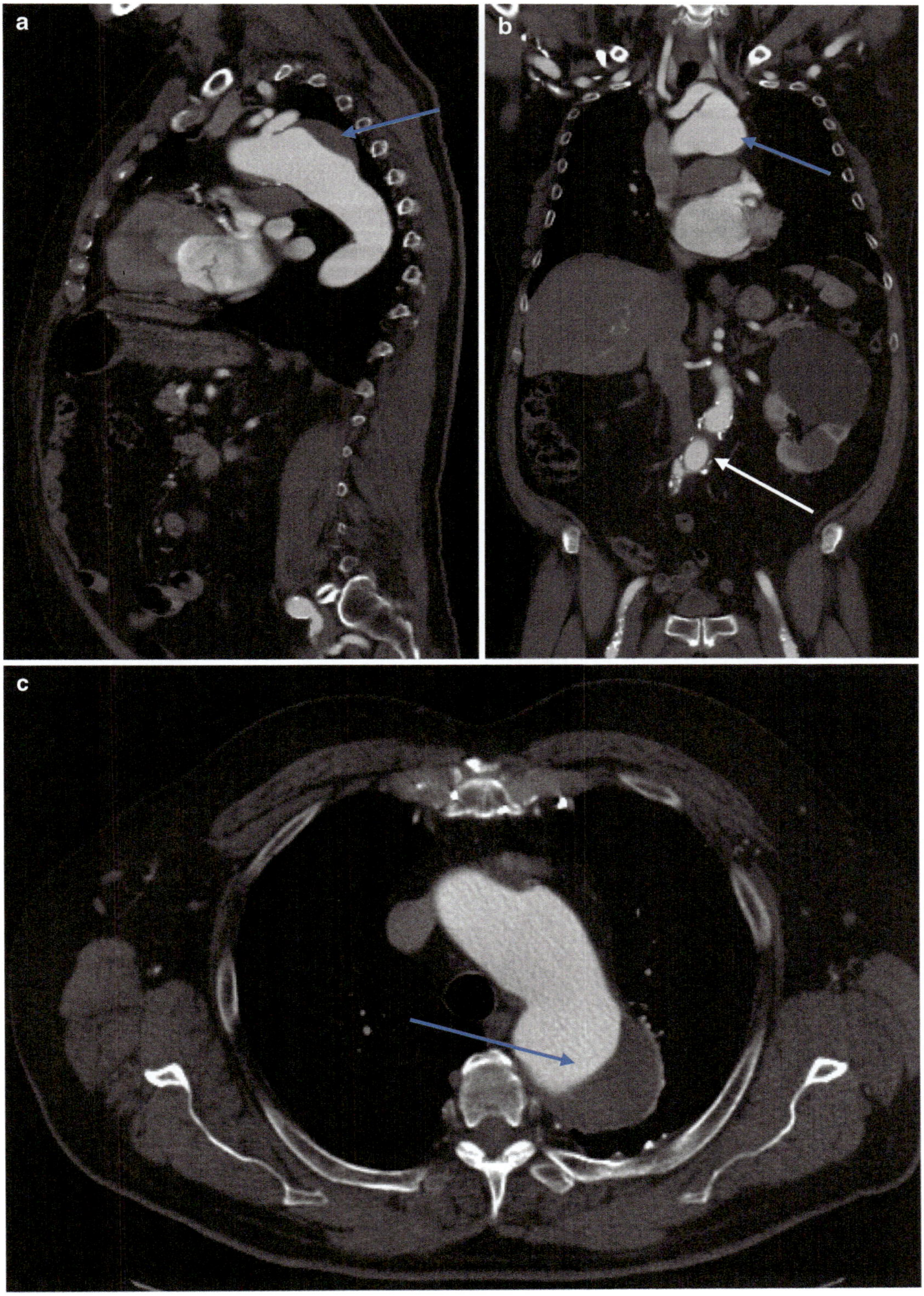

Fig. 3.45 (**a**) Sixty millimetre distal aortic arch aneurysm (blue arrows). The proximal part of the aortic arch also had a 40 m aneurysm. (**b**) White arrow indicates a previous abdominal aortic surgery. (**c**) Axial reconstruction and 60 mm distal aortic arch aneurysm

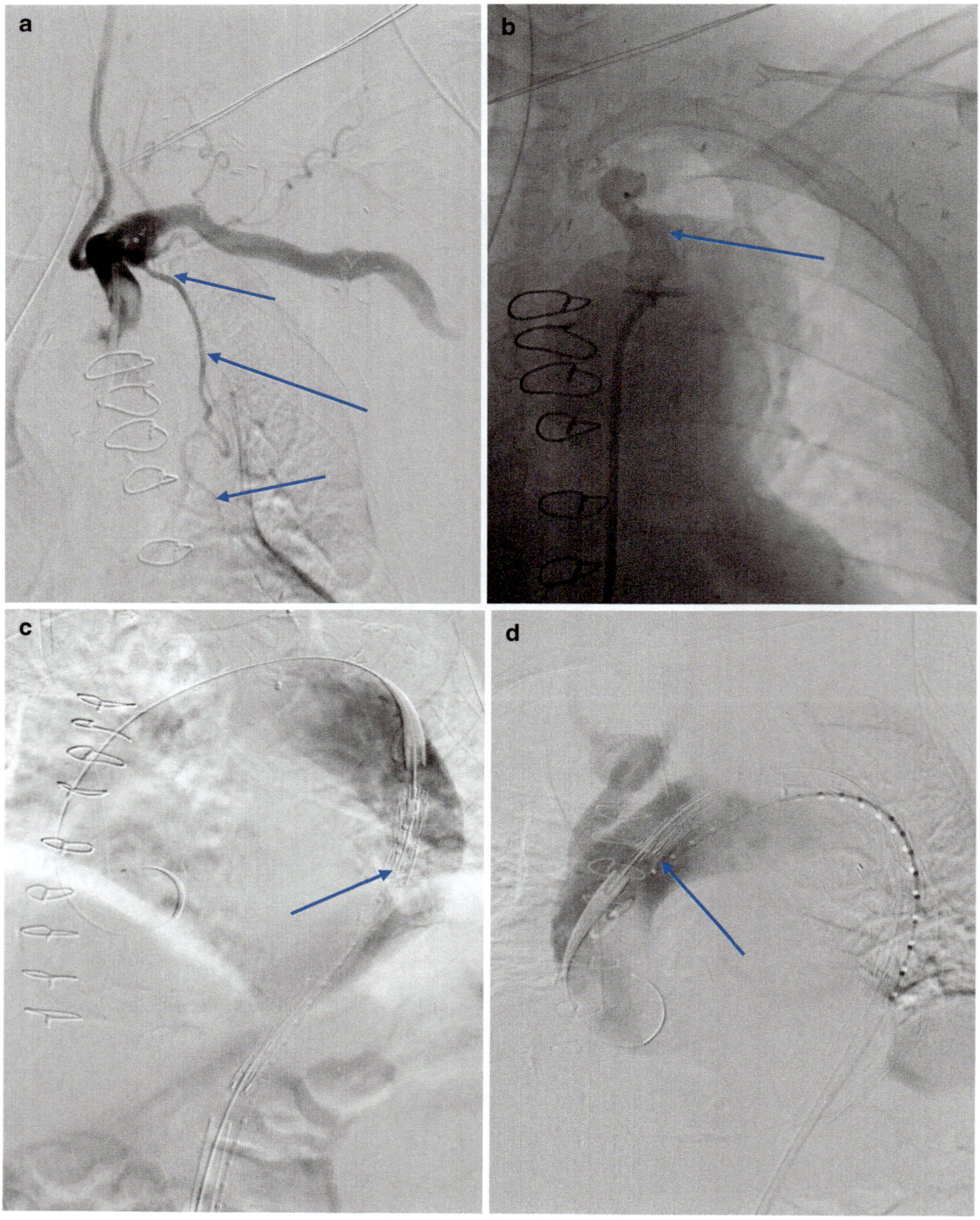

Fig. 3.46 Angiographic details. (**a**) blue indicate LIMA-LAD bypass. (**b**) deployment of the Amplatz plug into the pre-vertebral segment. (**c**) image; advancement of the distal tapered stent graft (arrow). (**d**) advancement of the proximal tapered stent graft (arrow)

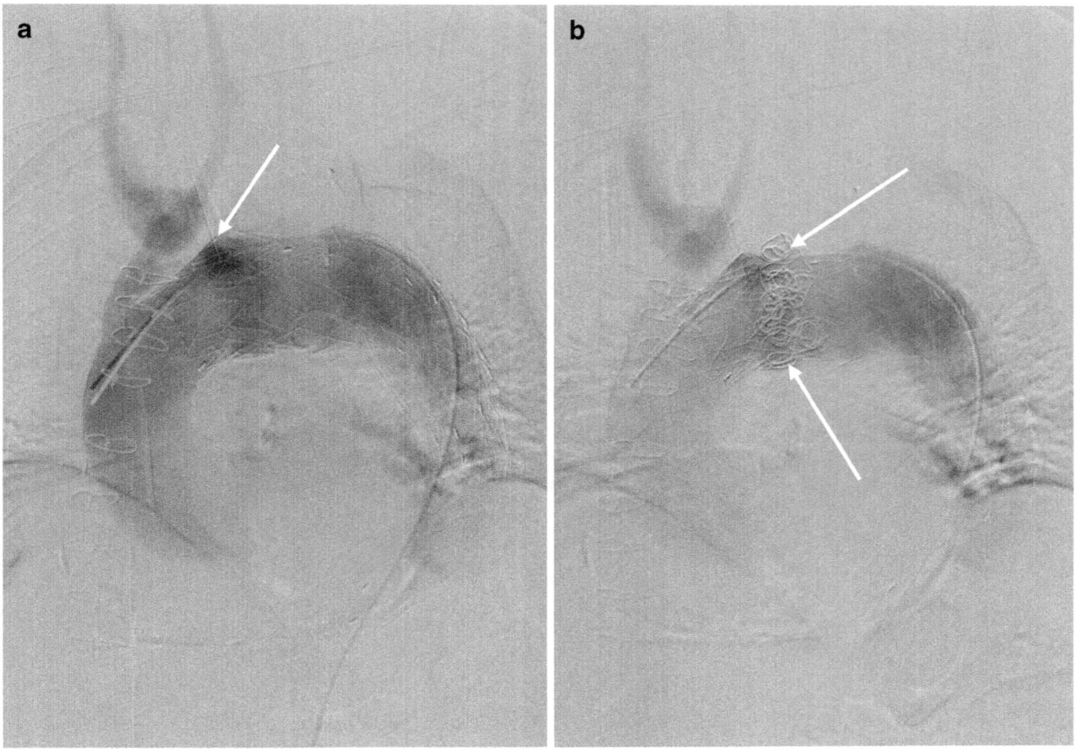

Fig. 3.47 Control angiography after stent graft deployment. Discrete type 1 endoleak was detected- (arrow) (**a**). (**b**) micro-coil embolization was performed. White arrows indicate deployment of micro-coils between the stent graft and aortic wall

3.2.4 Symptomatic Thoracoabdominal Aneurysm

Key Points

- It is often difficult to diagnose symptomatic aneurysms; in the present case, the pain could have also come from the stenosed superior mesenteric artery.
- Local puncture-related complications and pseudoaneurysms occur more frequently with brachial access than with femoral access.
- Severe stenosis of the visceral arteries should be treated electively prior to the complex aortic stent graft intervention, and acute situations involving occlusion of the vessels should be avoided.

3.2.4.1 Aetiology and Clinical Presentation

A 71-year-old patient had previously undergone acute surgery due to a ruptured abdominal aortic aneurysm and left kidney nephrectomy. Six years after the surgery, a 53 mm diameter thoracoabdominal aortic aneurysm was incidentally discovered. The patient had a long history of arterial hypertension. One year control CT was scheduled.

3.2.4.2 Pre-interventional Diagnosis

One year control CT showed enlargement of the aneurysm up to 60 mm, and the patient complained about abdominal pain (Fig. 3.50). The superior mesenteric artery showed significant stenosis, and the coeliac trunk was occluded. The patient did not have classical abdominal angina; therefore, we considered a diagnosis of symptomatic

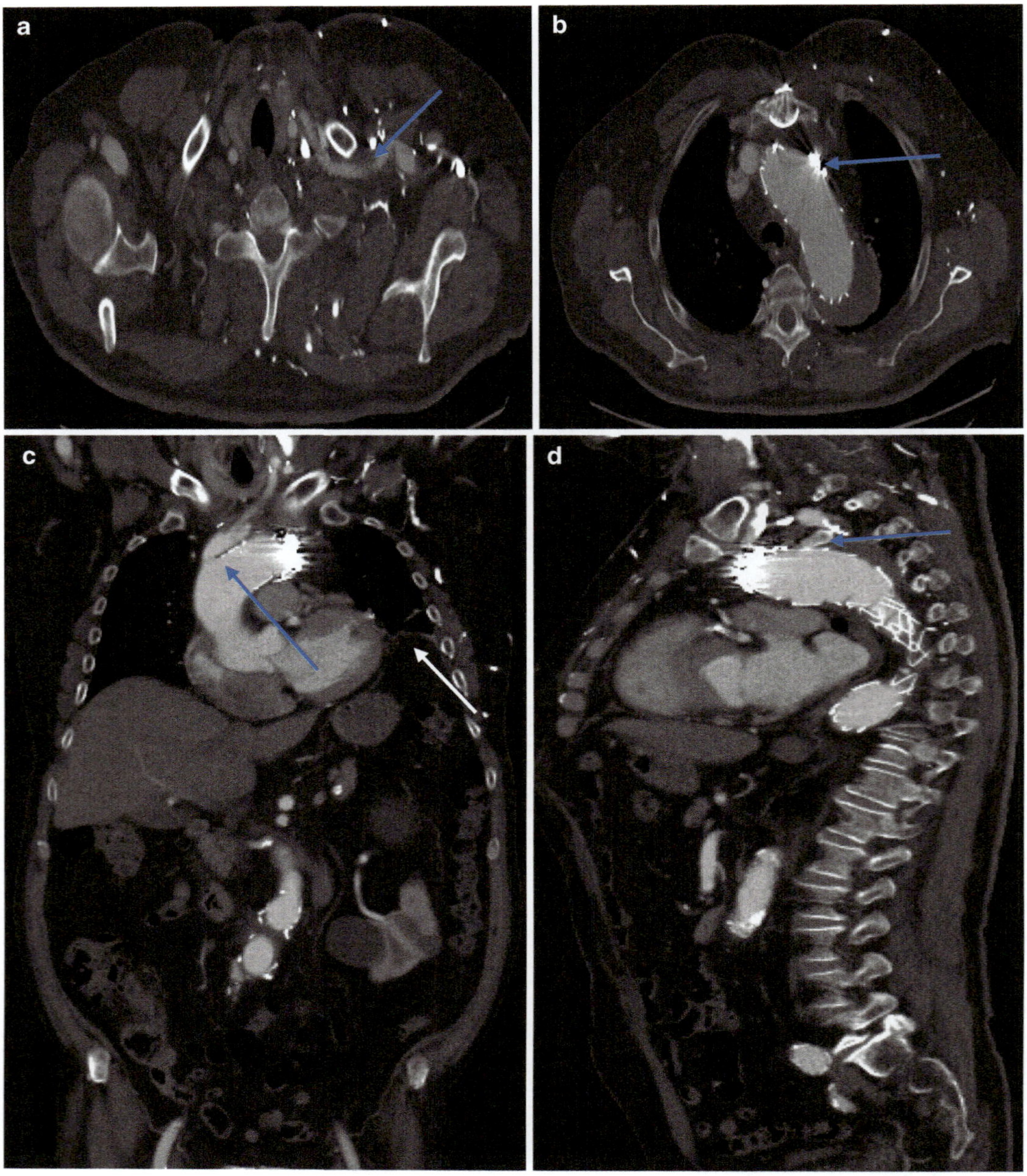

Fig. 3.48 Control contrast-enhanced CT 3 months after surgery. (**a**) blue arrow indicates patent left carotid-subclavian bypass. (**b**) arrow indicates micro-coils placed between the aortic wall and stent graft. (**c**) blue arrow indicates proximal part of the stent graft, showing good wall apposition with no endoleak. White arrow shows paralytic left diaphragm. (**d**) arrow indicates the Amplatz plug in the left subclavian artery

thoracoabdominal aneurysm. A branched custom-made stent graft (COOK, Bloomington, IN, USA) was ordered with two branches for the right renal and superior mesenteric arteries.

3.2.4.3 Endovascular Treatment

The patient was acutely admitted due to constant severe abdominal pain and diarrhoea that had begun 2 days prior. The patient did not have

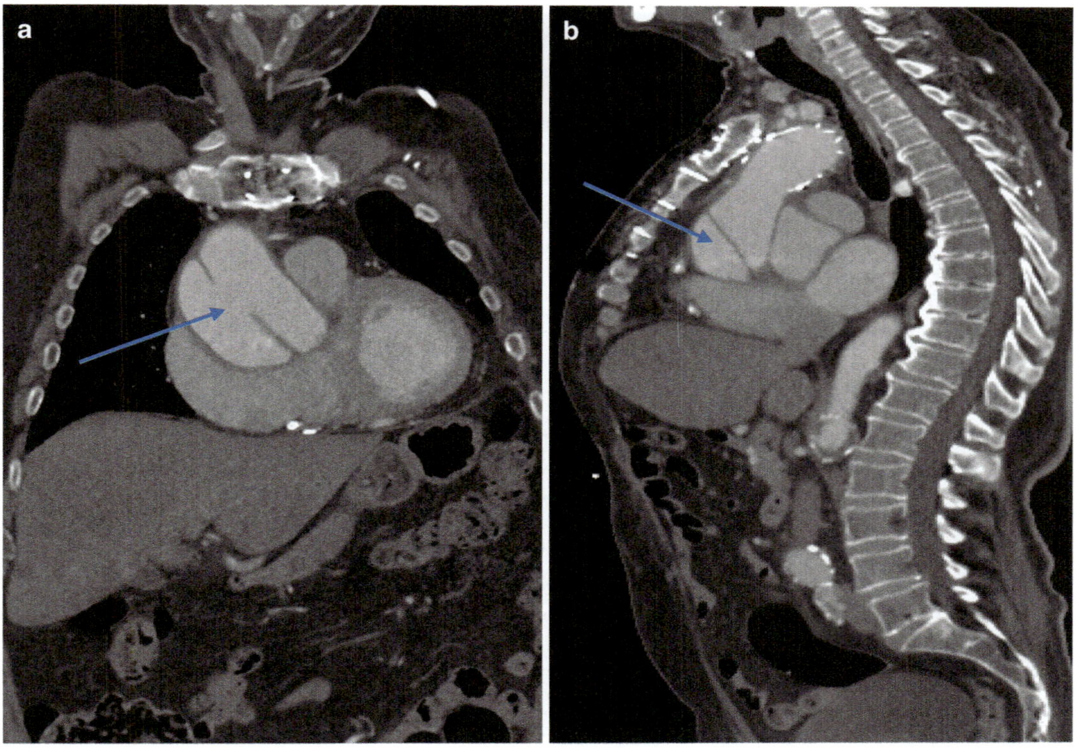

Fig. 3.49 Two years after the surgery, the ascending aorta was dilated, and a new aortic dissection type A had occurred (arrows). (**a**) coronal reconstruction with retrograde dissection in ascending aorta (arrow). (**b**) sagittal reconstruction with retrograde dissection in ascending aorta (arrow)

peritonitis on clinical examination. We suspected complete occlusion of the superior mesenteric artery due to known stenosis. Acute angiography via left brachial access confirmed occlusion of the superior mesenteric artery. Successful recanalization was performed, and a balloon-expandible stent were deployed, resulting in a good outcome and clinical improvement in the following days (Fig. 3.51). The patient then became asymptomatic again and was discharged 3 days after stenting. Plavix and aspirin were to be taken while the patient awaited the TEVAR stent graft operation.

The patient underwent the stent graft operation under general anaesthesia after the custom-made stent graft was produced. A spinal drainage catheter was prophylactically placed to minimize the risk for spinal ischaemia due to aortic coverage with the stent graft and previous aortic abdominal surgery. A bolus of 5000 IU heparin was injected, and ACT was kept >250 s during the intervention. First, the simple TEVAR stent graft was deployed proximally through the exposed right femoral artery. After that, a stent graft with branches for the right renal and superior mesenteric arteries was deployed. Via left trans-brachial access, the branched stent graft was advanced into the renal and superior mesenteric arteries (Fig. 3.52). Completion angiography demonstrated well-deployed stent grafts and open branches (Fig. 3.53).

3.2.4.4 Outcome

The patient showed no spinal ischaemia complications, and no drainage was used. There were no other complications, but the local left brachial artery was surgically repaired due to development of a pseudoaneurysm, with an excellent outcome. The patient was discharged from the hospital a few days later, asymptomatic and in good status. Contrast-enhanced control CT 1 month after the surgery showed well-deployed stent grafts. There

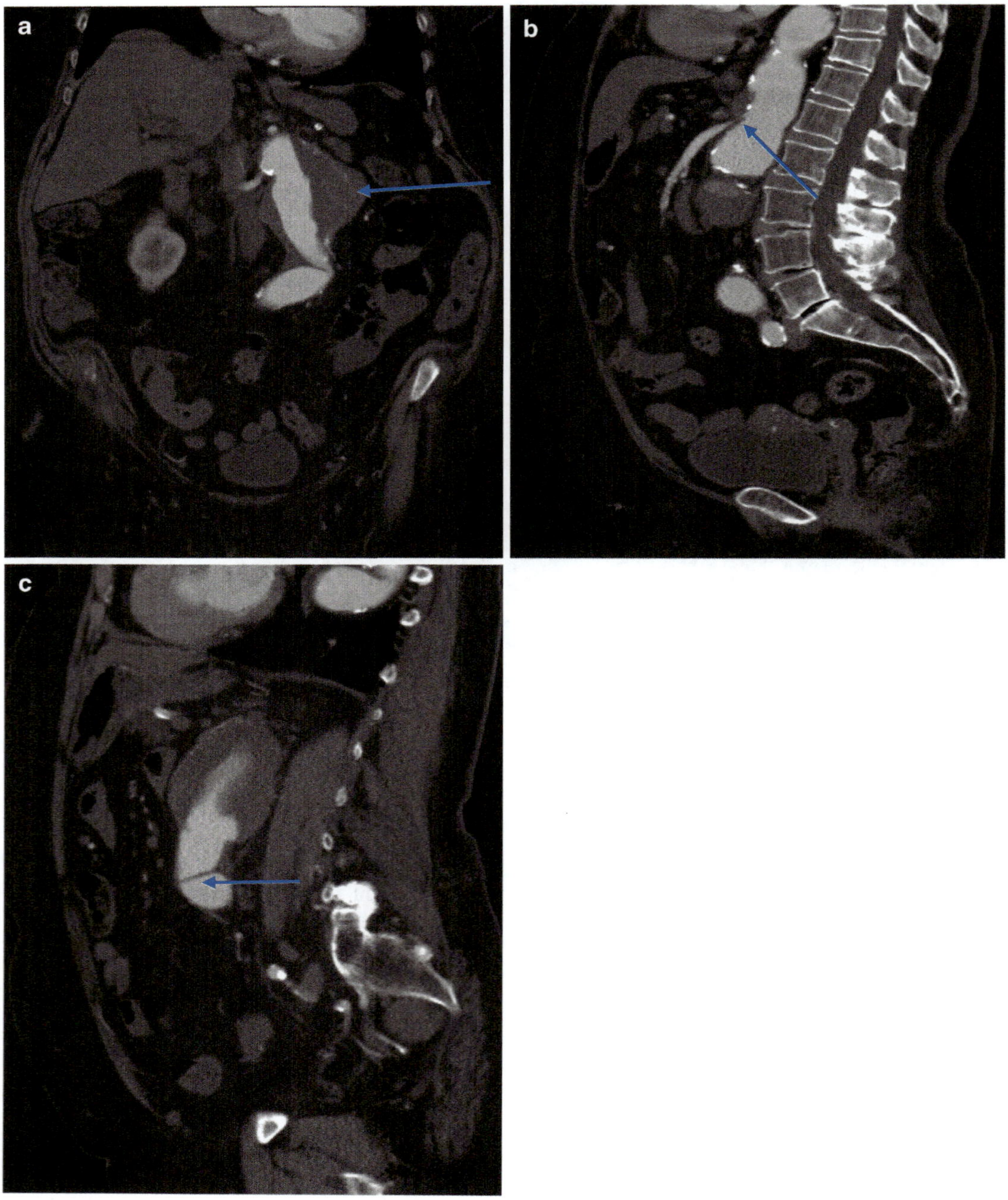

Fig. 3.50 Contrast-enhanced CT with a growing thoraco-abdominal aneurysm. The aneurysm was 60 mm in diameter –(arrow) (**a**). The coeliac trunk was occluded, and there was severe stenosis of the superior mesenteric artery (arrow) (**b**). The left kidney had been previously removed. Previously, aortic surgery was performed with aortic tube grafting and a proximal anastomosis sewn in the distal part of the infrarenal aorta (arrow) (**c**)

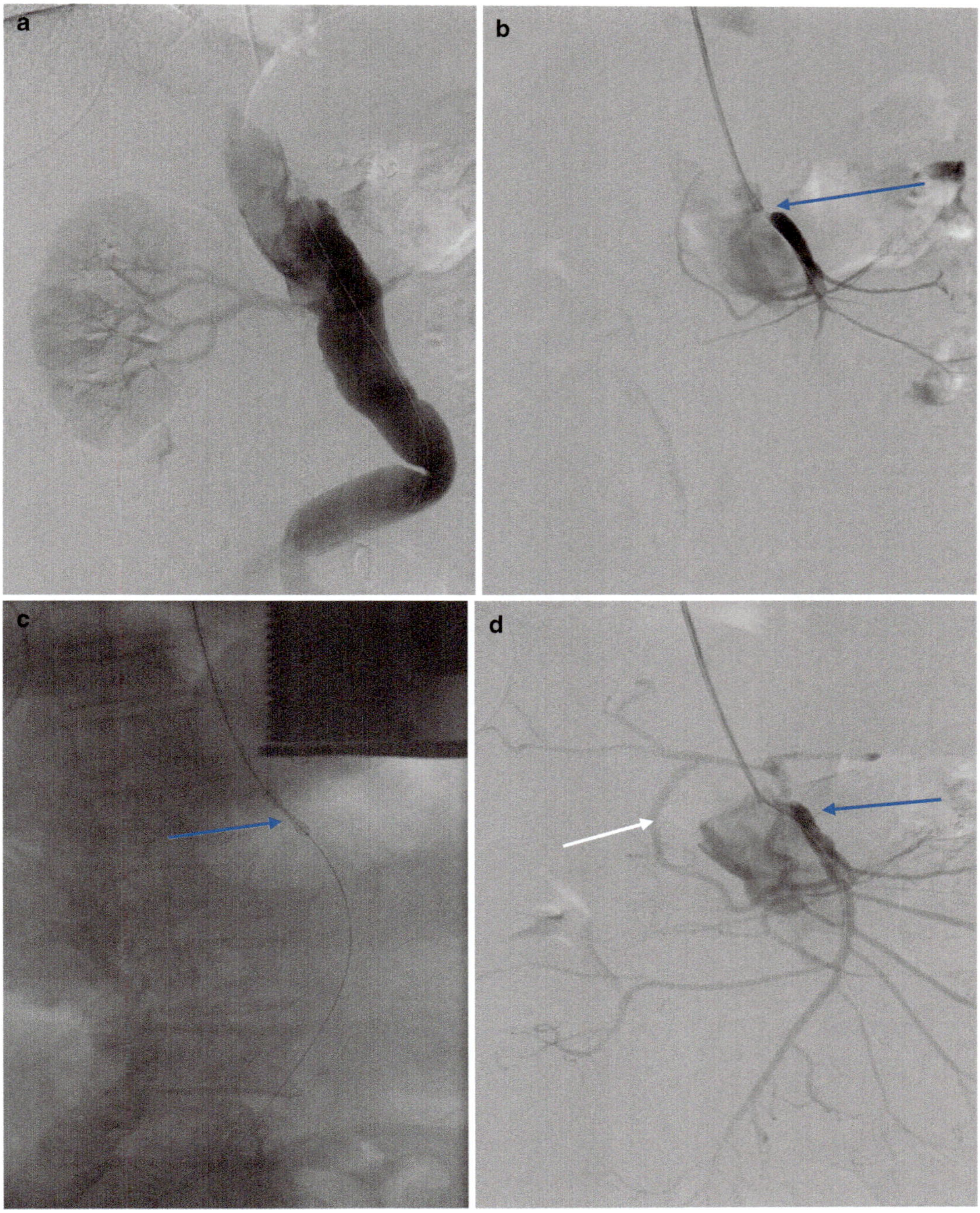

Fig. 3.51 Emergency angiography confirmed the clinical suspicion and occluded superior mesenteric artery (**a**). (**b**) selective catheterization and recanalization of the occluded superior mesenteric artery –(arrow). (**c**) balloon-expandible stent deployment (arrow). (**d**) control angiography showing a good result. Retrograde flow into the coeliac trunk via the pancreaticoduodenal artery indicated by the white arrow

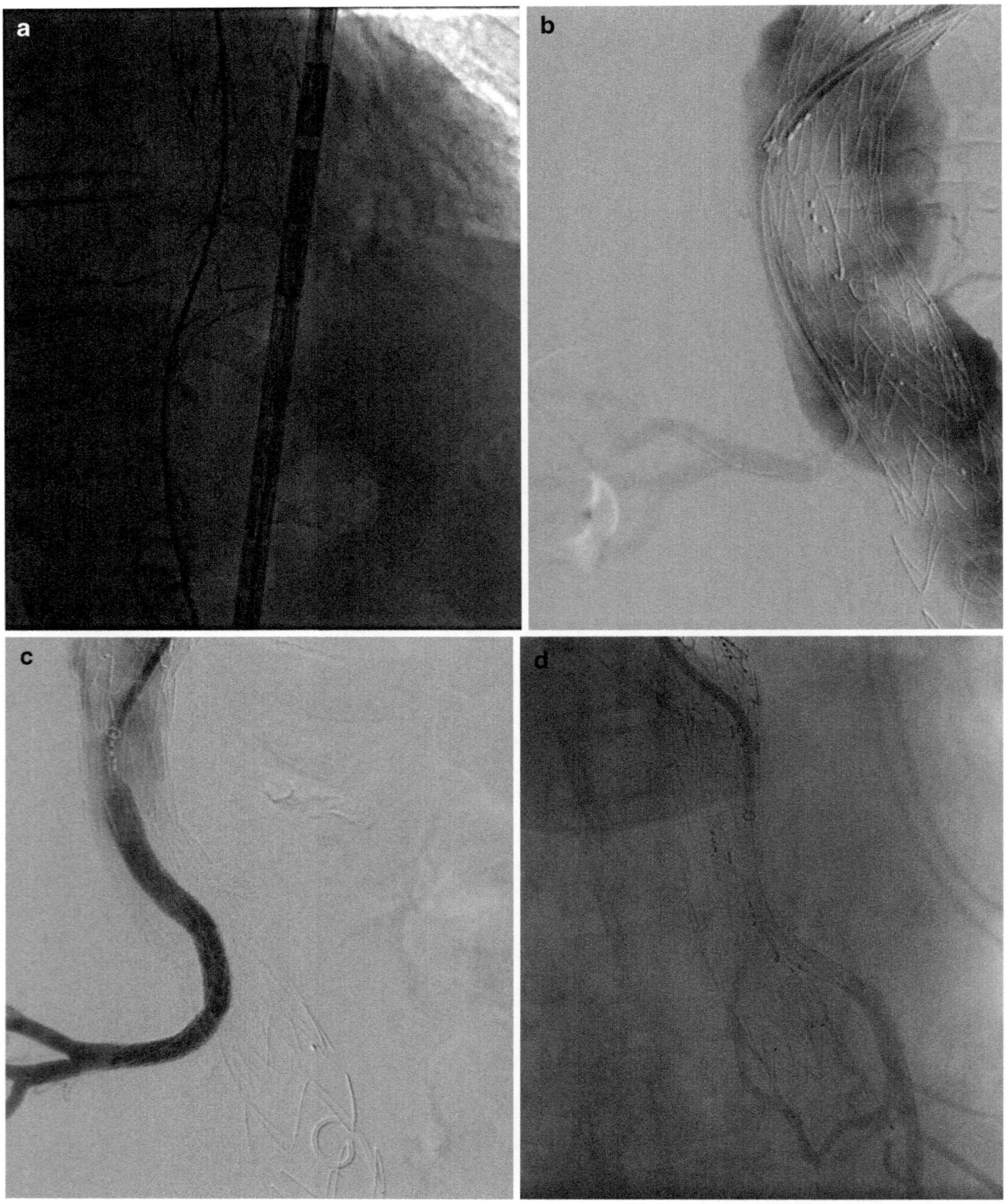

Fig. 3.52 Intraoperative details. (**a**) first, a standard TEVAR stent graft was deployed proximally, followed by orientation of a branched stent graft. (**b** and **c**) cannulation and advancement of the stent graft into the right renal artery. (**d**) deployment of the stent graft into the superior mesenteric artery

was local dissection in the superior mesenteric artery distal to the deployed stent graft (Fig. 3.54). The patient was asymptomatic, but we decided to place a self-expandable stent into the superior mesenteric artery to eventually avoid thrombosis. The intervention was performed under local anaesthesia via left trans-brachial access. The self-expandable stent was easily deployed across

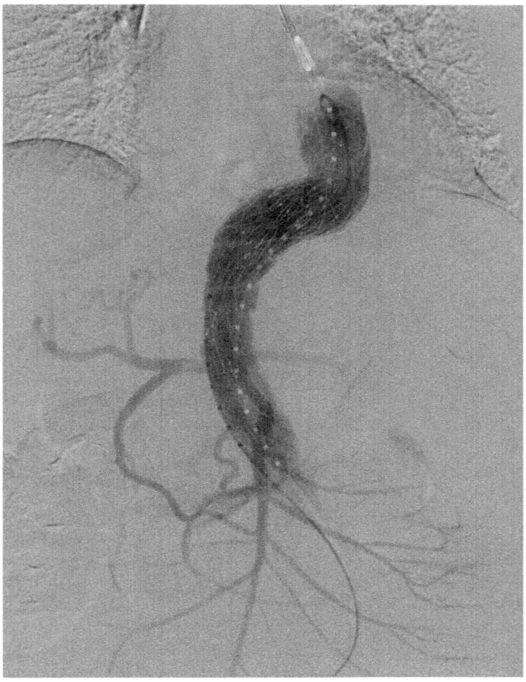

Fig. 3.53 Control angiography after completion of the intervention. A well-deployed stent graft and open right renal and superior mesenteric arteries can be seen

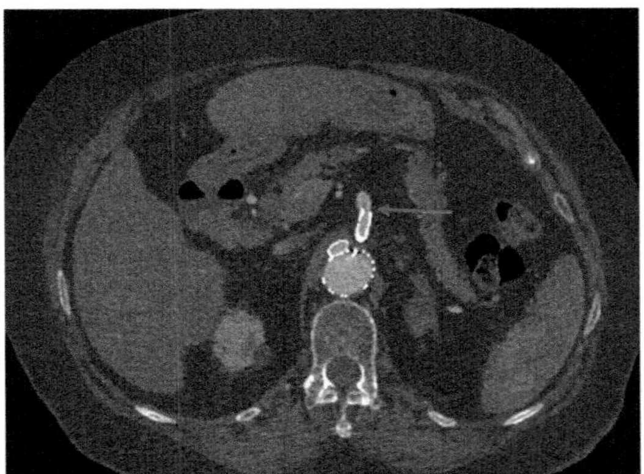

Fig. 3.54 Control contrast-enhanced CT 1 month after FEVAR showing dissection distally from the deployed stent in the superior mesenteric artery (arrow)

the dissection (Fig. 3.55). The patient was discharged the next day. Three month control CT showed a satisfactory result and open right renal and superior mesenteric arteries. There was no endoleak (Fig. 3.56). The patient remains asymptomatic.

3.3 Thoracic Aortic Intramural Haematomas

3.3.1 Intramural Haematoma Involving the Ascending and Descending Aorta

Key Points

- An intramural haematoma in the ascending aorta is an emergency in which acute open surgery is usually indicated, as in classically aortic dissection.
- There are reports that show a positive outcome following conservative treatment of intramural haematomas in some cases, bringing the patient into the subacute phase, where TEVAR is much safer than in the acute phase.
- Spinal ischaemia is a devastating complication.

3.3.1.1 Aetiology and Clinical Presentation

A 59-year-old patient experienced acute tearing and radiating retrosternal pain in the back during work. The pain was constant, and the patient was haemodynamically stable. The patient had a known history of arterial hypertension. There were no signs of coronary ischaemia. The patient soon developed symptoms of spinal ischaemia and lower bilateral extremity paralysis. Emergency contrast-enhanced CT scanning was ordered.

3.3.1.2 Pre-interventional Diagnosis

Contrast-enhanced CT scanning showed intramural haematoma in the ascending aorta, aortic arch and descending aorta. There was an aortic dissection in the descending aorta. In the ascending aorta, there was no intimal flap (Fig. 3.57). The dissection extended below the renal arteries. Antihypertensive and pain killer medications helped to bring the patient to the asymptomatic phase, but the lower limb paralysis was unchanged. The intramural haematoma

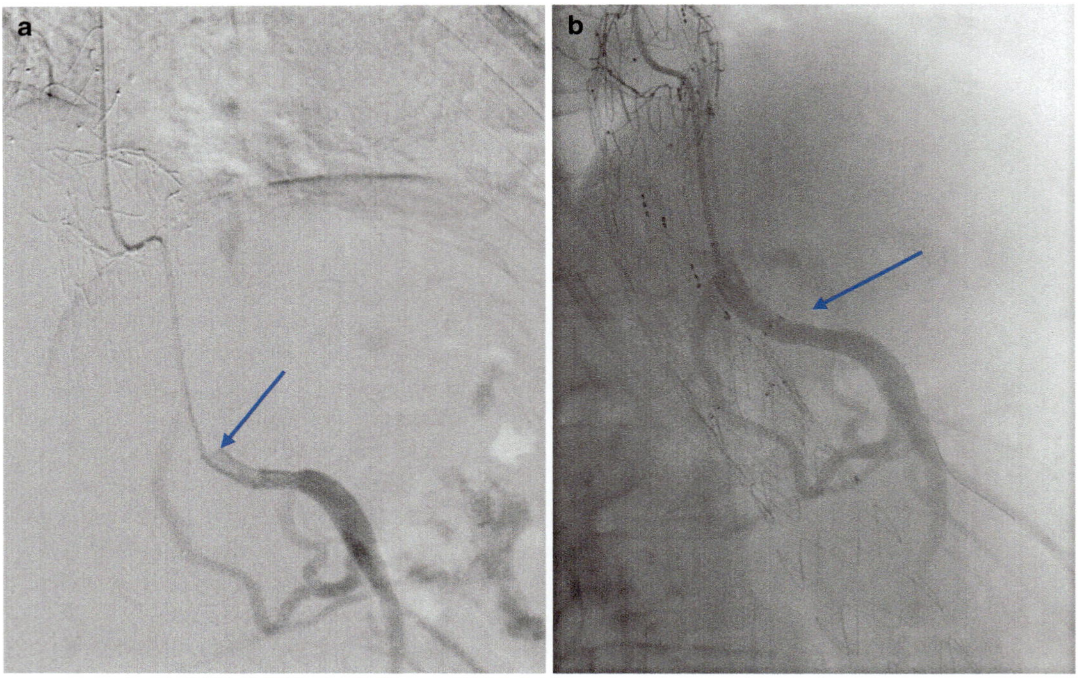

Fig. 3.55 Left trans-brachial access. (**a**) arrow indicates the dissection. (**b**) deployment of the self-expandible stent and satisfactory result (arrow)

in the ascending aorta was the reason for considering acute open surgery and ascending aorta reconstruction. Nevertheless, the risk for further worsening of spinal ischaemia during the open operation was too high. Therefore, it was decided to treat the patient conservatively and to keep the mean arterial pressure between 80 and 90 mmHg. Gradually, after a few days, the patient recovered some lower limb function following physiotherapy, showing impressive improvement. The patient was without pain and was discharged to the local hospital. Control contrast-enhanced CT 3 months after symptom onset revealed a normal status in the ascending aorta and aortic arch with intramural haematoma regression. In the descending aorta, the type B dissection was still present, and the intramural haematoma was unchanged (Fig. 3.58). The patient recovered very well and could walk without assistance. The ascending aorta was without haematoma and was not as fragile as it was at the beginning. It was decided to treat the dissection with a TEVAR stent graft.

3.3.1.3 Endovascular Treatment

The right femoral artery was exposed. The TEVAR stent graft was advanced over the super-stiff guidewire and was deployed without difficulty to intentionally cover approximately 30% of the left subclavian artery (Fig. 3.59). The stent graft had a diameter of 34 mm, which was an approximately 10% oversizing relative to the aortic diameter. There were no complications during the TEVAR intervention.

3.3.1.4 Outcome

The patient was discharged 2 days later without any complications or pain. Control contrast-enhanced CT 3 months and 1 year after TEVAR was uneventful and showed a satisfactory result with complete aortic remodelling of the proximal descending aorta (Fig. 3.59). The patient remains asymptomatic and without pain. The dissection in the distal descending aorta and abdominal aorta grew only a few millimetres 1 year after the control scan, but false lumen thrombosis occurred. The dissection in the abdominal aorta is still unsuitable for treatment. The patient is scheduled for yearly inspections.

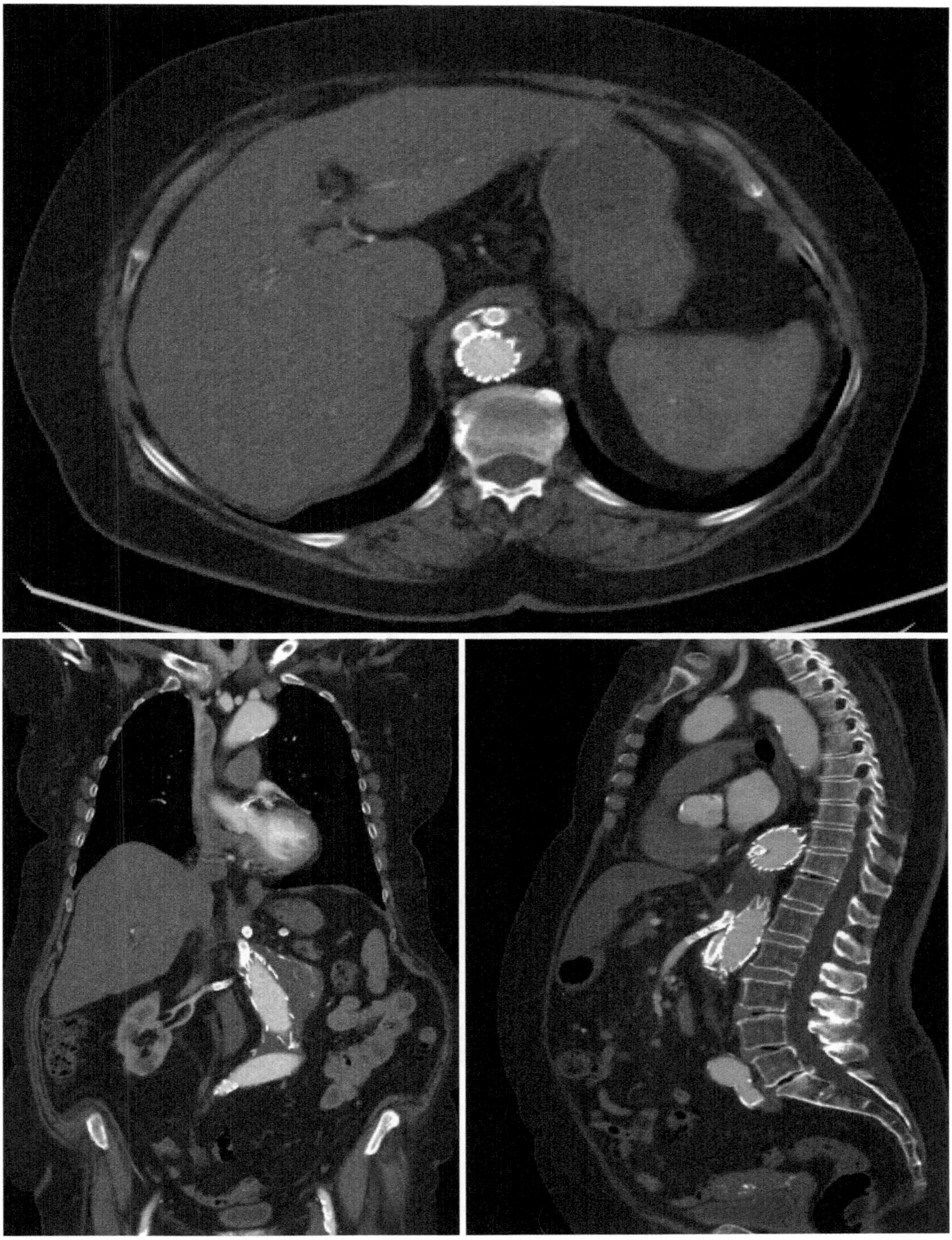

Fig. 3.56 Contrast-enhanced CT 3 months after surgery. Patent renal and superior mesenteric arteries. No endoleak was observed, and the aneurysm remained the same size

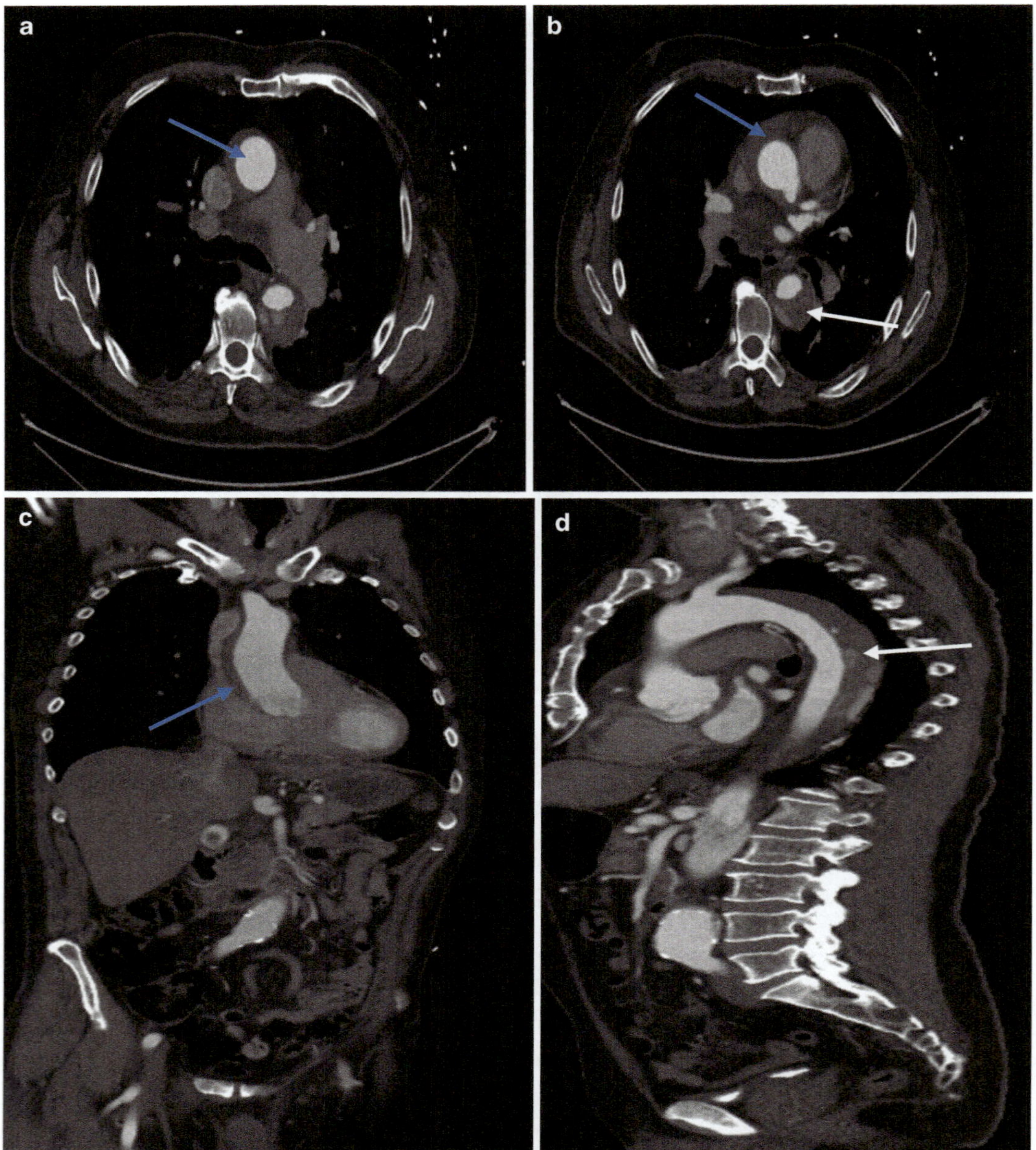

Fig. 3.57 (**a**) intramural haematoma in the ascending aorta without intimal tearing (arrow). (**b**) blue arrow indicates haematoma in the ascending aorta. White arrow indicates an intimal tear in the descending aorta. (**c**) blue arrow indicates intramural haematoma in the ascending aorta. (**d**) white arrow indicates the intimal tear in the descending aorta

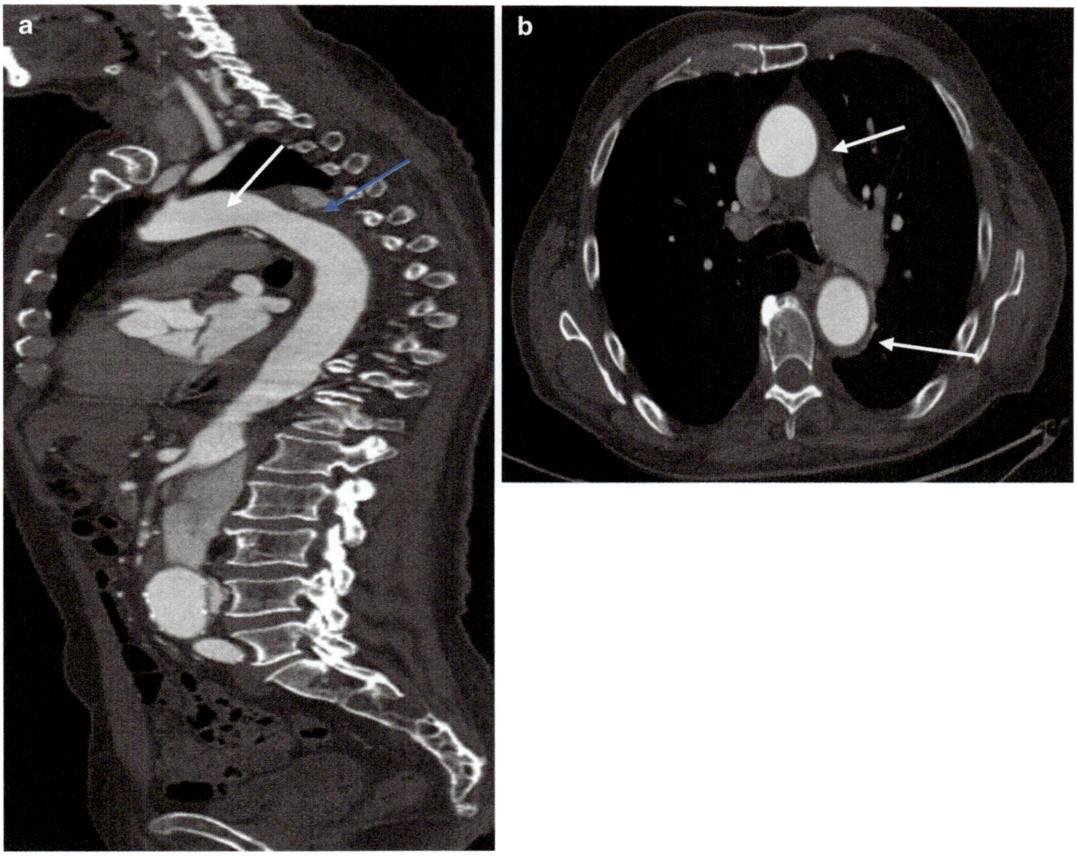

Fig. 3.58 Three month control CT control showed regression of the intramural haematoma in the ascending aorta – (white arrows). Blue arrows indicate the now-clear aortic dissection type B

3.3.2 Intramural Haematoma in the Descending Aorta-I

> **Key Points**
> - Frequent control imaging is needed for patients with intramural haematoma.
> - All effort should be devoted to treating intramural haematomas in the subacute phase to avoid possible complications.
> - Minimal stent graft oversizing and no post-dilatation are recommended.

3.3.2.1 Aetiology and Clinical Presentation

A 59-year-old patient with arterial hypertension complained of chest and back pain lasting for a few hours. Arterial hypertension was 175/100 mmHg. There were no signs of myocardial ischaemia. The patient did not have any other diseases.

3.3.2.2 Pre-interventional Diagnosis

Emergency contrast-enhanced CT was performed and showed an intramural haematoma in the descending aorta with a small ulcer-like lesion (Fig. 3.60a,b). Distally in the descending aorta, an intimal tear dissection was recorded. There was no haematoma in the ascending aorta or aortic arch. Intramural haematoma extended to the visceral artery level. The patient responded well to antihypertensive therapy and became asymptomatic. Arterial systolic pressure was maintained at approximately 110 mmHg. The patient was discharged 4 days later without pain. The next control CT was performed 1 month later,

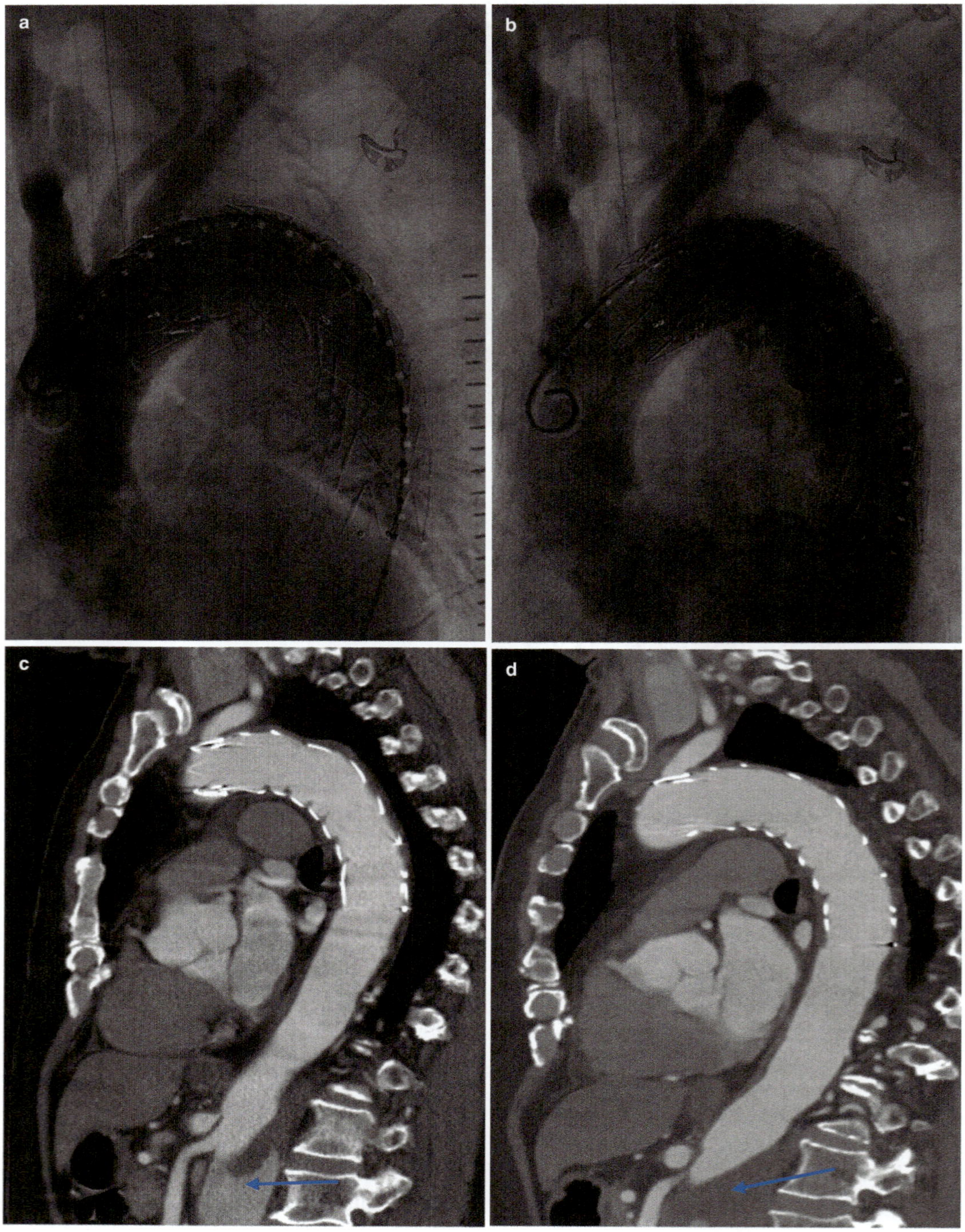

Fig. 3.59 (**a**, **b**) TEVAR stent graft deployment distally from the left subclavian artery. (**c**) control CT scan showing a satisfactory result 3 months after TEVAR. (**d**) one year control image showing a satisfactory result and complete aortic remodelling in the proximal thoracic aorta. The dissection in the distal thoracic and abdominal aorta showed slow growth but currently remains unsuitable for treatment (arrows)

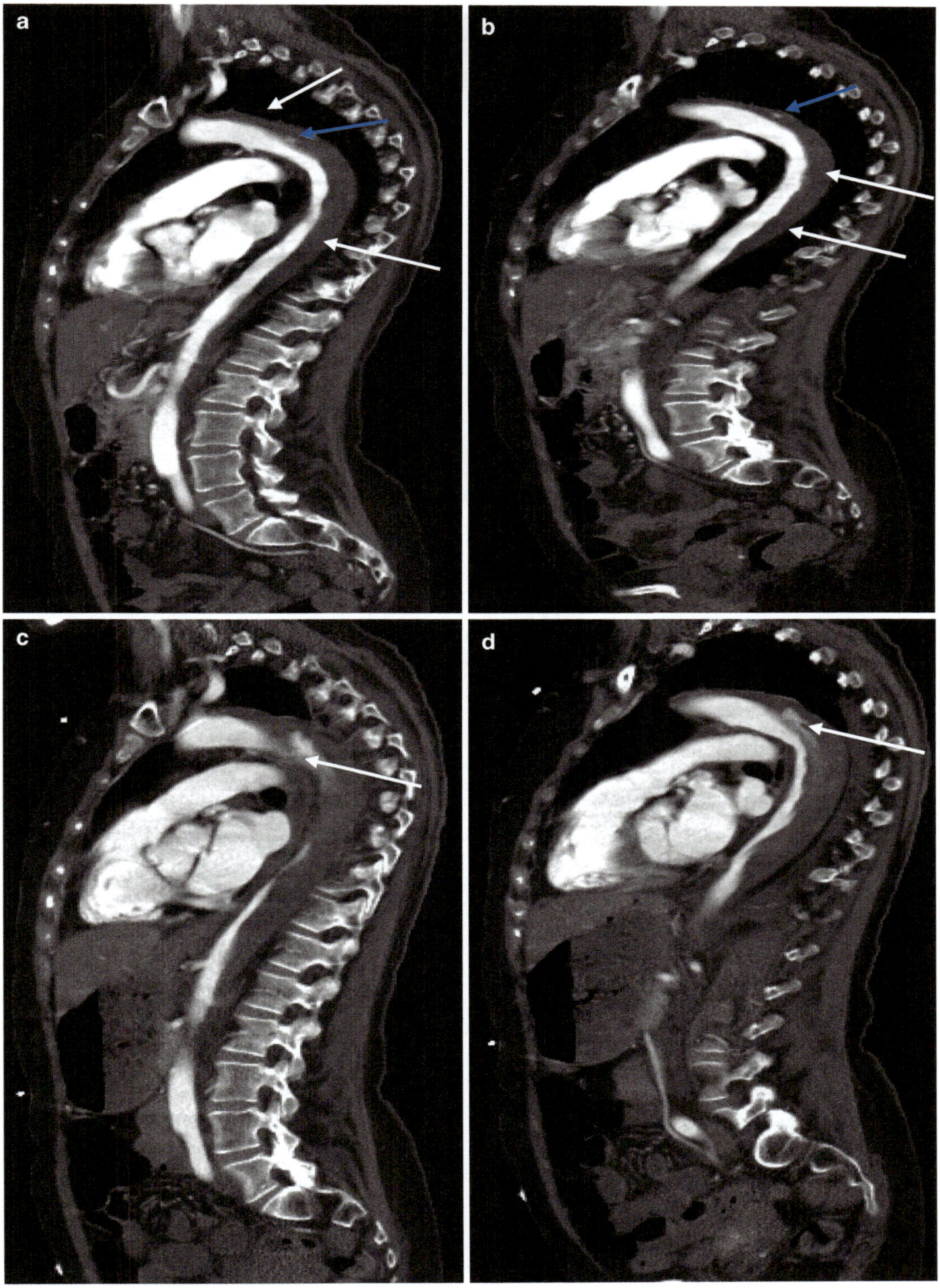

Fig. 3.60 Contrast-enhanced CT showing an intramural haematoma in the descending aorta. (**a** and **b**) white arrows indicate intramural haematoma. Blue arrows indicate a small ulcer-like lesion. (**c** and **d**) control CT showing increasing intramural haematoma in the descending aorta and a now clear aortic dissection. White arrows indicate an intimal tear

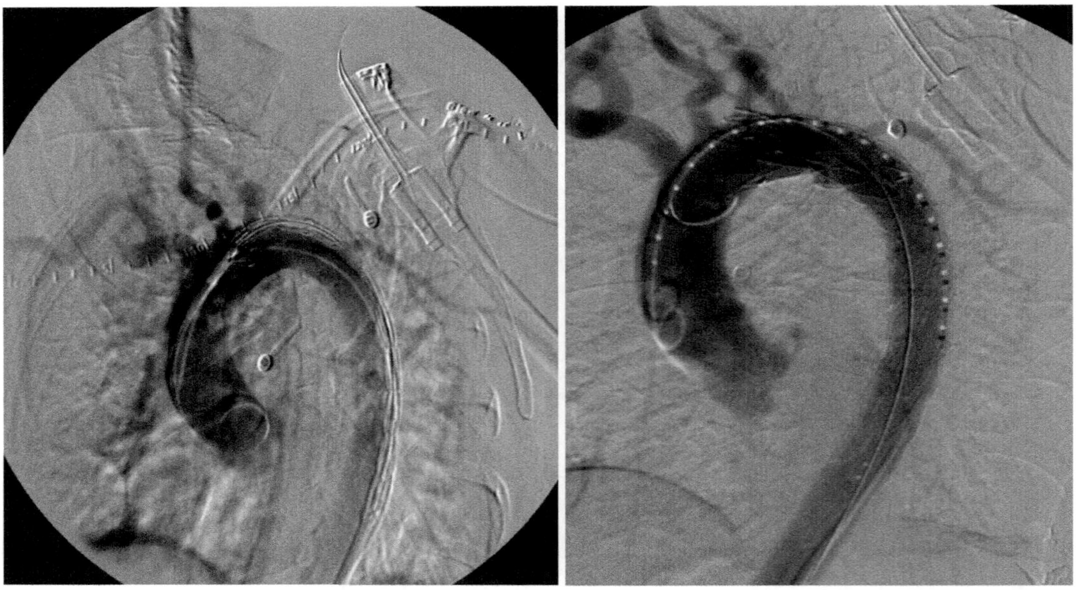

Fig. 3.61 Details from the TEVAR stent graft deployment. The stent graft was inserted without difficulties, leading to a satisfactory result

revealing progression of the intramural haematoma and a now clear dissection type B with an intimal tear (Fig. 3.60c,d). As this was considered rapid disease progression, TEVAR treatment was indicated.

3.3.2.3 Endovascular Treatment

The TEVAR stent graft, approximately 10% oversized and 20 cm in length, was advanced, deployed via the surgically exposed right femoral artery, and placed distally from the subclavian artery. No post-deployment balloon angioplasty was performed. Finally, control angiography showed a well-placed stent graft (Fig. 3.61). There were no complications.

3.3.2.4 Outcome

The patient was discharged from the hospital 2 days after TEVAR. Control contrast-enhanced CT 3 months later showed excellent results and complete aortic remodelling (Fig. 3.62). The patient showed no symptoms.

3.3.3 Intramural Haematoma in the Descending Aorta–II

Key Points

- Frequent control imaging is needed for patients with intramural haematoma.
- All effort should be devoted to treating intramural haematomas in the subacute phase to avoid possible complications.
- Minimal stent graft oversizing and no post-dilatation are recommended.

3.3.3.1 Aetiology and Clinical Presentation

A 65-year-old patient complained of an acute sharp onset of retrosternal pain. There were no ECG changes, and myocardial enzymes were within normal limits. The patient had well-controlled hypertension.

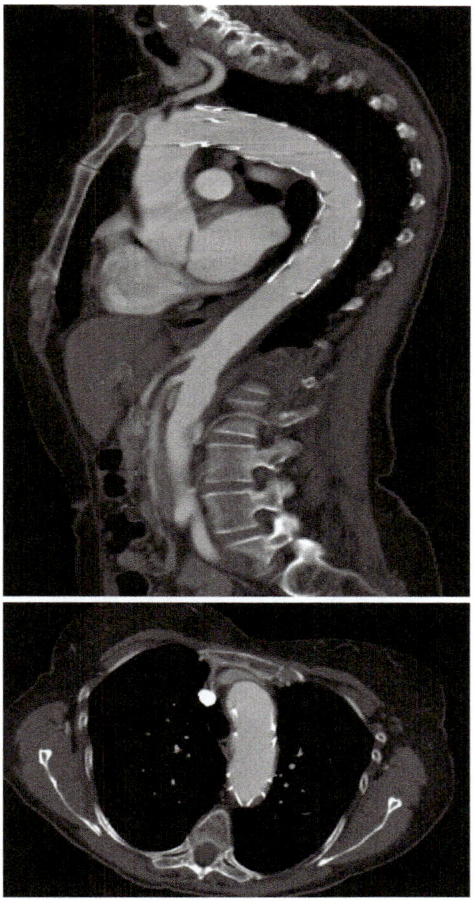

Fig. 3.62 Three month control CT showing complete aortic remodelling and excellent results. Full intramural haematoma regression occurred

3.3.3.2 Pre-interventional Diagnosis

Contrast-enhanced CT scanning was performed and showed intramural haematoma involving the descending aorta (Fig. 3.63). A small ulcer-like lesion was noticed. The patient was admitted and responded very well to medical therapy. Two days later, the patient remained asymptomatic and was discharged from the hospital without pain. Control CT was performed approximately 3 weeks later, and the patient complained of pain that was not as strong as the previous one. Control CT showed increasing intramural haematoma, and the ulcer-like lesions in the descending aorta had increased in size. The intramural haematoma started just distally from the left subclavian artery. (Fig. 3.64). There was no haematoma in the aortic arch or ascending aorta.

3.3.3.3 Endovascular Treatment

Under general anaesthesia, a TEVAR stent-graft with a diameter of 32 mm and length of 100 mm was deployed through the surgically exposed right femoral artery in the descending aorta to cover the ulcer-like lesion. The diameter of the aorta was between 30 and 31 mm, including 50% of the haematoma in the diameter calculation. The first stent graft was intentionally deployed in the mid-portion of the descending aorta. Control angiography showed a type 1 endoleak, and it appeared that the stent graft was undersized.

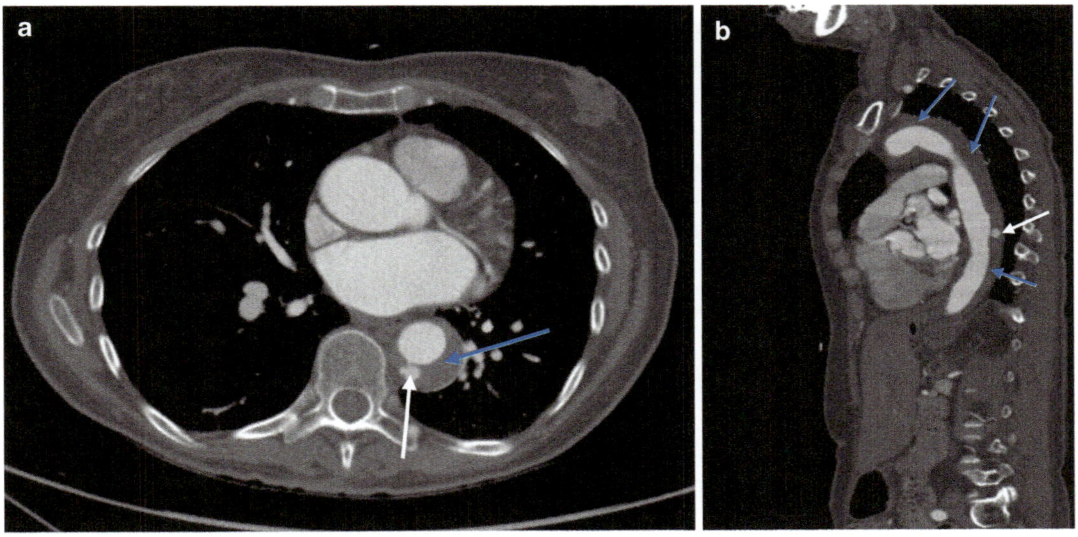

Fig. 3.63 Contrast-enhanced CT showing intramural haematoma (blue arrows) and a small ulcer-like lesion (white arrows)

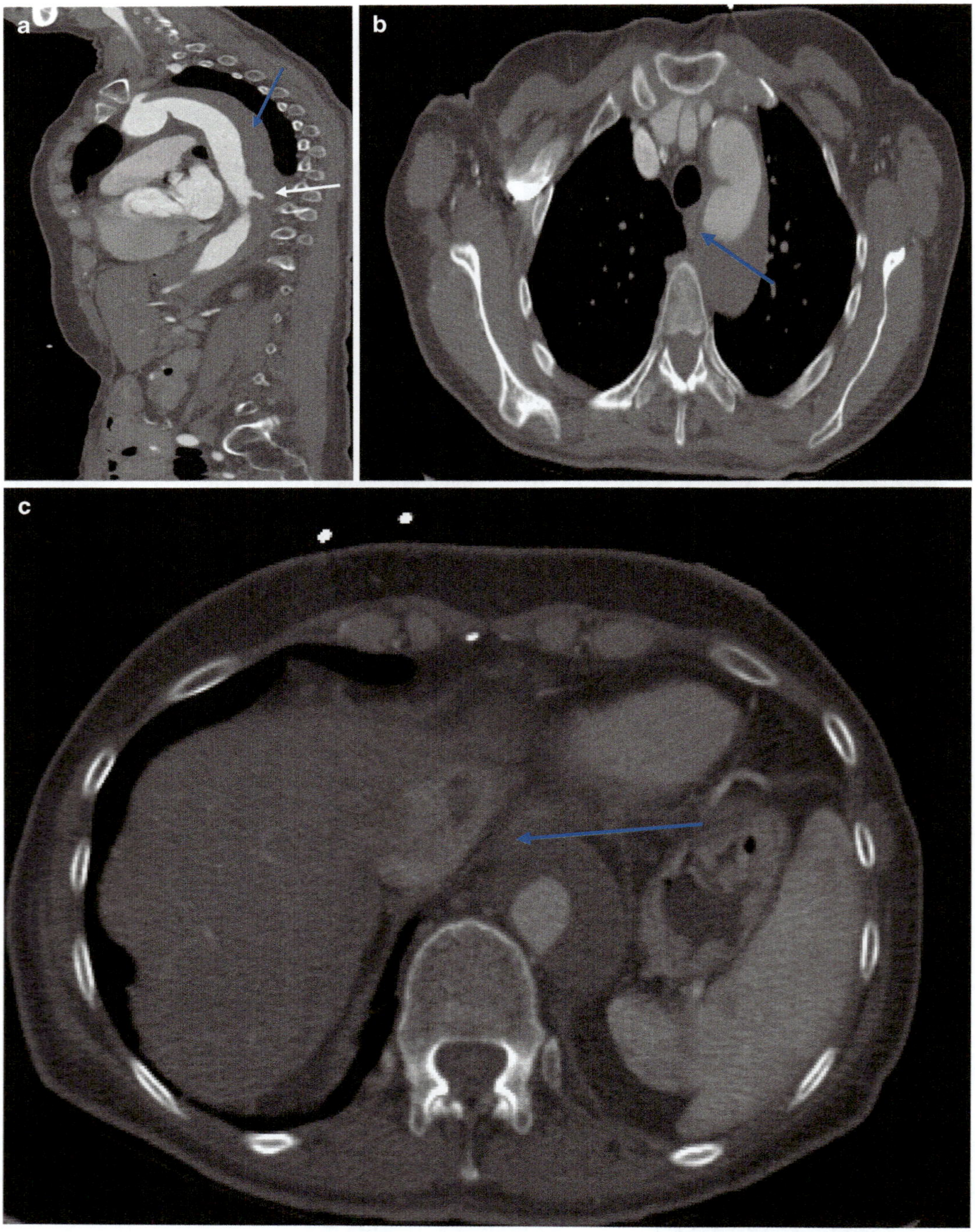

Fig. 3.64 Control contrast-enhanced CT showing an increasing intramural haematoma (blue arrows). The small ulcer-like lesion had increased in size as well. The aortic arch showed no haematoma

Therefore, an additional stent graft with a diameter of 34 mm was deployed, and control angiography showed satisfactory results (Fig. 3.65).

3.3.3.4 Outcome

The patient was discharged from the hospital 3 days after TEVAR in good health and with no

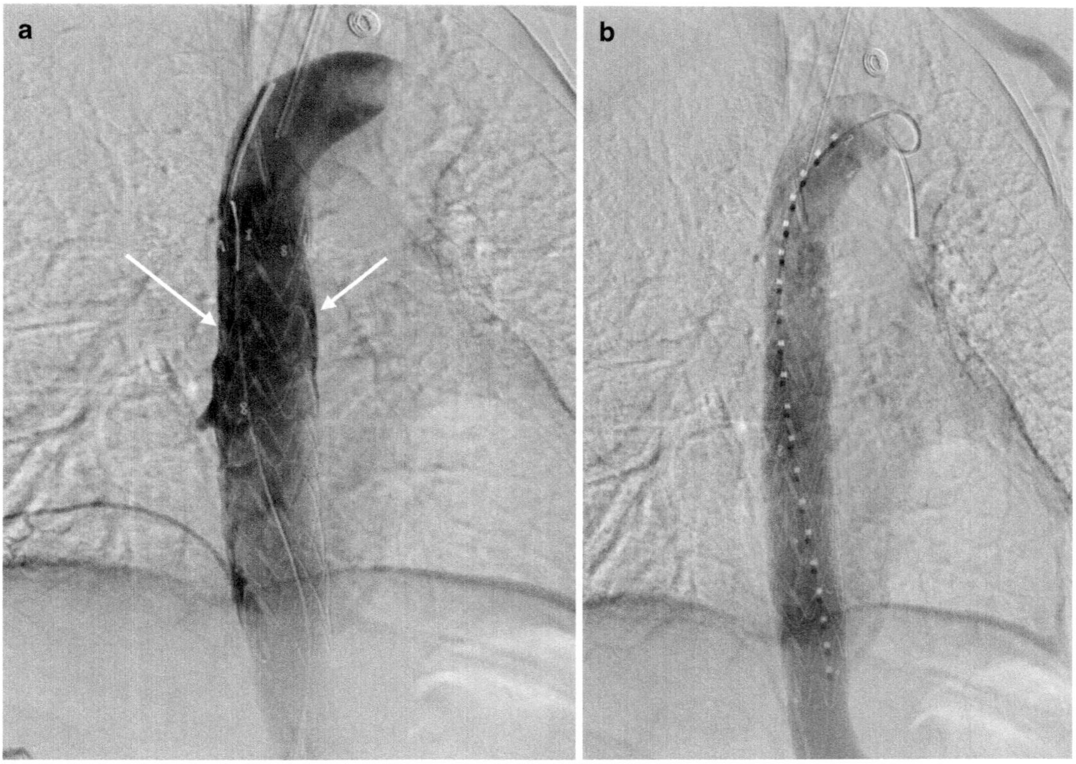

Fig. 3.65 (**a**) deployment of a stent graft with a diameter of 32 mm. Arrows indicate an endoleak resulting from the use of an undersized graft. (**b**) deployment of a second stent graft with a diameter of 34 mm, showing satisfactory results

symptoms. The first control scan was performed 3 months after discharge, showing resolution of the intramural haematoma. There were new stent graft-induced intimal lesions on the proximal and distal ends (Fig. 3.66). A subsequent control scan 1 year later showed slight progression of the intima lesions (Fig. 3.67). There were no symptoms or extension of either the proximal or distal intima lesion. The patient remains asymptomatic and is on a yearly control imaging regimen.

3.3.4 Intramural Haematoma in the Descending Aorta-III

Key Points
- Frequent control imaging is needed for patients with intramural haematoma.
- All effort should be devoted to treating intramural haematomas in the subacute phase to avoid possible complications.
- Minimal stent graft oversizing and no post-dilatation are recommended.

3.3.4.1 Aetiology and Clinical Presentation

A 53-year-old patient with hypertension and obesity was admitted to the emergency service due to chest pain. The patient was afebrile, and myocardial ischaemia was ruled out following negative ECG and normal coronary enzymes.

3.3.4.2 Pre-interventional Diagnosis

Contrast-enhanced CT showed intramural haematoma type B, starting distally from the left subclavian artery and extending to the diaphragm level (Fig. 3.68). There were no intimal tears and

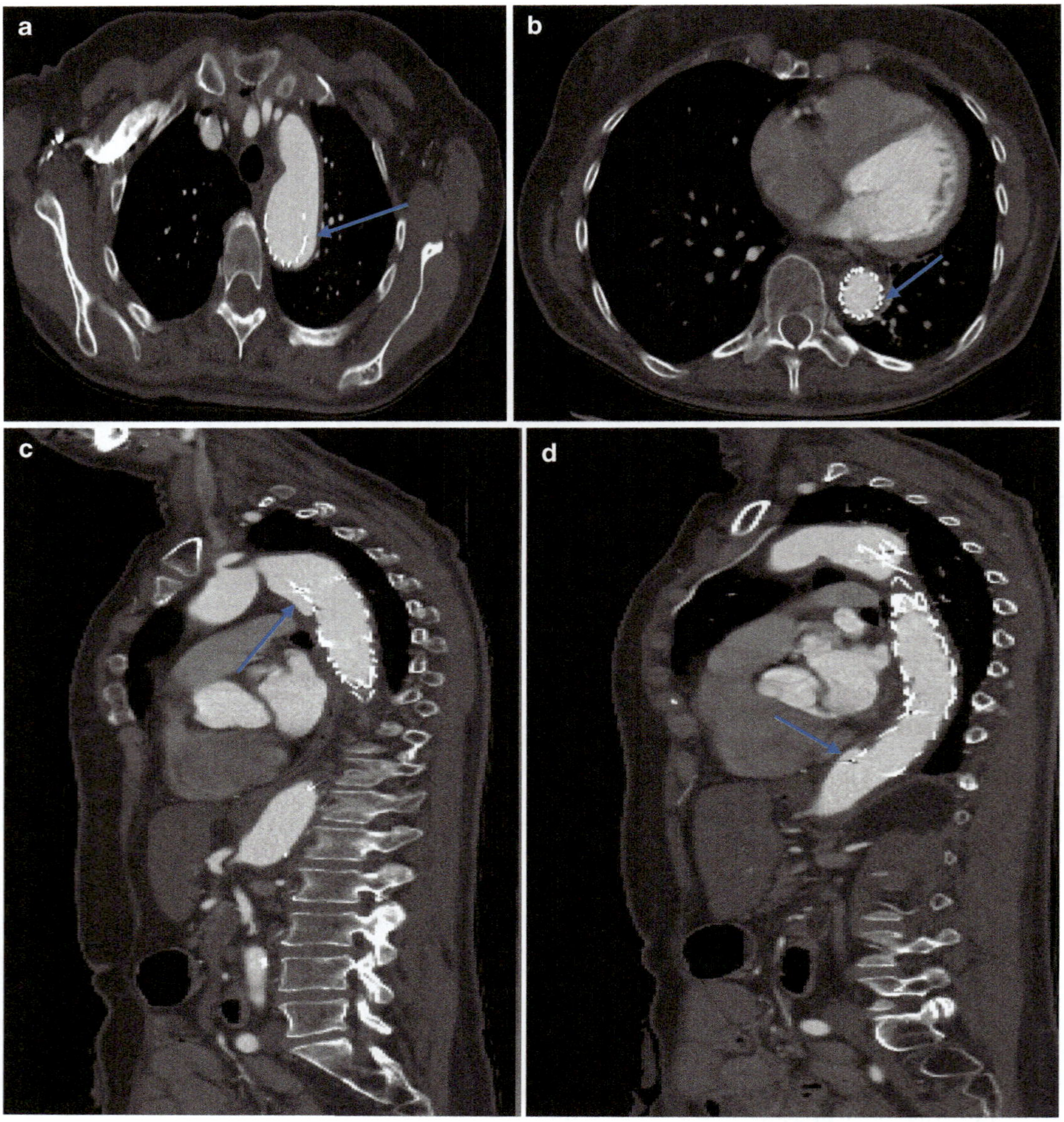

Fig. 3.66 Contrast-enhanced CT 3 months after TEVAR. Blue arrows indicate a new stent graft-induced aortic lesion: (**a**) proximal stent graft-induced aortic intima lesion. (**c** and **d**) distal stent graft-induced aortic intima lesion. (**b**) regression of the intramural haematoma (arrow)

no haematomas in the ascending aorta or aortic arch. The patient was treated conservatively with antihypertensive medicine with a good result. Two weeks later, emergency CT scanning was performed due to severe retrosternal pain. The control CT showed thoracic aorta dissection development and rupture (Fig. 3.69).

3.3.4.3 Endovascular Treatment

The right femoral artery was surgically exposed. A TEVAR stent graft was advanced over the super-stiff guidewire. A dissection stent graft was used with minimal oversizing of 10–12%. The stent graft was intentionally placed to cover the left subclavian artery to obtain at least a 20 mm proximal landing zone (Fig. 3.70). The blood pressure during deployment was kept below 90 mmHg. This is especially important in cases of rupture where an optimal sealing zone is imperative. Carotid-subclavian bypass is recommended in elective cases where the subclavian artery intends to be covered, but in acute situations, there is no time for

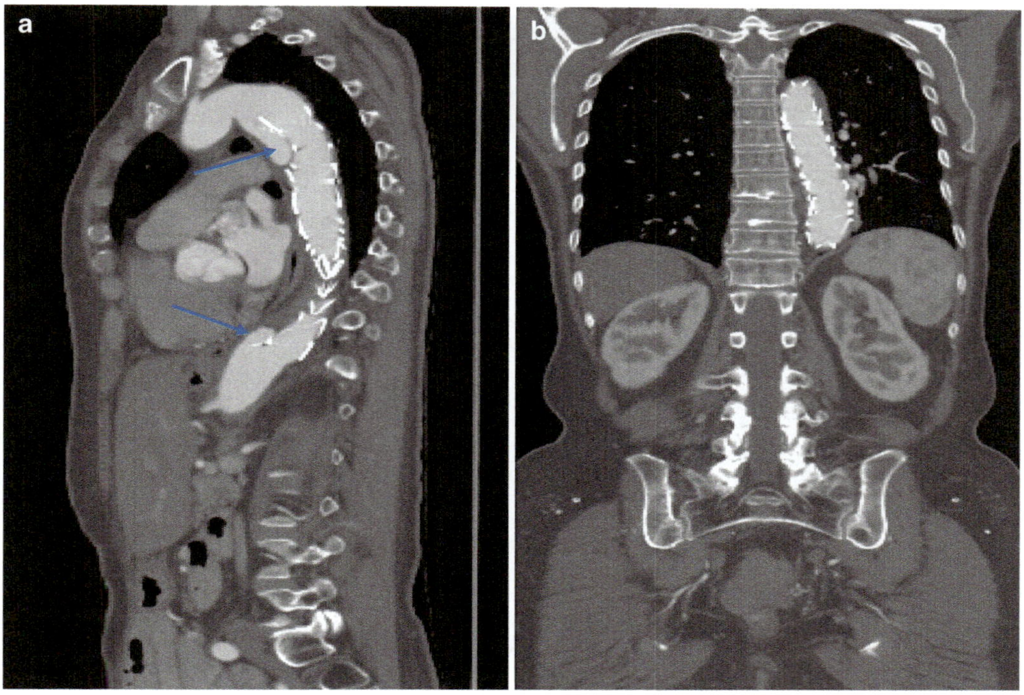

Fig. 3.67 Contrast-enhanced CT 1 year after TEVAR. Blue arrows indicate progression of the distal and proximal stent graft-induced aortic intima lesions (**a**). The patient remained asymptomatic. (**b**) complete regression of the intramural haematoma

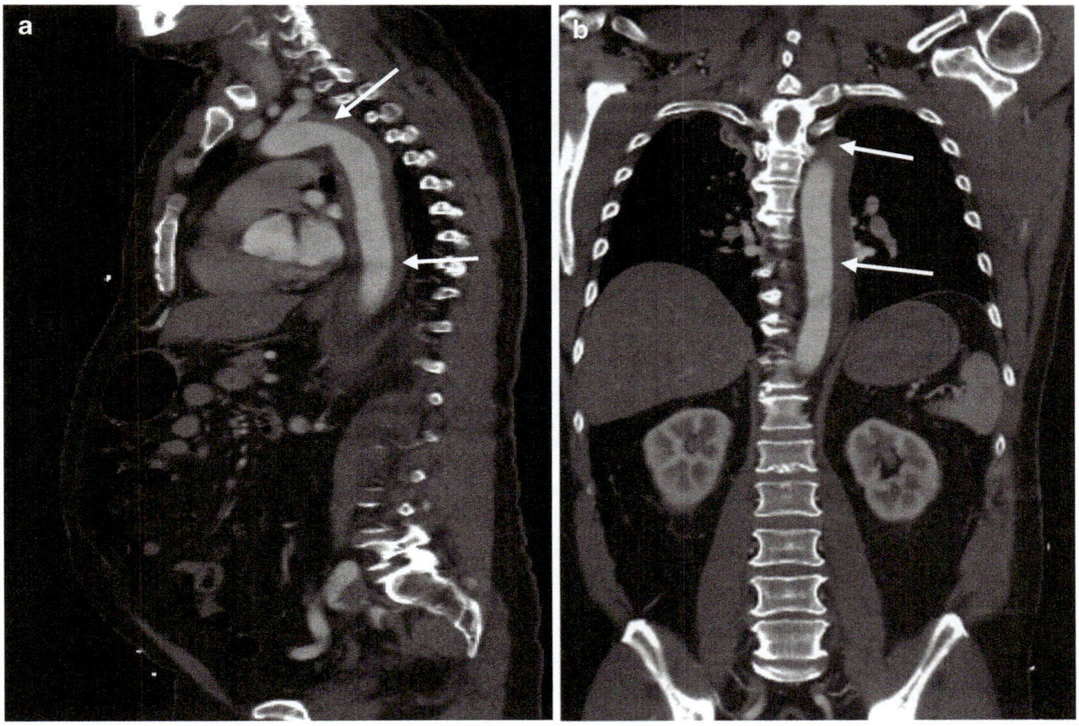

Fig. 3.68 Contrast-enhanced CT showing intramural haematoma type B, without intimal tears (arrows). The haematoma starts distally from the left subclavian artery

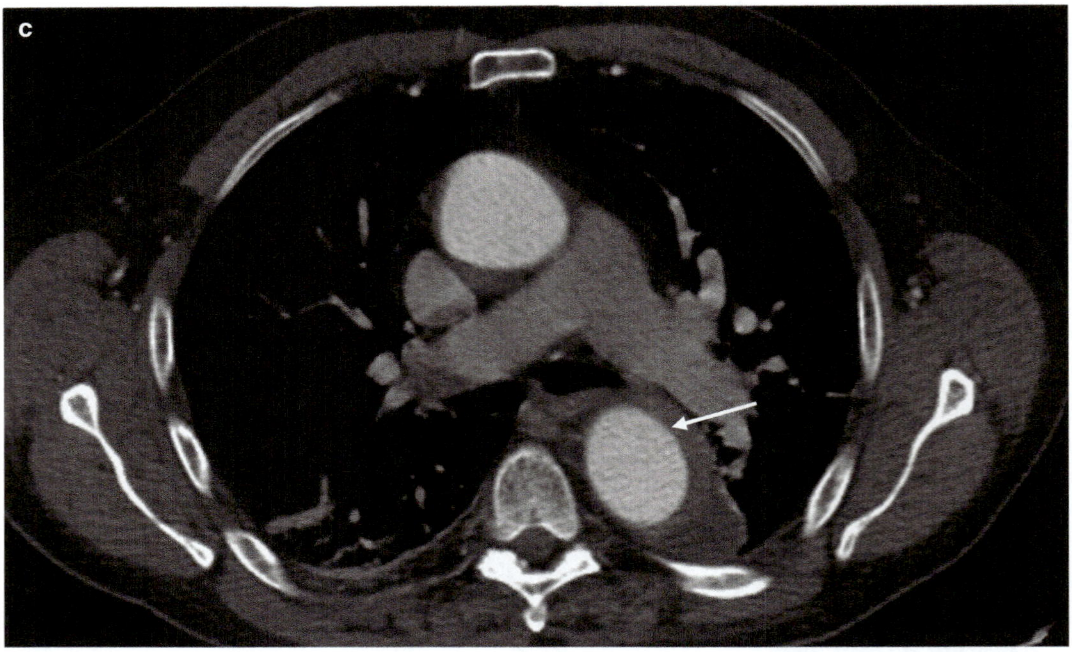

Fig. 3.68 (continued)

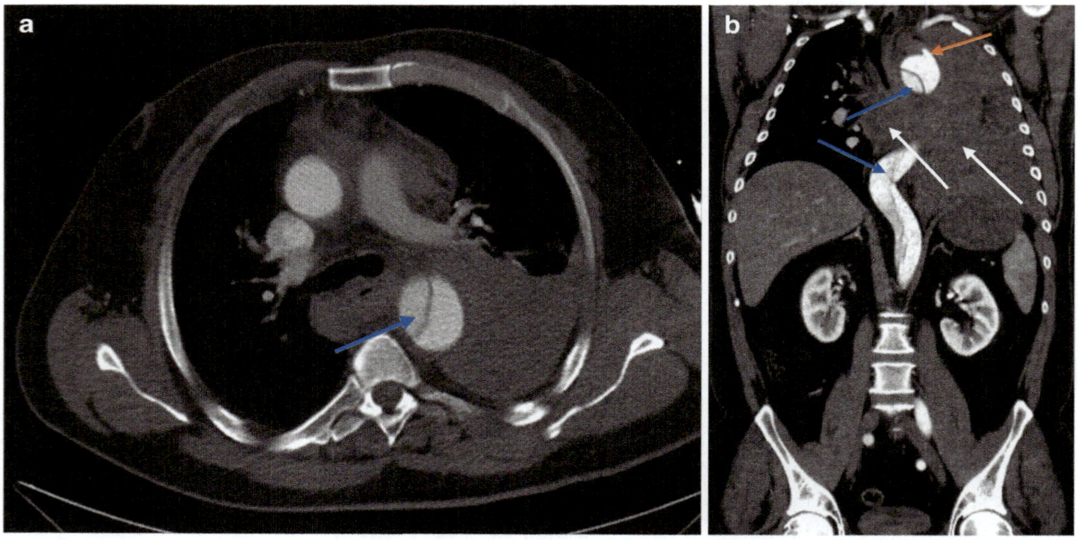

Fig. 3.69 Emergency contrast-enhanced CT 2 weeks after the first CT scan. Intramural haematoma progressed to an aortic dissection (blue arrows) and ruptured, leading to mediastinal haematoma and left haemothorax (white arrows). Orange arrow indicates the rupture site

surgery. In cases of off-arm ischaemia after TEVAR, carotid-subclavian bypass can be performed. The chimney stent graft technique is an option, but in cases of rupture, it is not advisable due to the risk of proximal seal compromise.

3.3.4.4 Outcome

The patient recovered gradually with some respiratory complications and remained haemodynamically stable. There was no sign of left-arm ischaemia or spinal ischaemia. Control

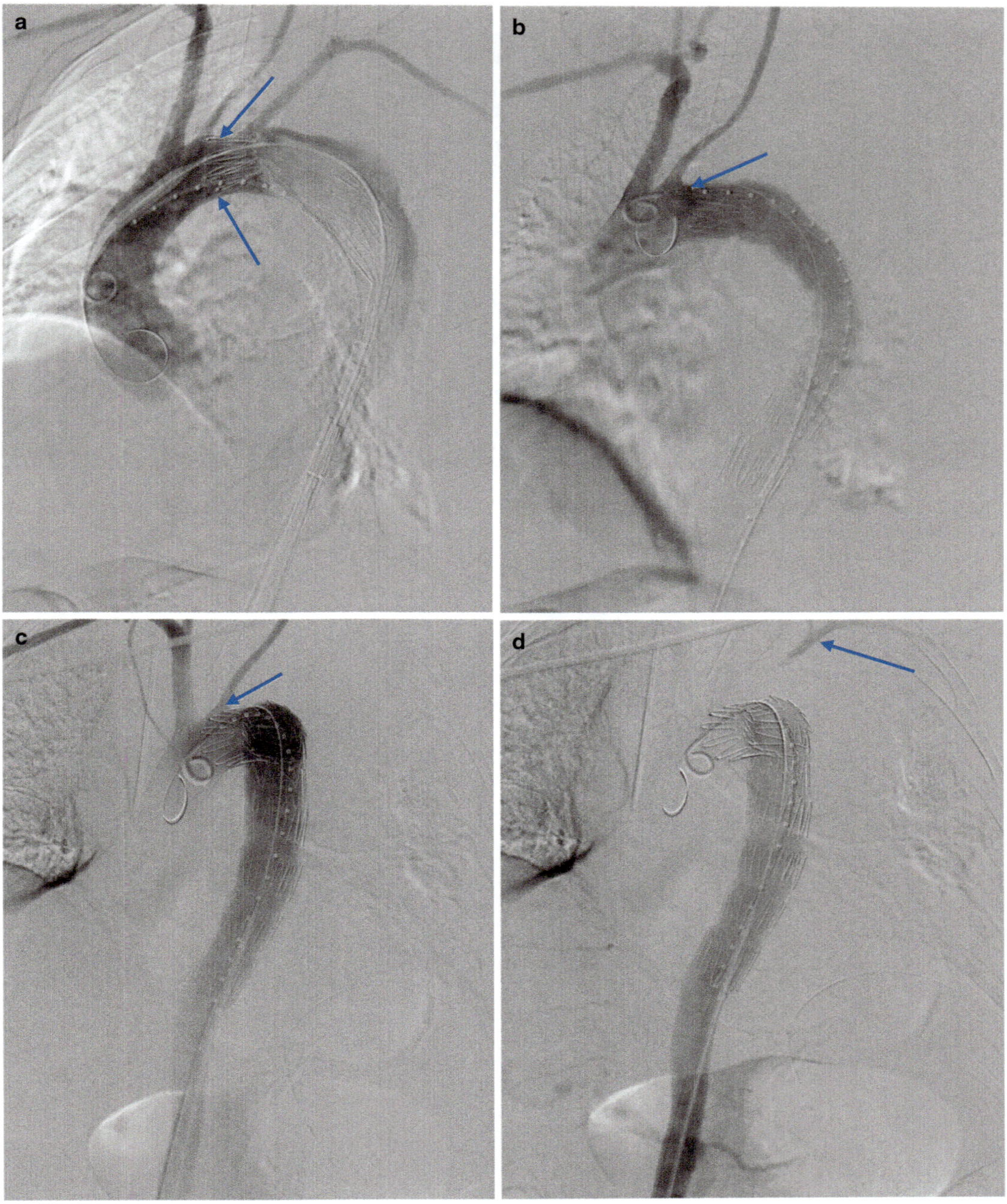

Fig. 3.70 Detail from the emergency TEVAR. Stent graft deployment close to the left carotid artery (arrows) (**a–c**), with intentional over-stenting of the left subclavian artery. Retrograde flow through the vertebral arteries to the left subclavian artery was observed (arrow) (**d**)

contrast-enhanced CT 3 months after TEVAR showed a well-deployed stent graft and satisfactory results (Fig. 3.71). The mediastinal haematoma and haemothorax had partially regressed. Subsequent control CT 1 year later showed complete aortic remodelling and haematoma regression (Fig. 3.72). The patient remains asymptomatic.

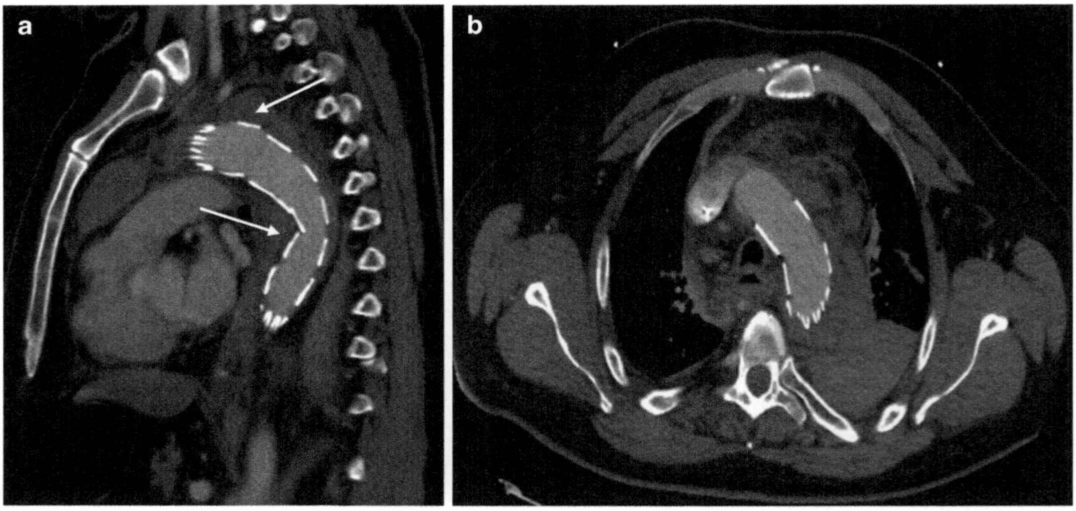

Fig. 3.71 Control contrast-enhanced CT 3 months after TEVAR showing a well-deployed stent-graft and no endoleak. Regression of the intrathoracic haematoma arrows

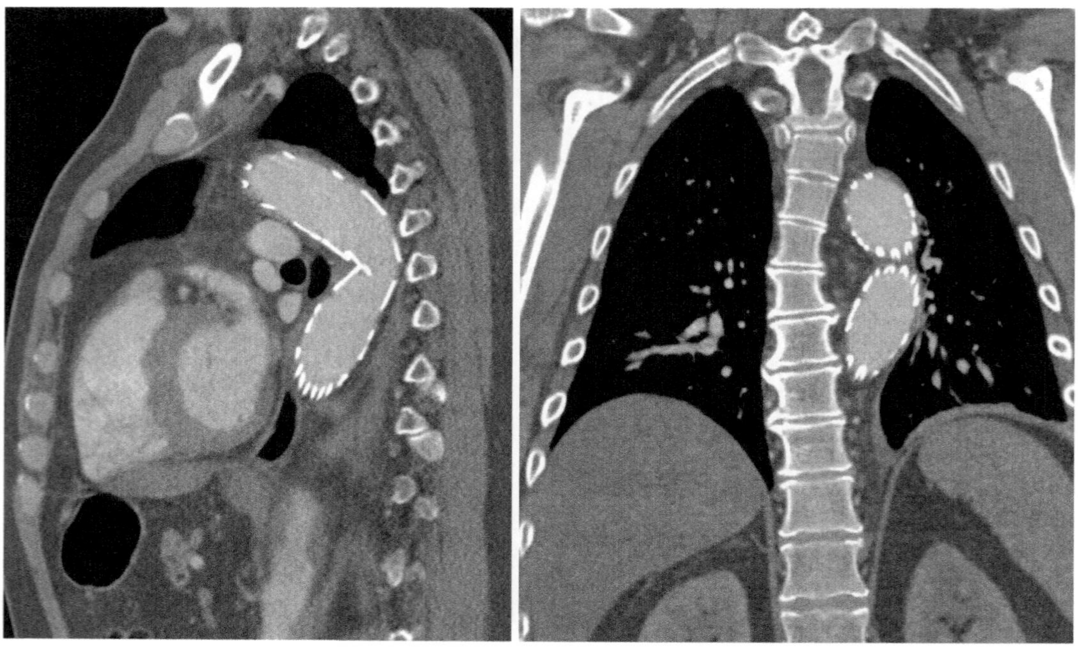

Fig. 3.72 Control contrast-enhanced CT 1 year after TEVAR showing a well-deployed stent-graft and no endoleak. Complete regression of the intrathoracic haematoma and complete aortic remodelling were observed

3.4 Penetrating Thoracic Aortic Ulcer

3.4.1 Penetrating Thoracic Ulcer in the Descending Aorta-I

Key Points

- PAUs have a high potential for developing complications such as rupture, progression to aortic dissection and pseudoaneurysm.
- PAUs >2 cm in diameter have a higher rate of complications.
- In cases with conservative treatment, frequent control is needed.

3.4.1.1 Aetiology and Clinical Presentation

A 75-year-old patient with cardiac insufficiency, myocardial diseases and hypertension complained of chest pain starting a few days prior. The patient was in pain but haemodynamically stable with oxygen saturation of 97% and average respiratory rate. ECG and coronary enzymes were not indicative of any acute myocardial problems. The patient had a temperature of 37.8 °C, a white blood cell count of $10/L \times 10^9/L$, and CRP of 42 mg/L. There were no signs of infection in the urine or blood culture.

3.4.1.2 Pre-interventional Diagnosis

Contrast-enhanced CT scan showed a penetrating aortic ulcer (PAU) in the descending aorta containing a heterogeneous mural thrombus (Fig. 3.73a). The aorta showed calcifications. The patient responded very well to conservative treatment with antihypertensive and pain medications and became pain-free. The temperature was still 37.8 °C, and the white blood cell count and CRP were unchanged. Infected atherosclerotic plaque and infective pseudoaneurysm could not be excluded entirely, and the patient remained in the hospital. Subsequent control CT 1 week later showed enlargement of the PAU up to 5 cm, a

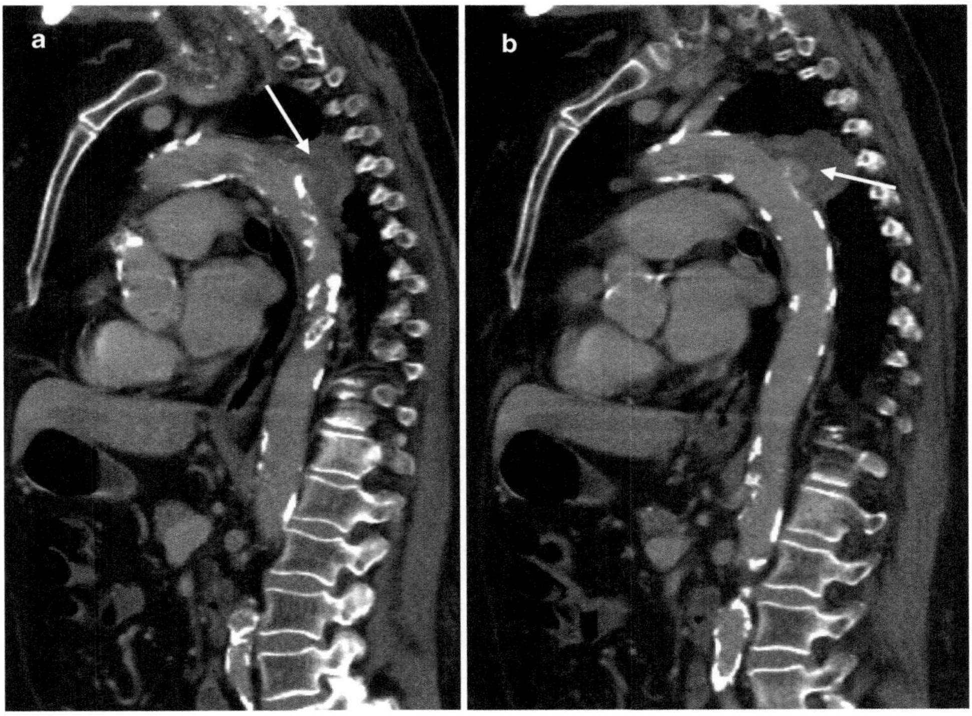

Fig. 3.73 Contrast-enhanced CT showing PAU. (**a**) PAU in the descending aorta showing a possible rupture or infective pseudoaneurysm (arrow). (**b**) control CT 1 week later showing growth in the PAU and pseudoaneurysm of approximately 1 cm (arrow)

growth of approximately 1 cm over 1 week (Fig. 3.73b). The patient was scheduled for TEVAR. Broad-spectrum antibiotics were administered before TEVAR and continuously for 2 weeks after TEVAR due to the possibility of an infective aetiology for the PAU/pseudoaneurysm.

3.4.1.3 Endovascular Treatment

Under general anaesthesia, the TEVAR stent graft was advanced through the surgically exposed right femoral artery and deployed distally to the left subclavian artery (Fig. 3.74). There was a sufficient proximal landing zone without the need to cover the subclavian artery. The stent graft was oversized between 15 and 20% and 100 mm in length. The intervention was performed without any difficulties.

3.4.1.4 Outcome

The patient did not experience any complications after TEVAR. The antibiotics were continued for 2 weeks, and the white blood cell count and CRP returned to normal. The patient was afebrile after a few days and currently remains asymptomatic. The first control imaging was performed 3 months later, showing shrinkage of the PAU and a well-deployed stent graft (Fig. 3.75a). The subsequent control CT 1 year later showed almost complete resolution of the PAU (Fig. 3.75b). There were no other signs of infection or reaction around the aortic wall. The fast growth of the PAU indicated the presence of an infective component in its development. Although the duration of antibiotic therapy is individualized, there is no consensus regarding this in the literature.

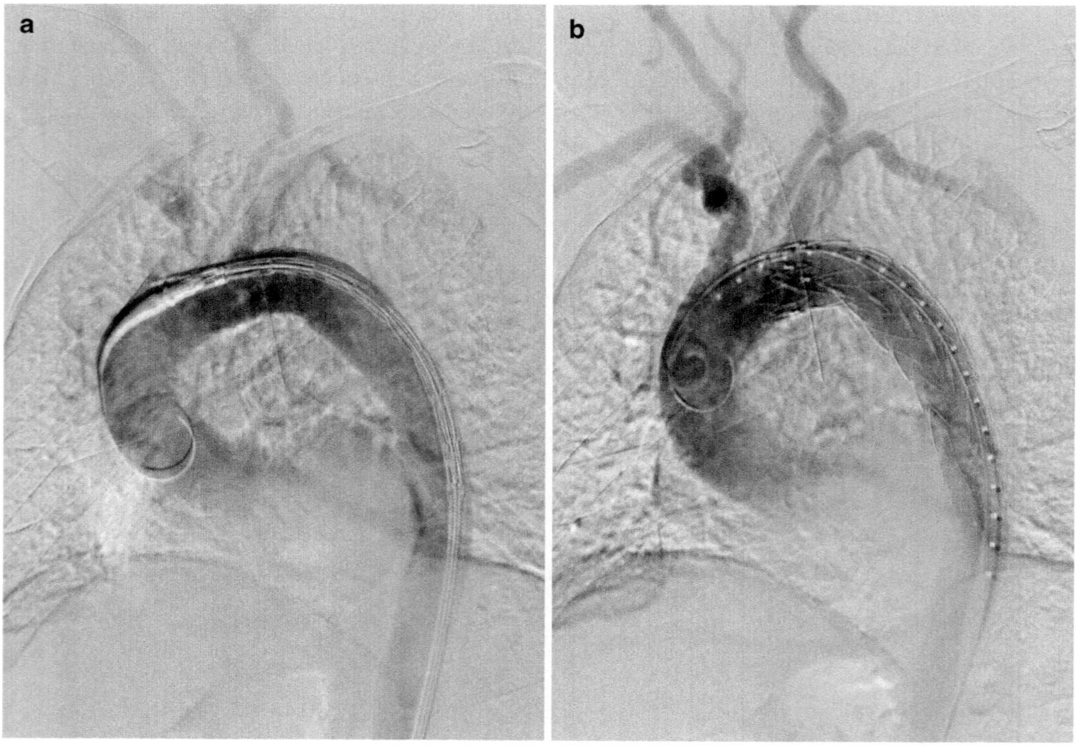

Fig. 3.74 Details from the TEVAR intervention. (**a**) advancement of the stent graft. (**b**) control image after stent-graft deployment distally from the left subclavian artery

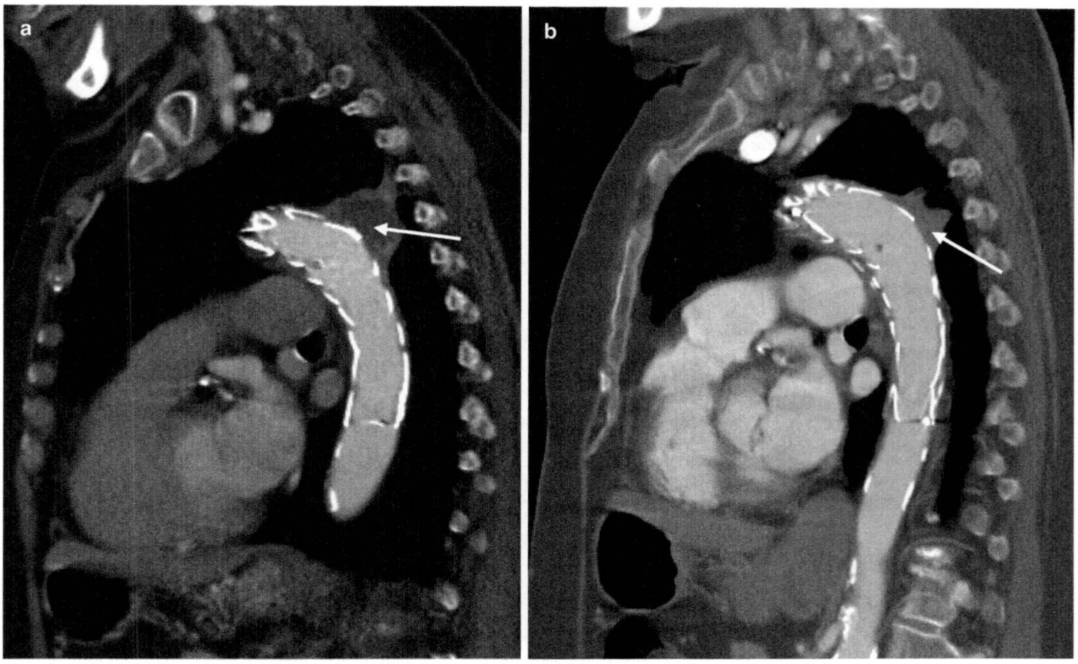

Fig. 3.75 Control contrast-enhanced CT. (**a**) three months after TEVAR, shrinkage of the PAU is observed (arrow). (**b**) one year control image after TEVAR showing almost complete regression of the PAU (arrow)

3.4.2 Penetrating Thoracic Ulcer in the Descending Aorta-II

> **Key Points**
> - PAUs have a high potential for developing complications such as rupture, progression to aortic dissection and pseudoaneurysm.
> - PAUs >2 cm in diameter have a higher rate of complications.
> - In cases with conservative treatment, frequent control is needed.

3.4.2.1 Aetiology and Clinical Presentation

A 73-year-old patient with well-controlled arterial hypertension complained of intermittent mild chest pain. No other significant comorbidities were present. ECG and blood tests were normal and showed no coronary ischaemic diseases. Contrast-enhanced CT was planned.

3.4.2.2 Pre-interventional Diagnosis

Contrast-enhanced CT (Fig. 3.76) showed a penetrating aortic ulcer (PAU) in the descending aorta measuring 23 mm × 12 mm in size with intramural haematoma (IM) around the proximal part of the descending aorta. There was no IM in the ascending aorta or aortic arch. The patient was frequently without pain, and it was decided to control the arterial hypertension. Control CT was scheduled 1 month later to wait for regression of the IM in the proximal part of the descending aorta. 1 month later, control CT showed significant enlargement of the PAU, now measuring 31 mm × 23 mm (Fig. 3.77), while the IM in the proximal portion of the descending aorta had slightly shrunk. The patient remained asymptomatic.

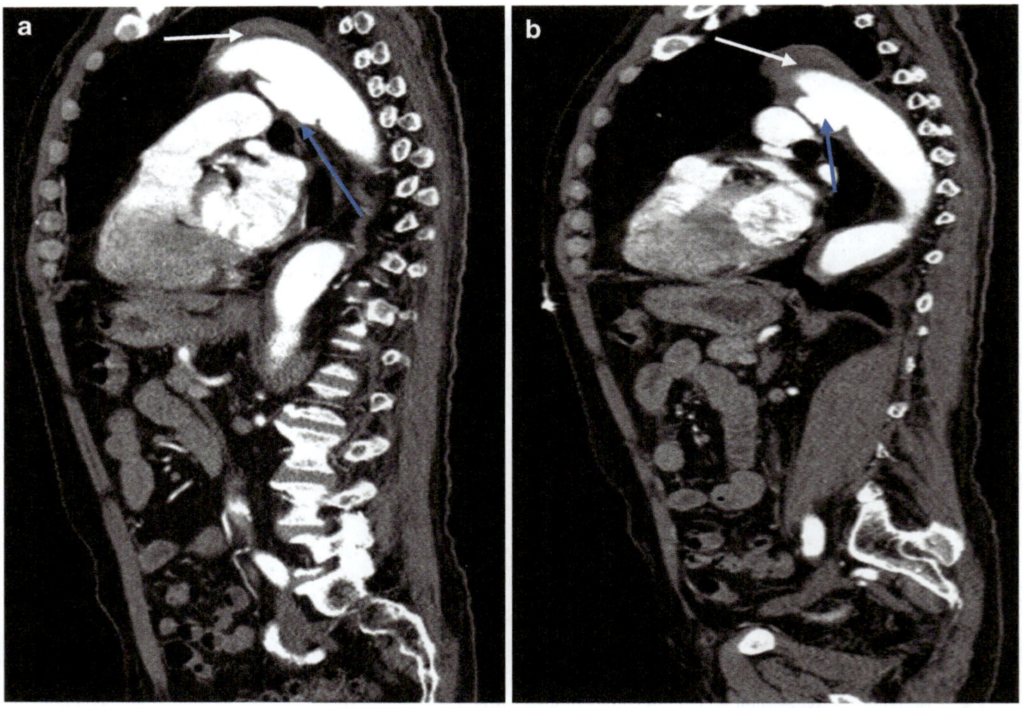

Fig. 3.76 Contrast-enhanced CT. Penetrating aortic ulcer (PAU) in the descending aorta- (blue arrows). White arrows indicate an intramural haematoma (IM)

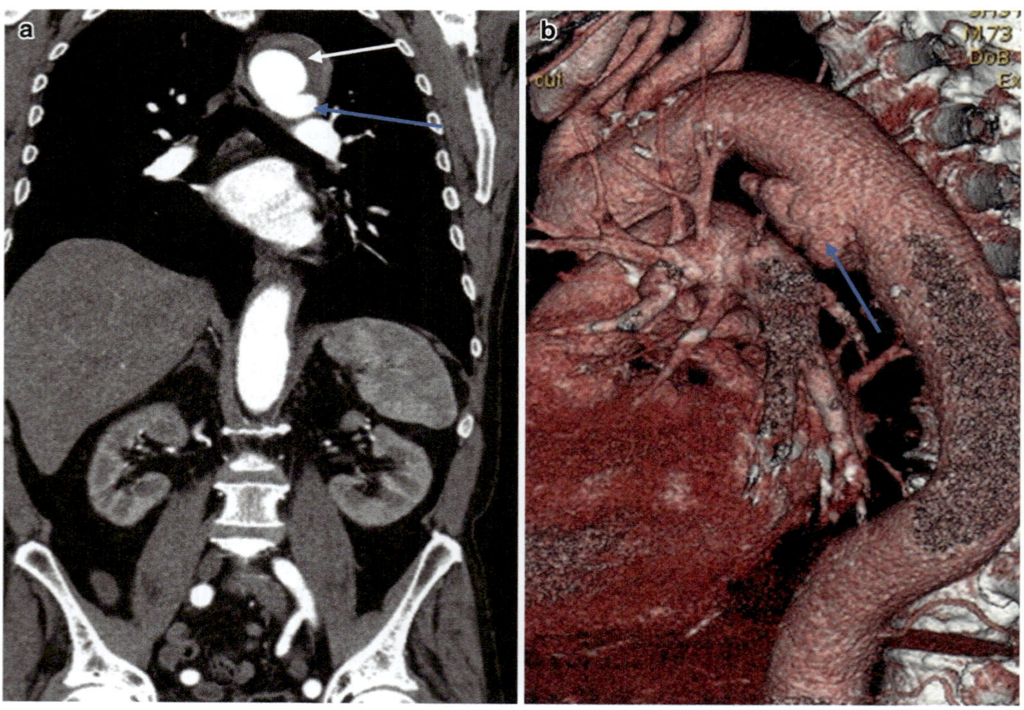

Fig. 3.77 Control contrast-enhanced CT 1 month later. The PAU had increased in size- (blue arrows). The IM was still present in the proximal portion of the descending aorta (white arrow)

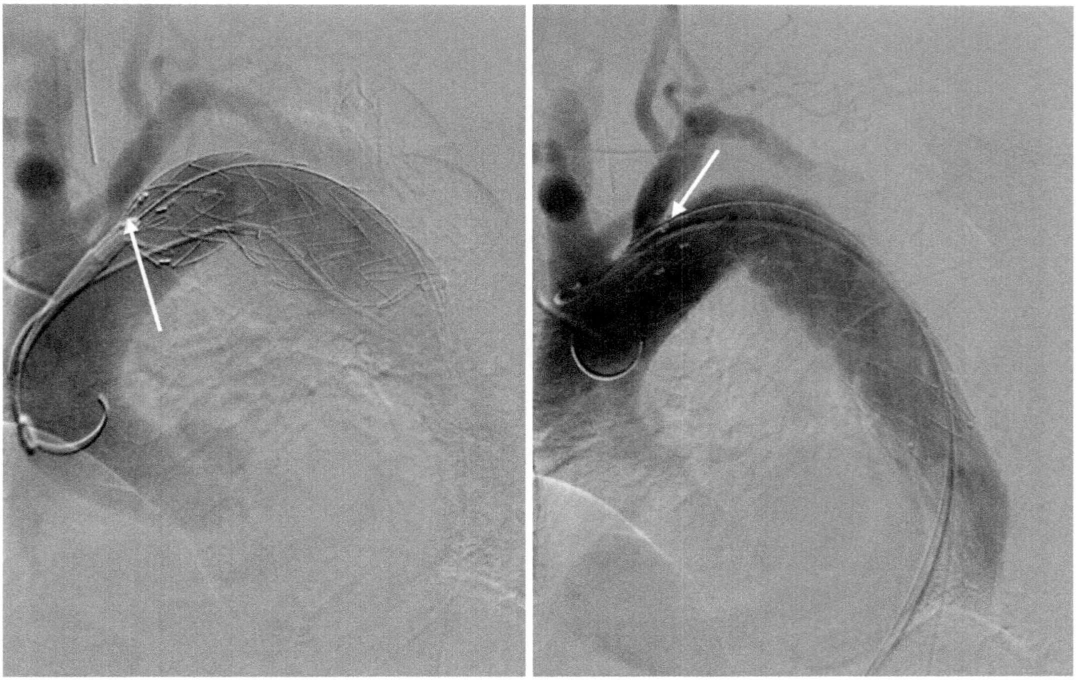

Fig. 3.78 TEVAR stent graft deployment. White arrows indicate the origin of the left subclavian artery. The stent graft was deployed distally from the left subclavian artery and covered the PAU satisfactorily

3.4.2.3 Endovascular Treatment

Under general anaesthesia, a TEVAR stent graft was advanced through the surgically exposed right femoral artery. There was an approximately 22 mm proximal landing zone, in which the aorta had a diameter of 30 mm, and there was no need to cover the left subclavian artery. A TEVAR stent graft measuring 34 mm × 150 mm was deployed distally from the left subclavian artery without difficulties, and an excellent result was obtained (Fig. 3.77).

3.4.2.4 Outcome

The patient did not experience any complications after TEVAR and was discharged from the hospital 2 days later without any symptoms (Fig. 3.78). The first control imaging was performed 3 months later, showing shrinkage of the PAU, a well-deployed stent graft and IM regression (Fig. 3.79). There were no new stent graft-induced intima lesions on control CT.

3.4.3 Penetrating Thoracic Ulcer in the Descending Aorta-III

Key Points

- PAU have a high potential for developing complications such as rupture, progression to aortic dissection and pseudoaneurysm.
- PAUs >2 cm in diameter have a higher rate of complications.
- Awareness of neurological complications is important during manipulation with diverse materials.

3.4.3.1 Aetiology and Clinical Presentation

A 78-year-old patient with cardiac insufficiency, diabetes mellitus and significant chronic obstructive pulmonary disease was admitted due to

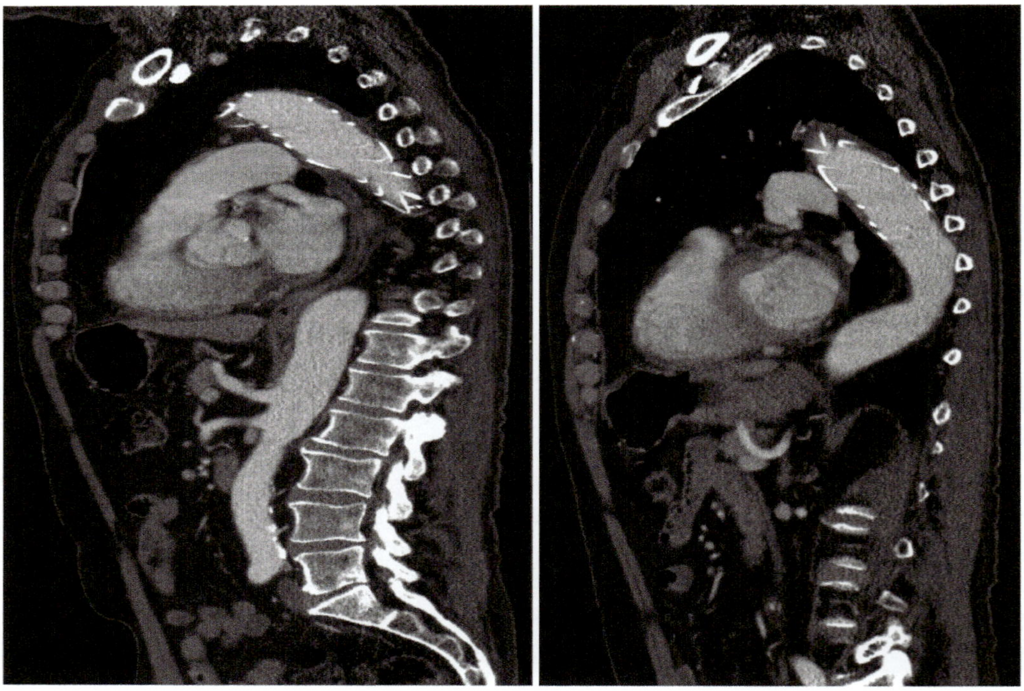

Fig. 3.79 Control contrast-enhanced CT after TEVAR showing shrinkage of the PAU and IM regression. Good stent graft apposition with the aortic wall was observed

constant chest pain radiating into the back. The patient had suffered a few neurologic ischaemic events without permanent sequelae and a history of chronic abdominal angina. The patient was not interested in treatment involving carotid and mesenteric arterial stenosis. There were no signs of acute coronary ischaemia, and the patient was afebrile.

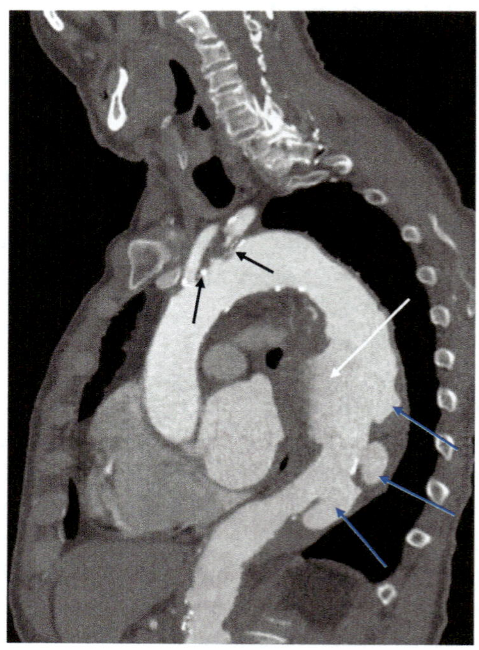

Fig. 3.80 Contrast-enhanced CT showing multiple PAUs-(blue arrows) in the descending aorta. White arrow shows a descending thoracic aorta aneurysm. Aortic arch showed calcifications and stenosis of the supra-aortic arteries- (black arrows)

3.4.3.2 Pre-interventional Diagnosis

Contrast-enhanced CT of the aorta showed multiple penetrating aortic ulcers (PAUs) and intramural haematomas (IMs) in the descending aorta. The descending aorta demonstrated an aneurysm measuring 58 mm in length (Fig. 3.80). After speaking with the patient, it was decided to treat the PAUs with TEVAR stent grafts. There was sufficient proximal and distal landing zone without the need for additional surgery.

3.4.3.3 Endovascular Treatment

Under general anaesthesia, two TEVAR stent grafts were advanced over a super-stiff guidewire through the surgically exposed right femoral

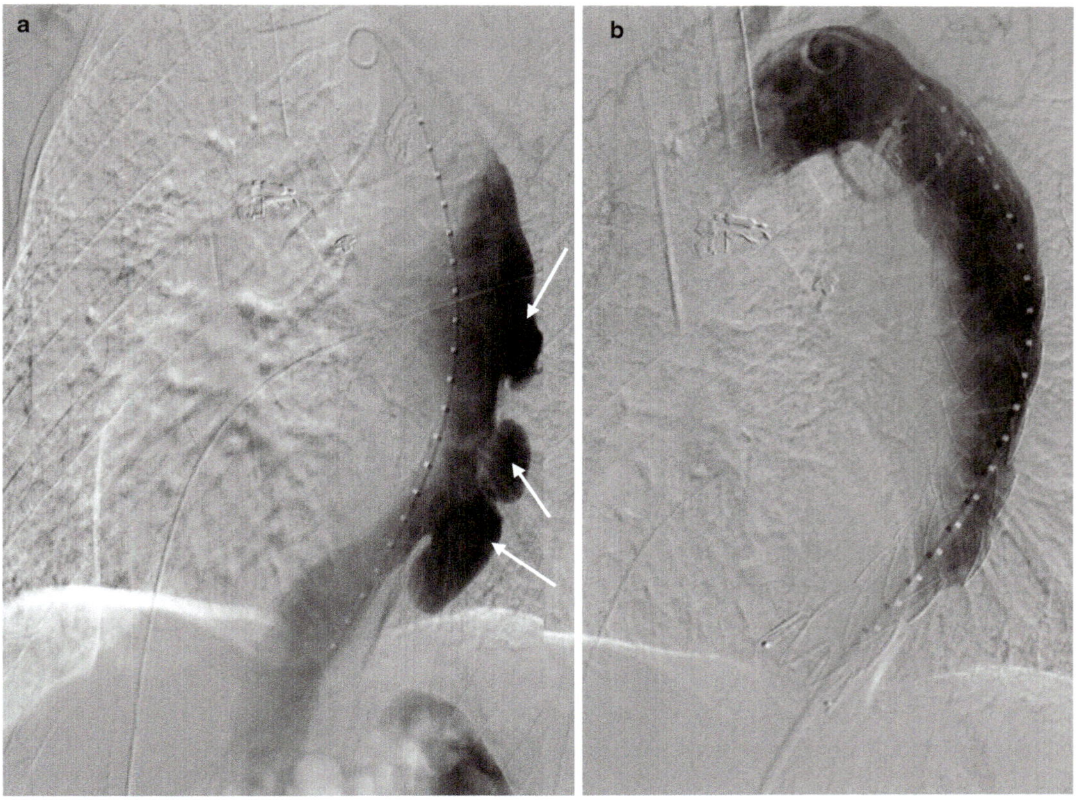

Fig. 3.81 Details from the TEVAR intervention. (**a**) multiple PAUs (arrows). (**b**) two well-deployed stent grafts with overlap of at least 5 cm

artery and placed into the ascending aorta. First, the proximal stent graft was deployed distally from the left subclavian artery. After that, the second stent graft was placed distally with at least 5 cm overlap between the stents (Fig. 3.81). The final control images showed a satisfactory result.

3.4.3.4 Outcome

The patient experienced a severe permanent neurological complication, which led to prolonged stay in the intensive care unit. CT of the brain a few days after TEVAR showed an infarct in the right posterior fossa (Fig. 3.82). The calcifications in the aortic arch and manipulations with the guide wire and stent graft caused the distal cerebral emboli and infarct. It is of utmost importance to be aware and very careful during the intervention to minimalize the possibility of complications.

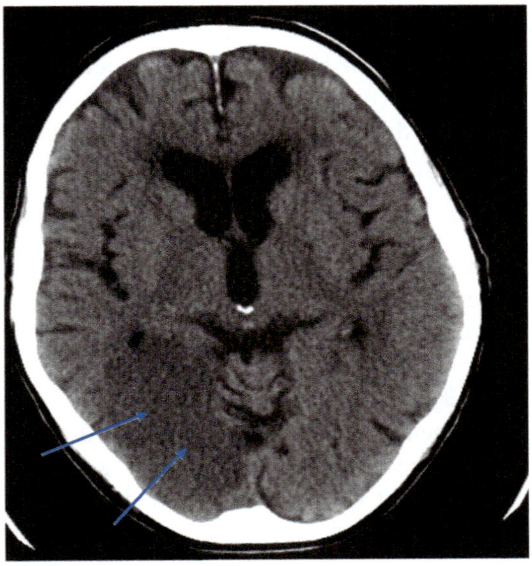

Fig. 3.82 Axial computed tomography of the brain showing infarction of the right posterior fossa (arrows)

3.5 Thoracic Aortic Trauma

3.5.1 Thoracic Aortic Trauma-I

> **Key Points**
> - It is usually straightforward to treat traumatic aortic lesions with TEVAR.
> - In an emergency, coverage of the left subclavian artery is usually well-tolerated.
> - Care should be taken regarding the size of the stent graft; for young patients with aorta diameters of 21–22 mm, TEVAR stent grafts with diameters of 25–26 are generally sufficient.

3.5.1.1 Aetiology and Clinical Presentation

A 20-year-old patient was admitted to the emergency department after a traffic accident. The patient was in shock and hypotensive and showed an oxygen saturation of 92%. After resuscitation and intubation trauma, contrast-enhanced CT was performed.

3.5.1.2 Pre-interventional Diagnosis

Acute CT showed a traumatic aortic lesion classically positioned distally from the left subclavian artery with haemothorax and mediastinal haematoma (Fig. 3.83). There was an intimal lesion just distal to the left subclavian artery, and it was decided to extend the proximal landing zone by covering the left subclavian artery without previous revascularization due to the emergency nature of the injury. Haemothorax was bilateral. There were multiple rib fractures and lung injuries.

3.5.1.3 Endovascular Treatment

Under general anaesthesia, two TEVAR stent grafts were advanced through the surgically exposed right femoral artery over a super-stiff guidewire placed into the descending aorta across the traumatic lesion. The first stent graft was intentionally deployed to cover the left subclavian artery and obtain a sufficient landing zone. After that, the second stent graft was placed distally with at least 5 cm overlap between the stents (Fig. 3.84). The patient had insufficient blood return into the right heart and hypotension due to haemothorax compression on the vena cava, and an emergency chest tube was deployed with a rapid positive outcome. Chest X-ray showed mediastinum displacement to the right (Fig. 3.84c), and a later control scan showed the chest tube placement (Fig. 3.84d).

3.5.1.4 Outcome

The patient recovered gradually without any complications. There was no problem with the left arm and no signs of ischaemia. There were no neurological complications. The rib fractures were conservatively treated.

3.5.2 Thoracic aortic trauma-II

> **Key Points**
> - It is usually straightforward to treat traumatic aortic lesions with TEVAR.
> - In an emergency, coverage of the left subclavian artery is usually well-tolerated.
> - Care should be taken regarding the size of the stent graft; for young patients with aorta diameters of 21–22 mm, TEVAR stent grafts with diameters of 25–26 are generally sufficient.

3.5.2.1 Aetiology and Clinical Presentation

A 48-year patient fell from a 5 m height while performing construction work and was brought to the emergency department. The patient was haemodynamically stable but in severe pain and had difficulty breathing. Oxygen saturation was 92%.

3.5.2.2 Pre-interventional Diagnosis

Emergency CT trauma was performed and showed a traumatic aortic lesion in the mid-portion of the descending aorta with mediastinal haematoma. There was haemothorax on the left

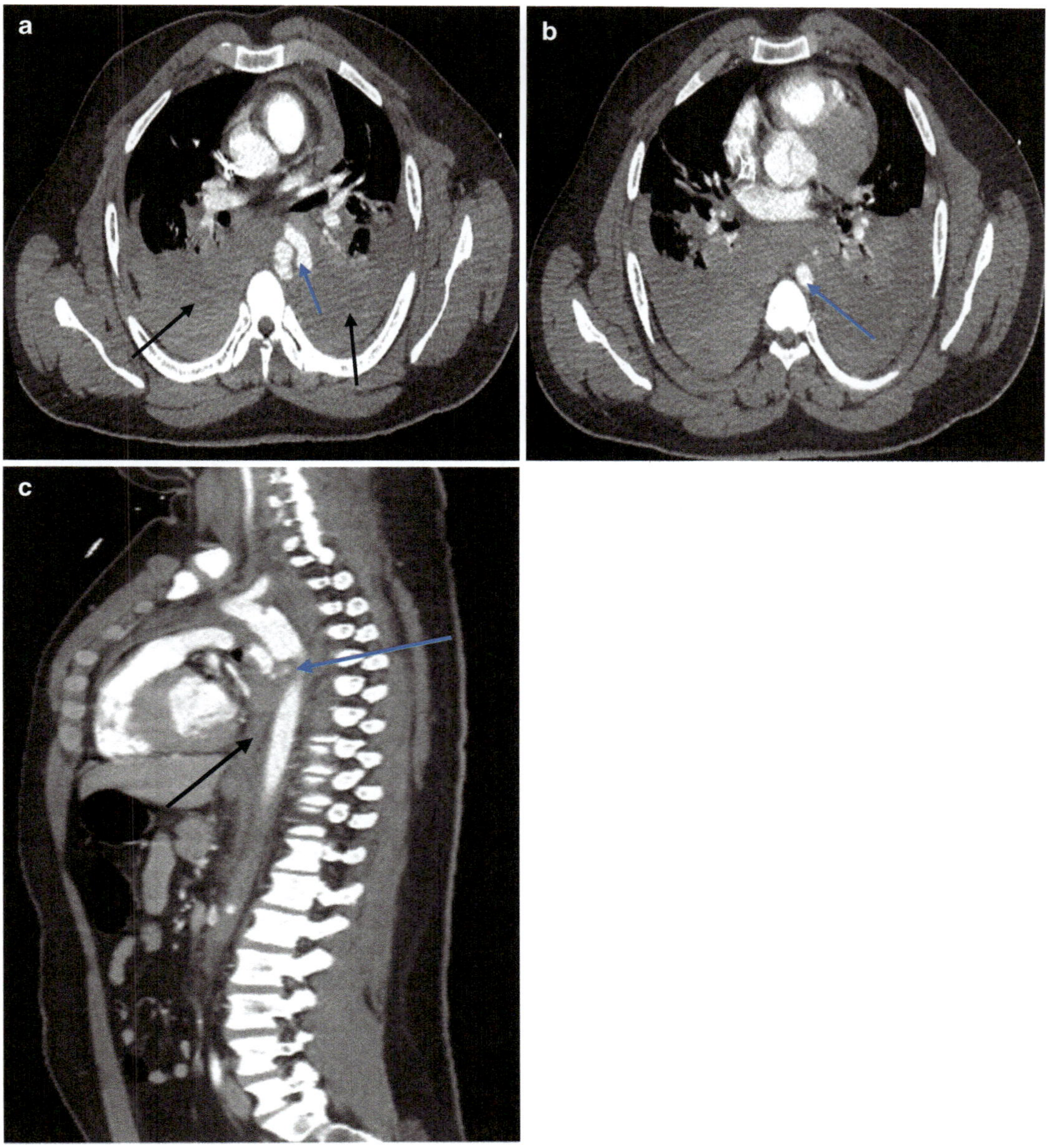

Fig. 3.83 Computed tomography of the chest and abdomen with traumatic aortic lesions (blue arrows) and bilateral haemothorax (black arrows)

side and lung atelectasis (Fig. 3.85). Multiple thoracic vertebrae had traumatic fractures.

3.5.2.3 Endovascular Treatment

Under general anaesthesia, a TEVAR stent graft was advanced over a super-stiff guidewire placed into the descending aorta across the traumatic lesion very quickly and without difficulty. There was sufficient proximal and distal landing zone, and there was no need to cover the left subclavian artery (Fig. 3.86). There were no complications during the intervention.

3.5.2.4 Outcome

The patient underwent spinal surgery and stabilization of the vertebral fractures after TEVAR and complete recovery. Control computed tomography was performed 3 months after TEVAR,

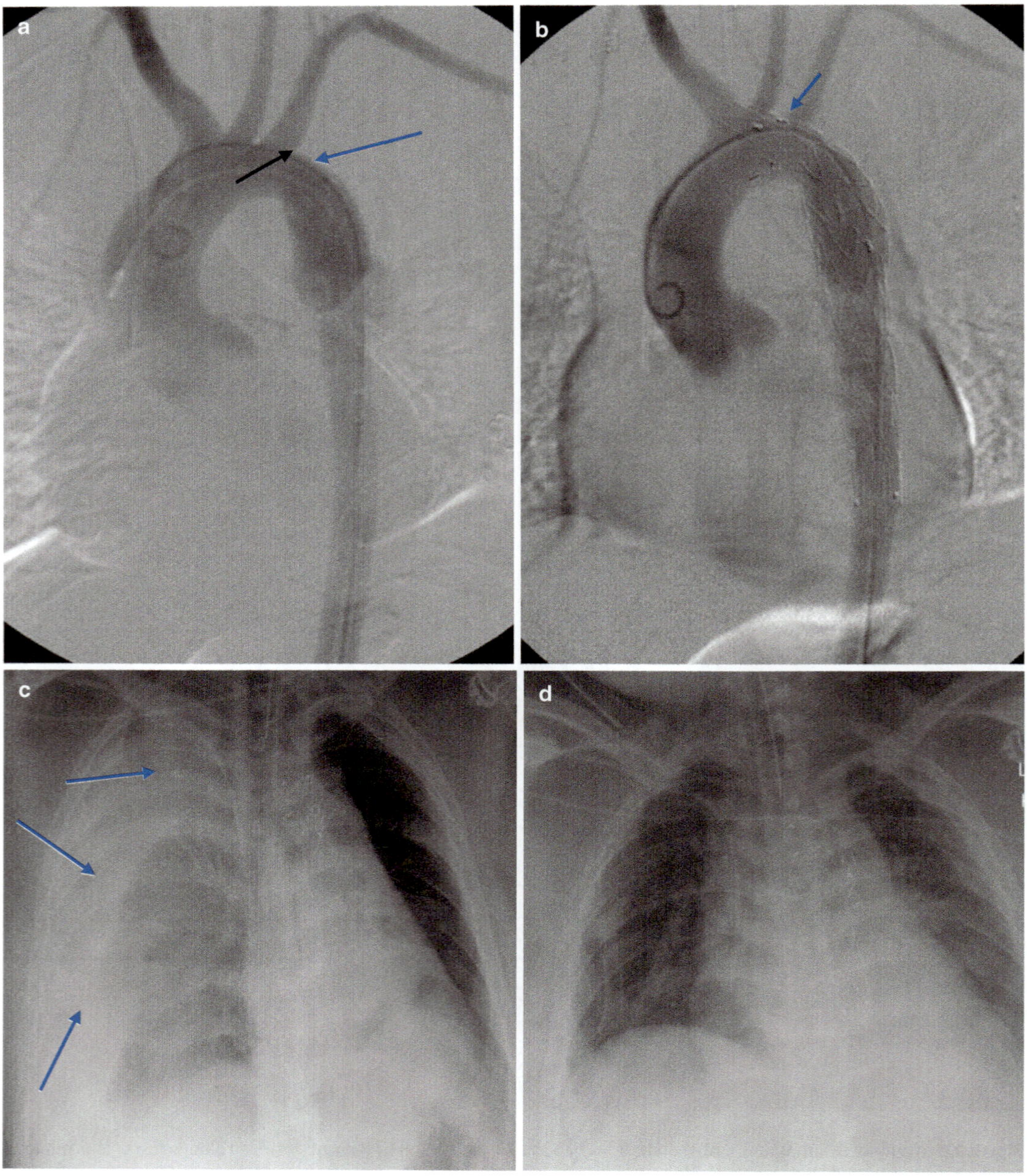

Fig. 3.84 Acute TEVAR stent graft deployment. (**a**) black arrow indicates the left subclavian artery. Blue arrow indicates the transection site. (**b**) deployed stent graft intentionally covering the left subclavian artery. Blue arrow indicates the covered portion of the stent graft. (**c**) chest X-ray showing right haemothorax (arrows). (**d**) scan following haemothorax drainage and placement of the chest tube

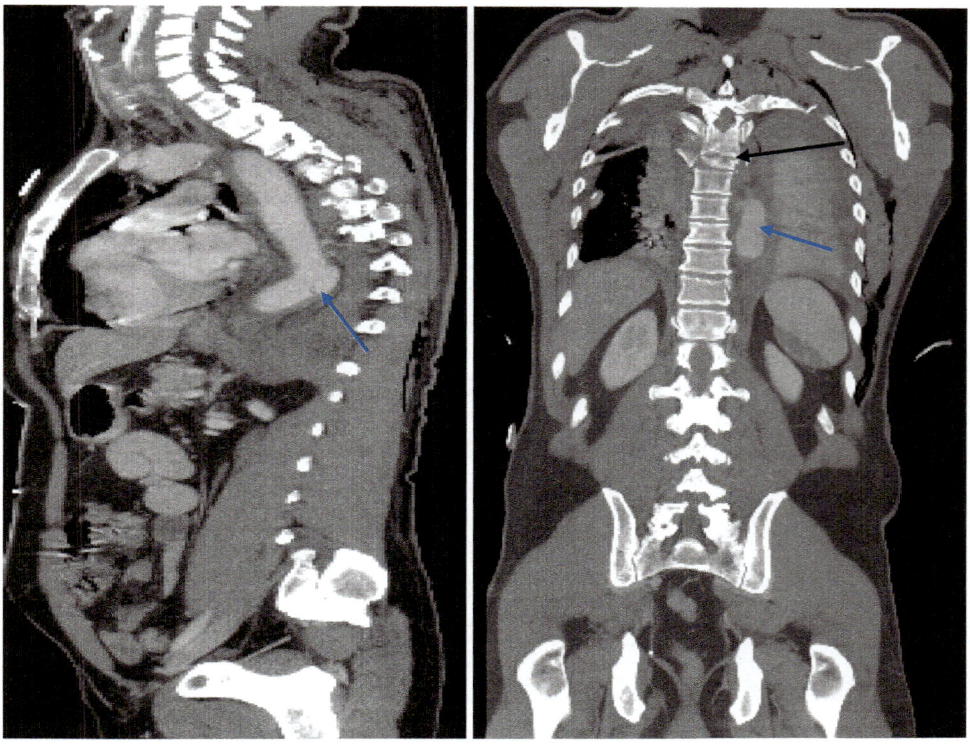

Fig. 3.85 Contrast-enhanced CT showing a traumatic descending aorta lesion–(blue arrows). Black arrow indicates a thoracic vertebral fracture

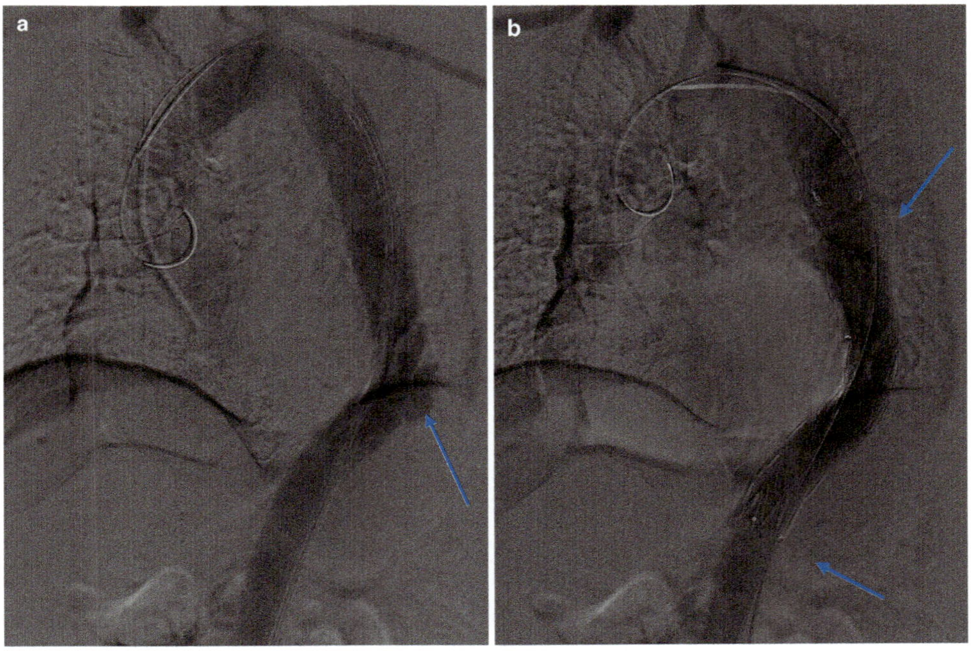

Fig. 3.86 TEVAR stent graft deployment. (**a**) advancement of the stent graft. Arrow indicates traumatic aortic lesion. (**b**) well-deployed stent graft covering the traumatic injury (arrows)

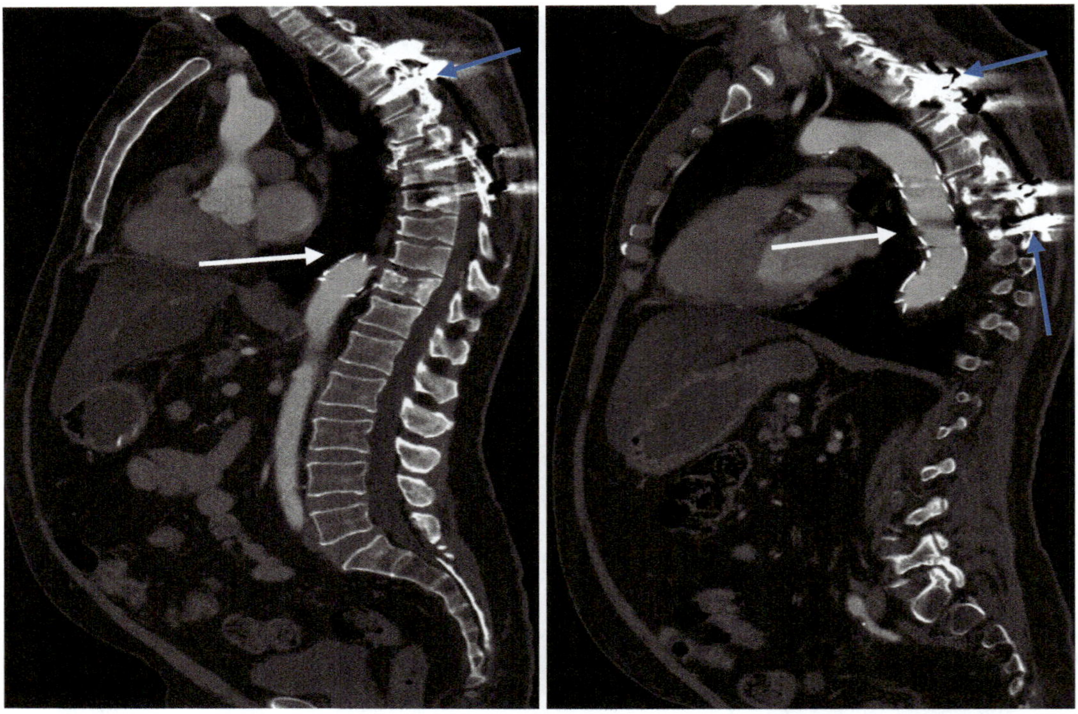

Fig. 3.87 Control computed tomography scan showing complete aortic remodelling and a well-deployed stent graft – (white arrows). Spinal surgery treated the vertebral fractures (arrow)

showing complete aortic remodelling and a well-deployed stent graft (Fig. 3.87).

3.5.3 Thoracic Aortic Trauma-III

Key Points

- An iatrogenic aortic lesion should be considered in cases of massive bleeding.
- A "larger arterial bleeding source" should be suspected when massive bleeding occurs.
- Stent graft deployment is a fast, easy treatment in an emergency.

3.5.3.1 Aetiology and Clinical Presentation

A 78-year-old patient presented with a history of haematemesis over 1 year and a diagnosis of Barret oesophagitis (Fig. 3.88). The patient had a

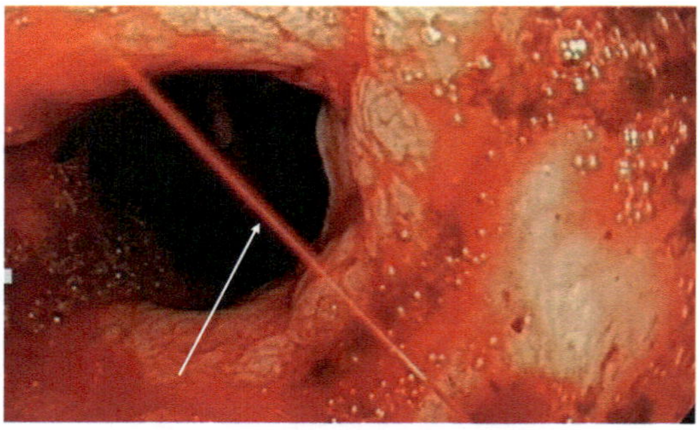

Fig. 3.88 Massive oesophageal bleeding during endoscopy (arrow). Endoscopic haemostasis was not possible

new episode of haematemesis this time with more bleeding than usual. Oesophagoscopy was difficult and identified a large ulcer at the distal part of the oesophagus and hiatus hernia. Contrast CT showed oesophageal wall thickening. The patient was admitted to the gastroenterological department. Endoscopic biopsy and ulcer treatment were performed. During the endoscopy, massive bleeding occurred, but it was not possible to stop the procedure. The patient was transferred to the angiographic unit for embolization based on the endoscopic colleagues describing bleeding from the distal oesophageal ulcer. The patient was haemodynamically unstable but responded to massive transfusion.

3.5.3.2 Pre-interventional Diagnosis

A CT scan performed some months prior showed oesophageal wall thickening and hiatus hernia. The aorta lacked ulcerations and pseudoaneurysms (Fig. 3.89).

3.5.3.3 Endovascular Treatment

The patient was intubated due to the risk of massive aspiration, and under general anaesthesia, aortography and selective angiography of the visceral arteries were performed (Fig. 3.90). The aim was to embolize the left gastric artery based on the endoscopic description and bleeding localization. Aortography was unable to reveal the source of bleeding, and selective angiography of the left gastric artery showed spastic changes but no active bleeding. Embolization with micro coils was performed rapidly (Fig. 3.90e, f). For a few minutes, the patient responded very well, but massive bleeding was soon observed. The patient was transferred to the CT unit and underwent CT of the thoracic and abdominal aorta.

Contrast-enhanced CT of the aorta showed contrast inside the oesophagus and ventricle. An aorto-oesophageal fistula was present on sagittal reconstruction and was one source of massive bleeding (Fig. 3.91b). The patient returned to the angiographic unit, and an aortic tube graft measuring 36 mm in diameter and 70 mm in length was deployed percutaneously through the right femoral artery (Fig. 3.92). The stent graft was deployed fast and had a rapid haemodynamic effect.

3.5.3.4 Outcome

Over the following days, the patient remained in the intensive unit, showing gradual recovery, and started on antibiotic treatment due to the presence of the fistula. There were no new bleeding episodes, and a control CT scan showed a well-deployed stent graft (Fig. 3.93).

3.6 Thoracic Arterial Bleeding

3.6.1 Pulmonary Artery Bleeding

3.6.1.1 Bleeding from a Pulmonary Arteriovenous Malformation

Key Points
- A ruptured PAVM is a very rare presentation
- In children, unexplained long-term respiratory and physical difficulties could be signs of PAVM
- Embolization is the first-line treatment

Aetiology and Clinical Presentation

A 5-year-old, previously healthy patient experienced a few episodes of massive haemoptysis and oxygen desaturation suddenly down to 88%. The patient was admitted to the specialized department with a further decrease in oxygen saturation and respiratory failure. Specialized venovenous extracorporeal membrane oxygenation (ECMO) treatment was initiated, and the patient was fully heparinized. Bedside echocardiography revealed a massive right-left shunt and no congenital heart anomaly. The family of the patient was not known to have hereditary haemorrhagic telangiectasia (HHT)/Osler-Weber-Rendu disease.

Pre-interventional Diagnosis

Non–contrast-enhanced CT scanning revealed a large ruptured pulmonary arteriovenous malformation (PAVM) on the left side (Fig. 3.94). Left haemothorax and right segmental atelectasis were present.

Endovascular Treatment

Due to a previously placed 10 Fr sheath in the right femoral vein, a 7 Fr guiding catheter was advanced into the left main pulmonary artery percutaneously through the left femoral vein, and angiography showed at least two large, complex PAVMs with feeding arteries measuring 8 mm

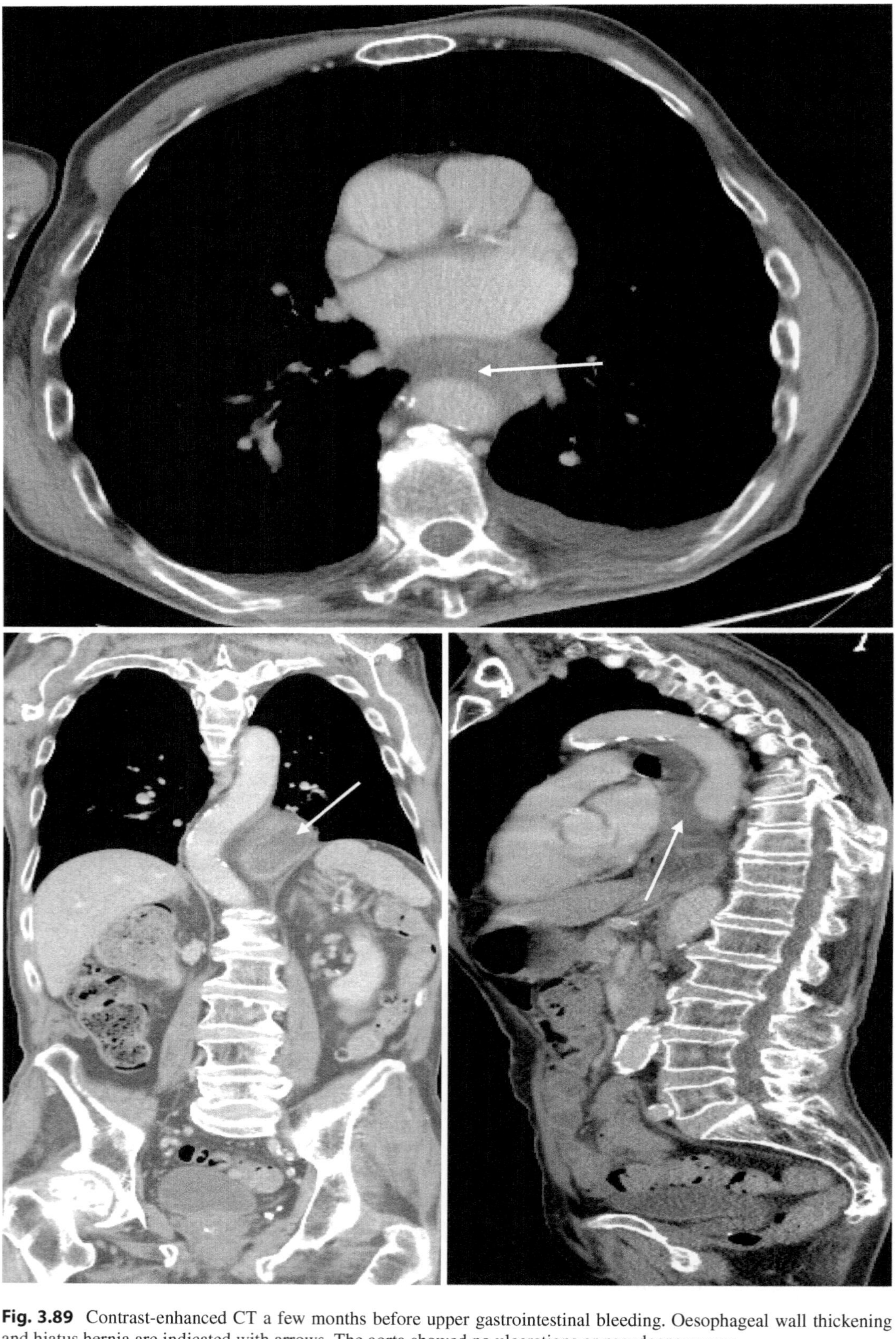

Fig. 3.89 Contrast-enhanced CT a few months before upper gastrointestinal bleeding. Oesophageal wall thickening and hiatus hernia are indicated with arrows. The aorta showed no ulcerations or pseudoaneurysms

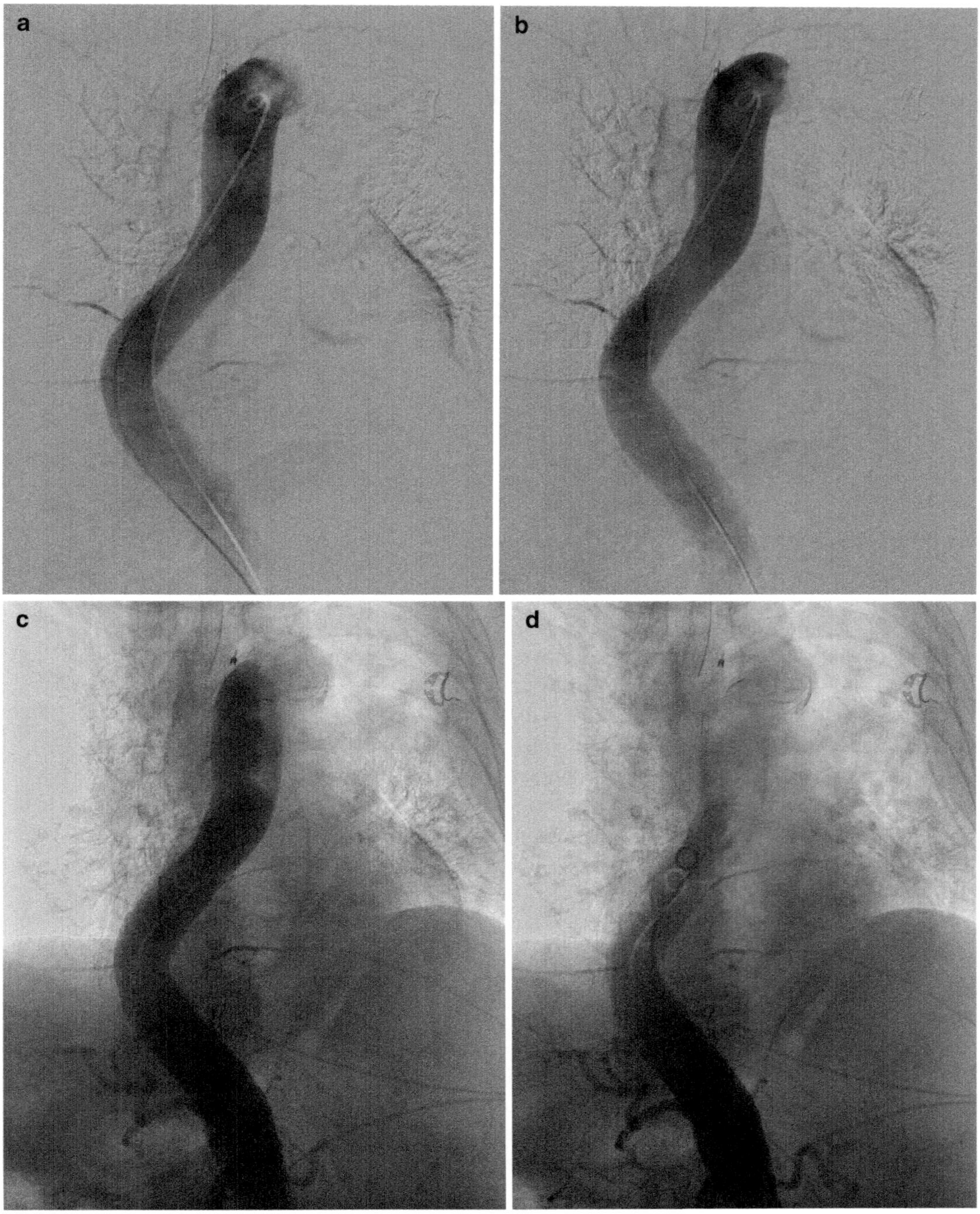

Fig. 3.90 Aortography was unable to show a bleeding source (**a–d**). Selective angiography of the left gastric artery showing spasm and no bleeding (**e**). Control image after embolization with micro coils (arrow) (**f**)

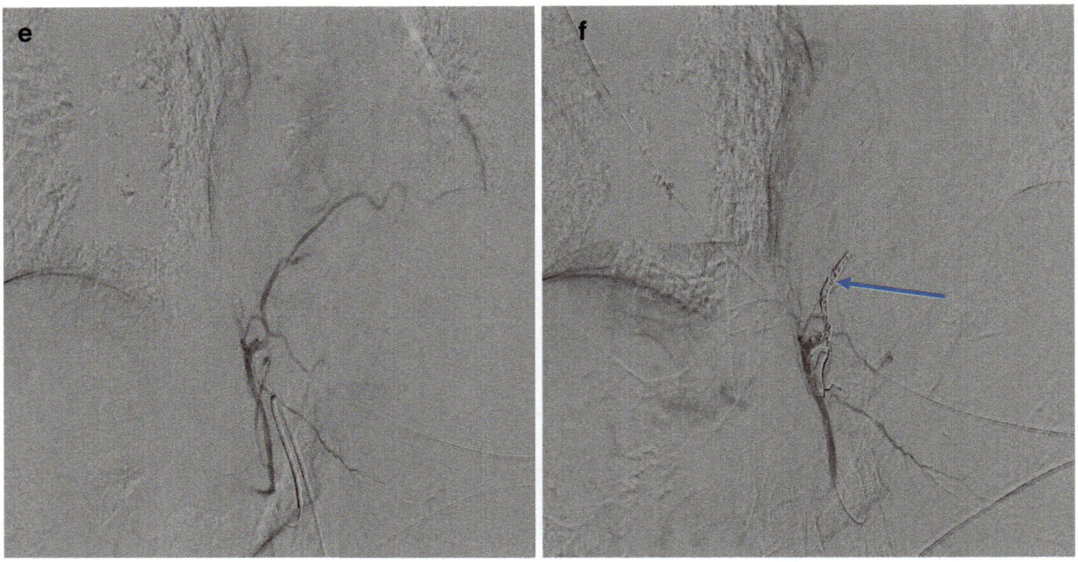

Fig. 3.90 (continued)

(Fig. 3.95a, b). Amplatz plugs with diameters of 10 mm and 8 mm and detachable micro coils with diameters of 10 mm and 8 mm were deployed into both PAVMs with good result (Fig. 3.95c, d). Finally, one more PAVM was discovered and occluded with detachable micro coils measuring 6 mm in diameter and an Amplatz plug measuring 6 mm in diameter. Control angiography showed a satisfactory result, and no additional PAVMs were seen during the scan (Fig. 3.95e, f).

Outcome

The patient recovered very well, and ECMO treatment was stopped after successful embolization. The patient did not experience any complications, and oxygen saturation increased to 98% with normal respiration. Following genetic testing, it was found that the family has Osler-Weber-Rendu disease. Additionally, contrast-enhanced CT of the cerebrum was eventually performed but found no brain malformations. CT showed well-deployed micro coils and Amplatz plugs no new PAVMs (Fig. 3.96).

3.6.1.2 Bleeding from a Pulmonary Artery Aneurysm/Pseudoaneurysm

Key Points

- Ruptured PAVMs are a very rare presentation
- In a majority of cases, the patient had Osler-Weber-Rendu disease (HHT)
- Embolization is the first-line treatment

Aetiology and Clinical Presentation

A 62-year-old healthy patient was admitted due to acute onset of haemoptysis and chest pain. The patient had never been ill and never had any kind of surgery or interventions. There were no signs of a lung infection, and the patient did not have chronic obstructive pulmonary disease. There was no history of smoking. Haemoptysis was massive, >500 mL in the last 24 h. The patient was haemodynamically stable, but the risk for aspiration was high.

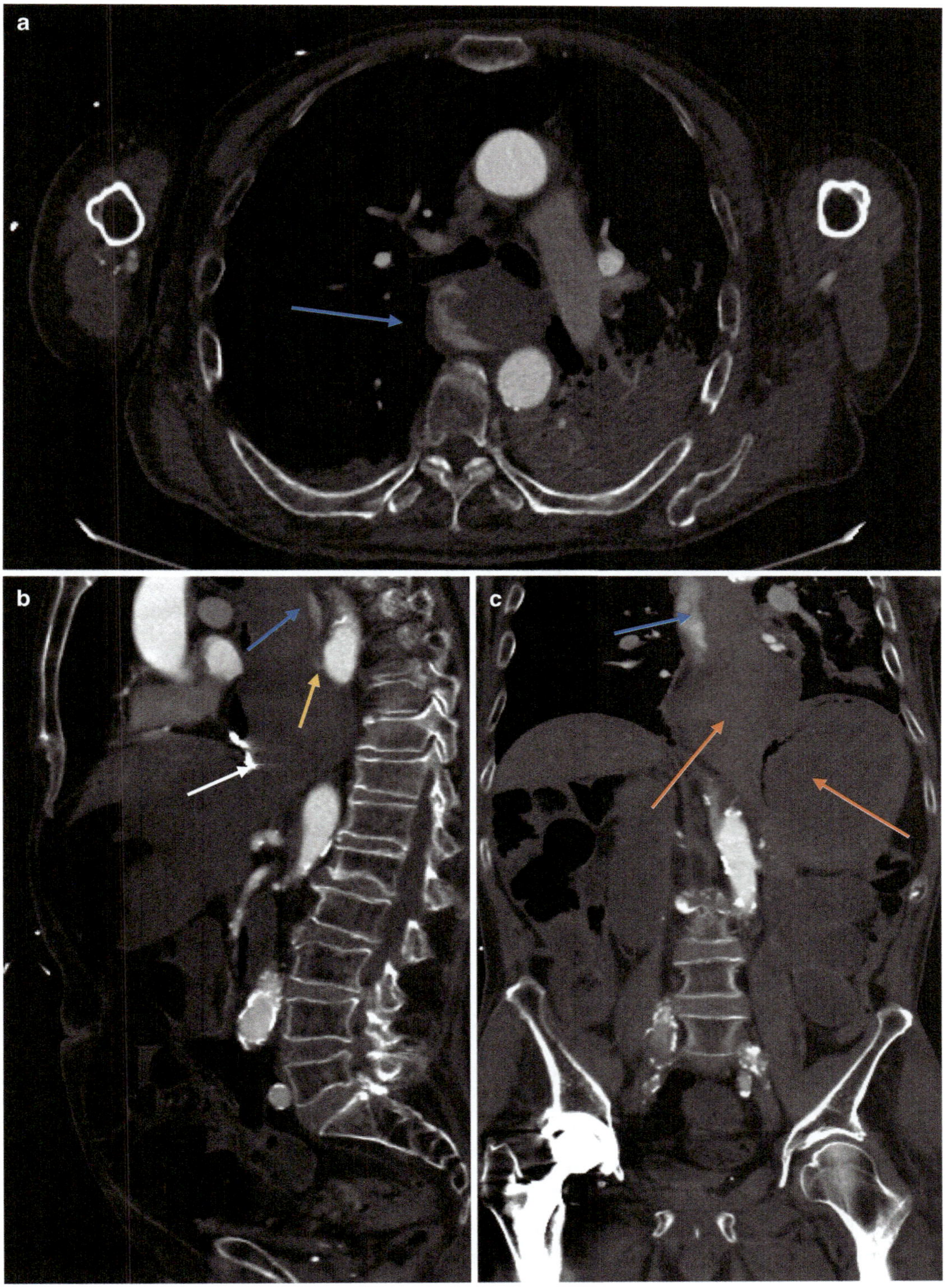

Fig. 3.91 Contrast-enhanced CT showing contrast agent inside the oesophagus (**a**) (blue arrows). Orange arrows indicate haematoma in the oesophagus and ventricle (**c**). Yellow arrow on sagittal reconstruction (**b**) shows aorto-oesophageal fistula. White arrow indicates micro coils in the left gastric artery

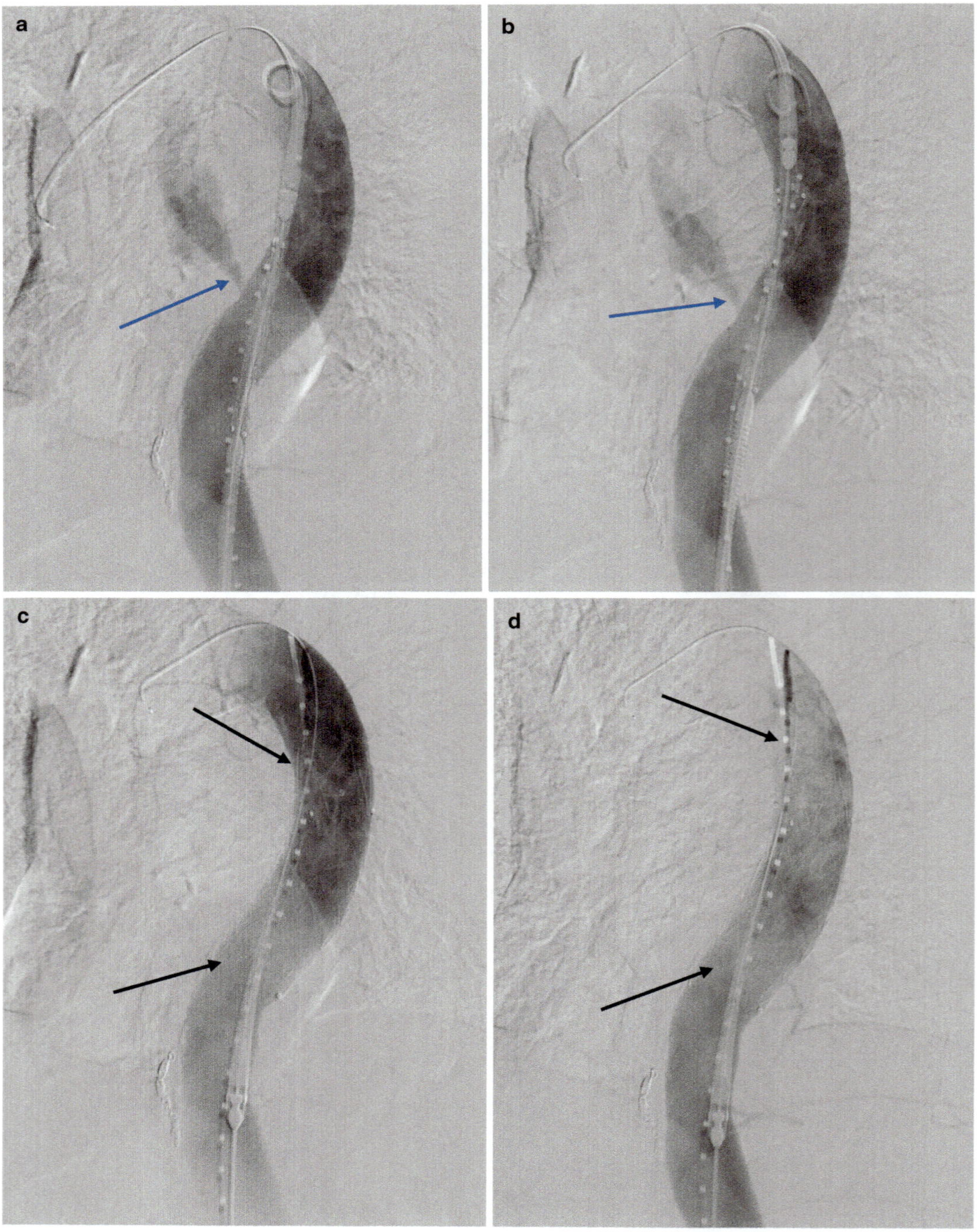

Fig. 3.92 Repeat aortography shows massive bleeding and aorto-oesophageal fistula- (blue arrows) (**a**, **b**). The bleeding was arrested after stent graft deployment as shown on early- and late-phase control angiography (black arrows) (**c**, **d**)

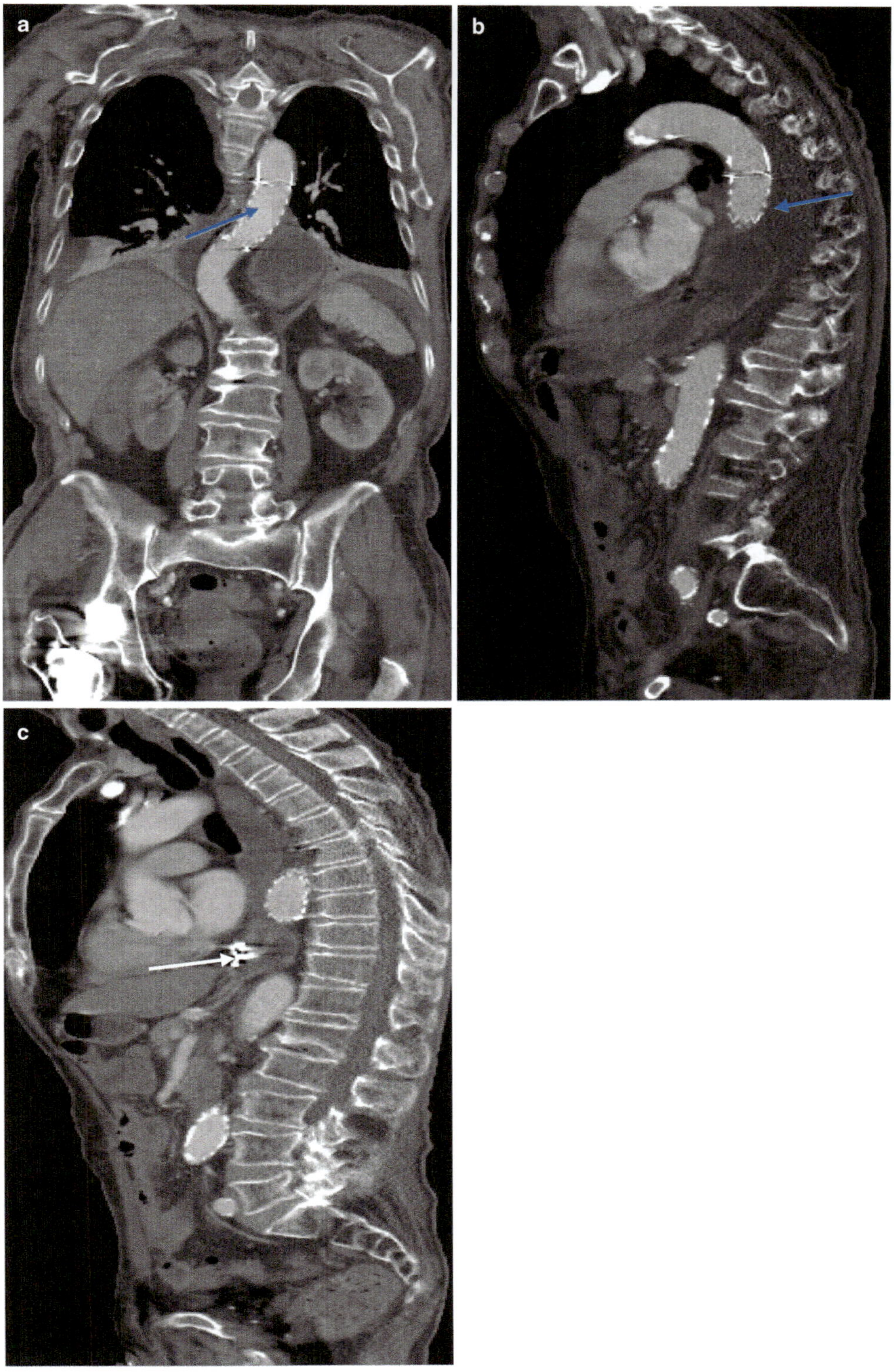

Fig. 3.93 Control contrast-enhanced CT showing a well-deployed stent graft –(blue arrows) and no bleeding. White arrow indicates micro coils in the left gastric artery

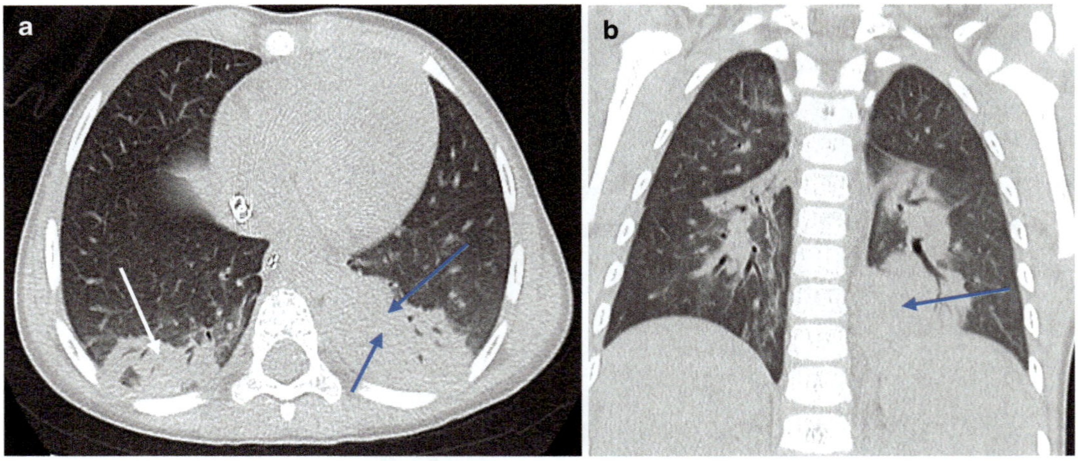

Fig. 3.94 Non–contrast-enhanced CT showing a ruptured left arterio-pulmonary-venous malformation (blue arrows) (**a**, **b**). Right lower lobe atelectasis is indicated by the white arrow (**a**)

Pre-interventional Diagnosis

Emergency angiography through the right renal vein was performed (Fig. 3.97a, b). Angiography showed an aneurysmatic PAVM with a feeding artery 6 mm in diameter. The aneurysmatic PAVM showed no sharp edges.

Endovascular Treatment

An Amplatz plug measuring 10 mm in diameter was advanced through a 7 Fr sheath into the PAVM and deployed with complete exclusion of and no flow through the aneurysmatic PAVM after deployment (Fig. 3.97c, d).

Outcome

The patient recovered very well and presented with no new bleeding problems. The patient was discharged from the hospital 2 days after embolization. Control CT one (Fig. 3.98) and 5 years (Fig. 3.99) after embolization showed satisfactory results with almost complete resolution of the aneurysmatic PAVM. The patient's family had been diagnosed with HHT/Osler-Weber-Rendu disease.

3.7 Intercostal/Bronchial Artery Bleeding

3.7.1 Bleeding from the Intercostal-Bronchial Artery

Key Points

- The bronchial artery is the most frequent bleeding source in cases of haemoptysis.
- Sometimes bleeding from the pulmonary artery can occur; therefore, it is important to exam the artery.
- Embolization is very useful and is the first-line treatment choice.

3.7.1.1 Aetiology and Clinical Presentation

A 69-year-old patient with non-small-cell lung cancer (NSCLC) treated with stereotactic radiotherapy was admitted to our institution. The

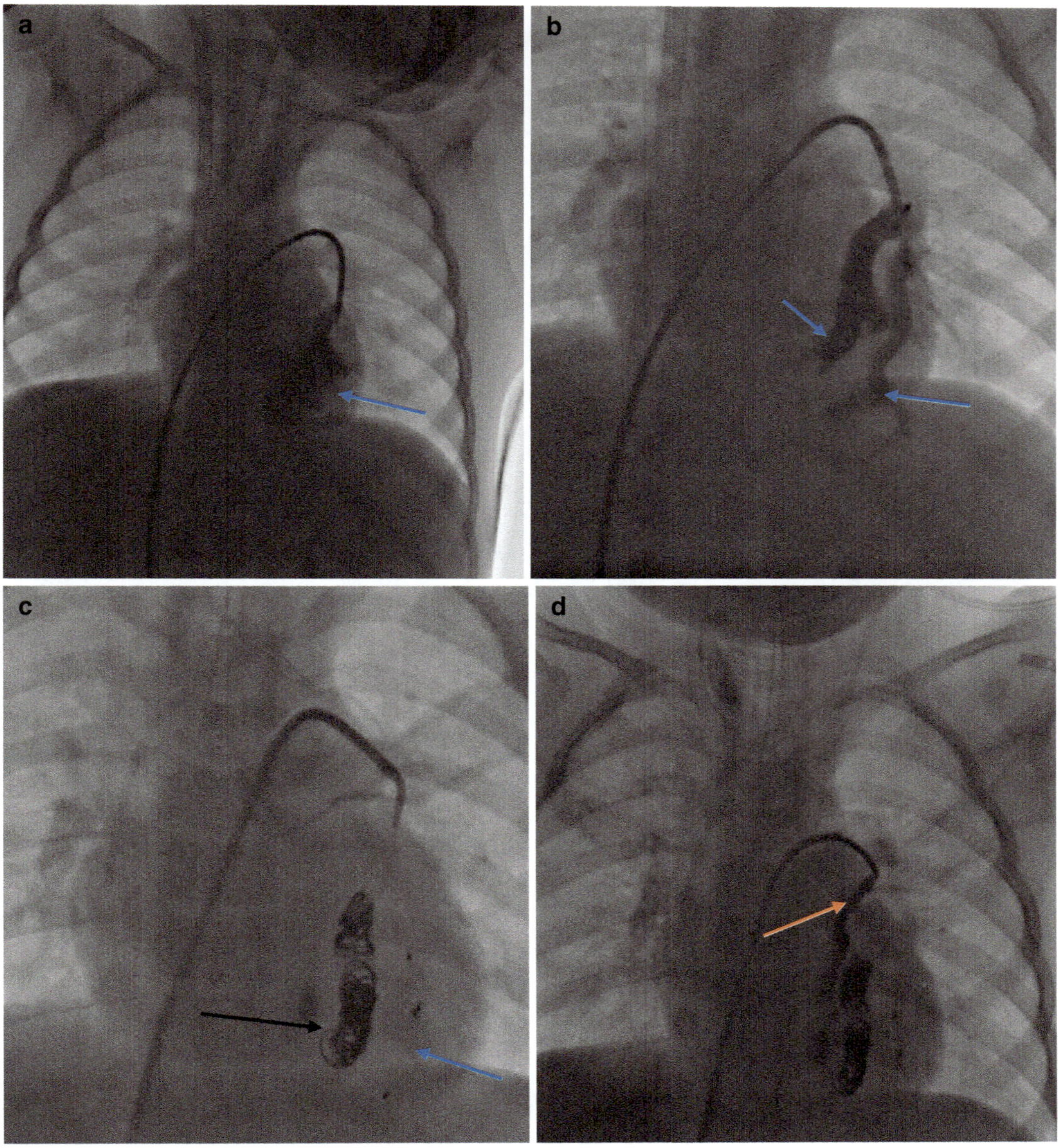

Fig. 3.95 Angiography through a 7 Fr guiding catheter showed at least two complex PAVMs with feeding arteries measuring 8 mm (blue arrows) (**a**, **b**). (**c**) black arrow indicates micro coils in one PAVM. Blue arrow indicates an Amplatz plug in another PAVM. (**d**) orange arrow indicates a smaller PAVM occluded with 6 mm micro coils and an Amplatz plug. (**e** and **f**) control angiography showing a satisfactory result. There were no PAVMs in the right lung

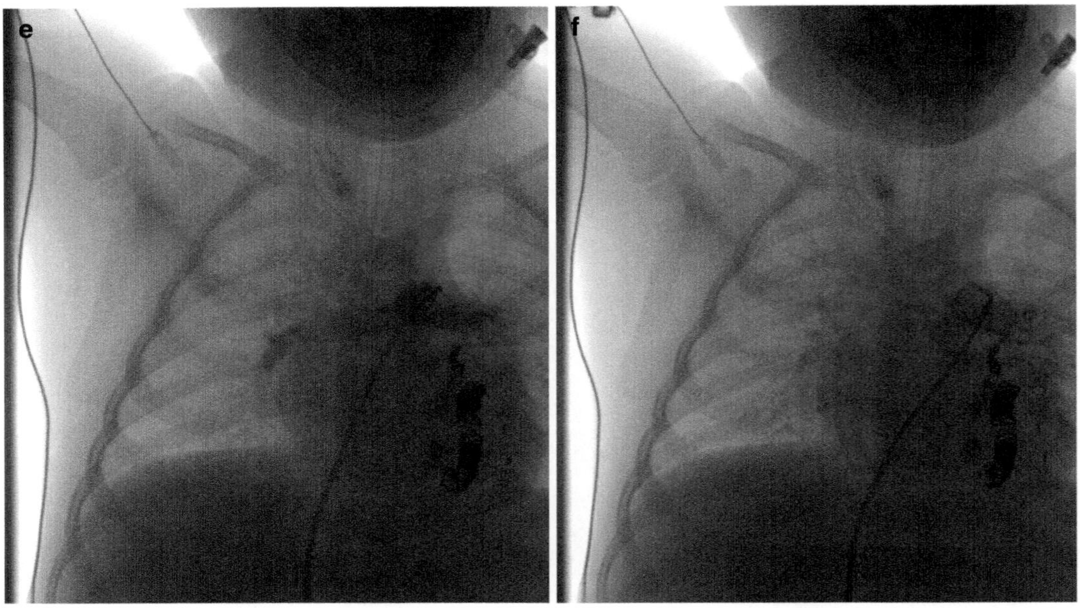

Fig. 3.95 (continued)

patient developed haemoptysis a few days after the last treatment. Bronchoscopy was unable to identify the source of bleeding, and thus it could not be treated endoscopically. The patient was haemodynamically stable, but the haemoptysis was ongoing.

3.7.1.2 Pre-interventional Diagnosis

Contrast-enhanced CT of the chest was performed (Fig. 3.100b, c). The previous CT (Fig. 3.100a) only showed NSCLC in the right upper lung, whereas the latest CT showed bleeding into the central lung parenchyma and in the right upper lobe. CT showed an intercostal-bronchial artery on the right side and consolidation and ground glass opacifications in the artery irrigation zone, which was described as bleeding. A nasogastric sonde was advanced into the stomach, and the patient was intubated to prevent aspiration.

3.7.1.3 Endovascular Treatment

A 5 Fr diagnostic catheter was used for selective catheterization of the right hypertrophic intercostal-bronchial trunk via percutaneous insertion through the right femoral artery. Furthermore, the microcatheter was advanced distally into the bleeding arteries (Fig. 3.101). Embolization of the bleeding arteries was performed first with 300–500 μm microspheres and then 3 mm diameter micro-coils. There were no complications during the intervention.

3.7.1.4 Outcome

The patient was extubated the day after the haemoptysis ceased. No complications occurred during the stay in the hospital. No new episode of haemoptysis was recorded. Control contrast-enhanced CT 3 months after embolization showed satisfactory results and

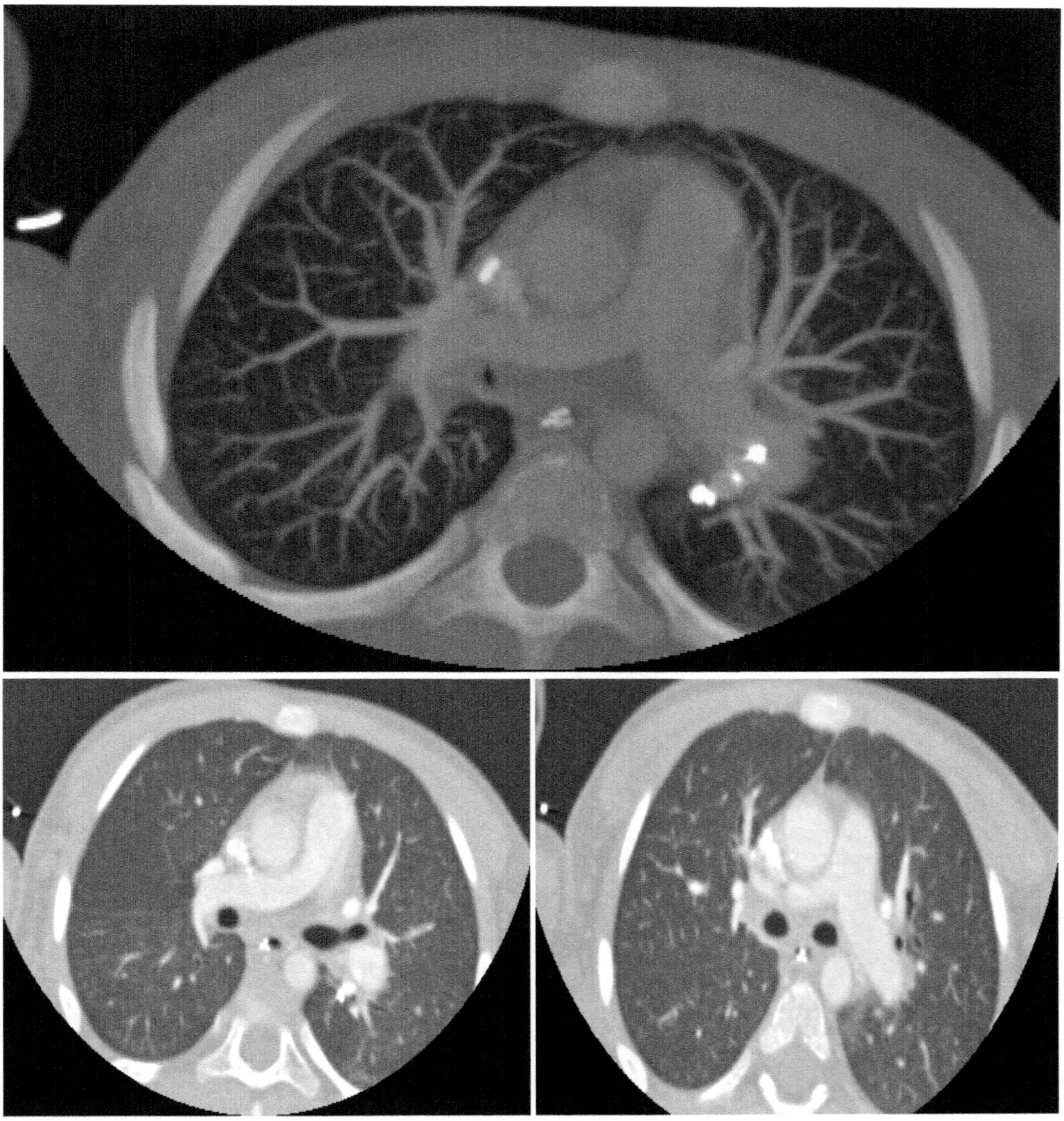

Fig. 3.96 Contrast-enhanced CT showing a satisfactory result and no new PAVMs

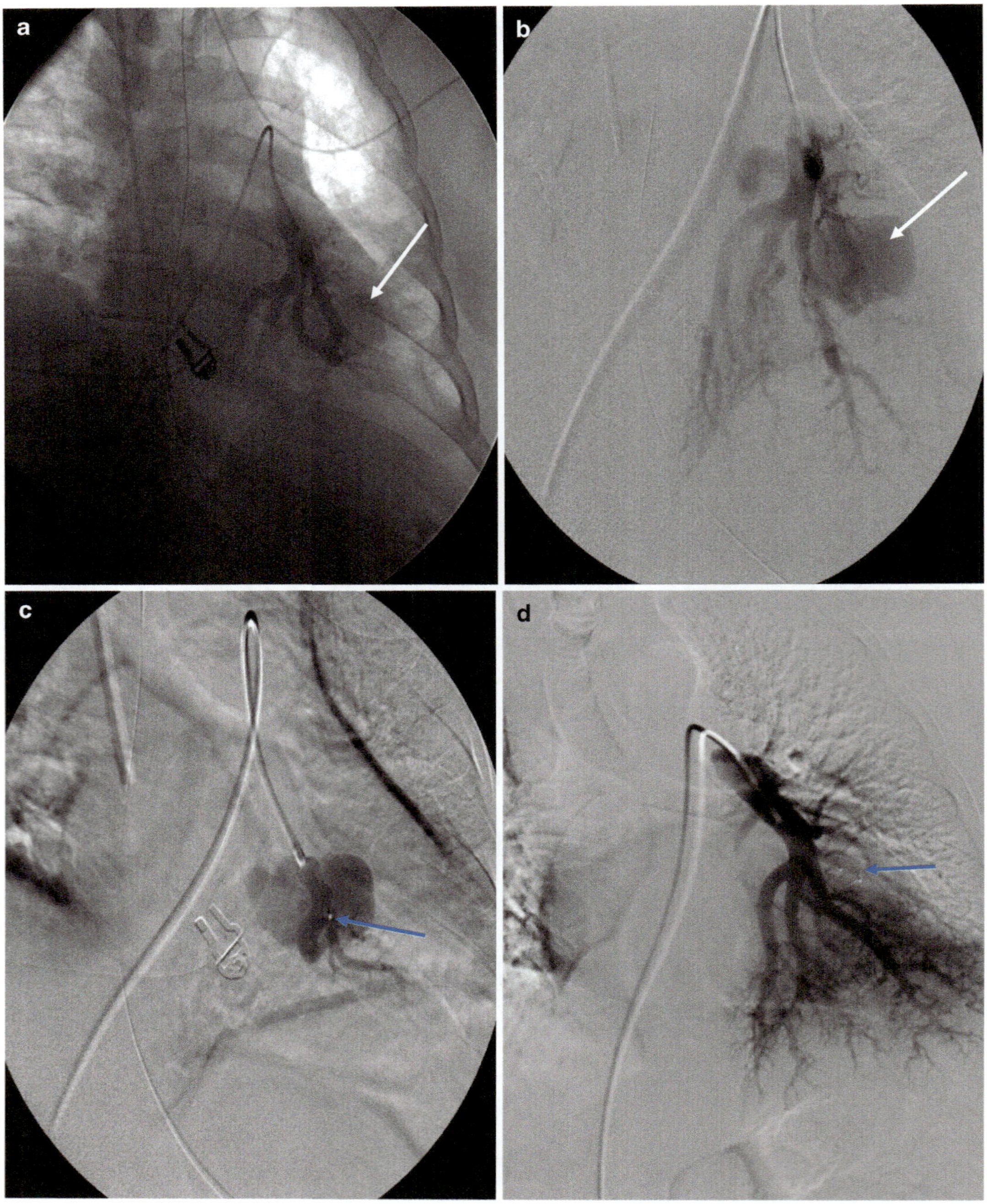

Fig. 3.97 Angiography revealed a single PAVM in the left lung with a 6 mm feeding artery. White arrows indicate the aneurysmatic PAVM (**a**, **b**). (**c**) advancement of a 10 mm Amplatz through a 7 Fr guiding catheter (blue arrow). (**d**) control angiography after Amplatz plug deployment showing immediate occlusion of the PAVM (blue arrow)

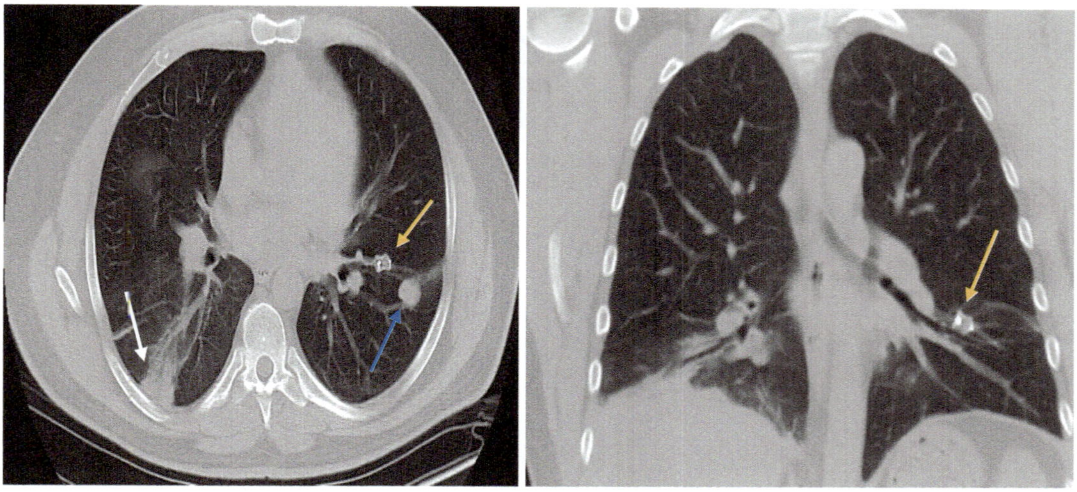

Fig. 3.98 One year control showed a decrease in the size of the PAVM (blue arrow). Yellow arrows indicate the Amplatz plug. In the basal part of the right lung, atelectasis is indicated with a white arrow

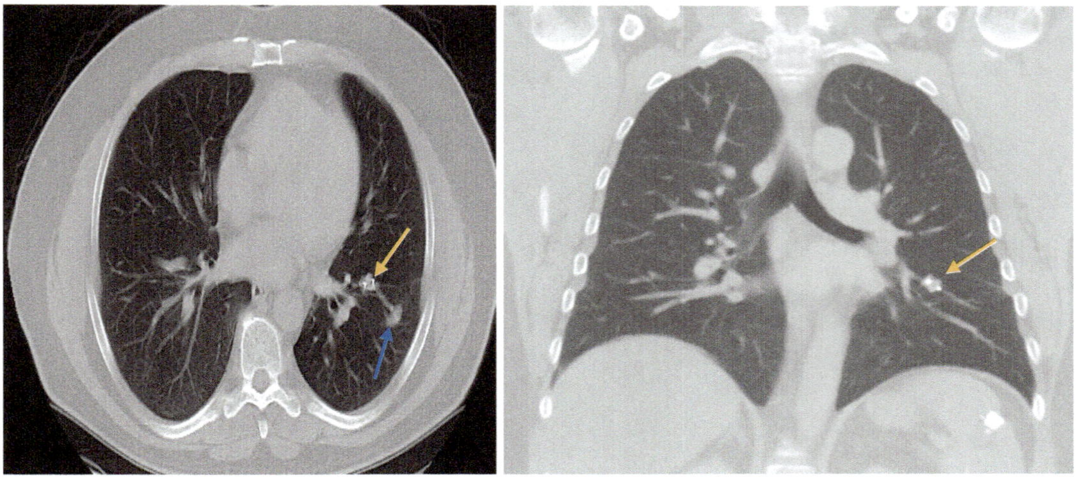

Fig. 3.99 Five-year control showed almost complete resolution of the PAVM (blue arrow). Yellow arrows indicate the Amplatz plug

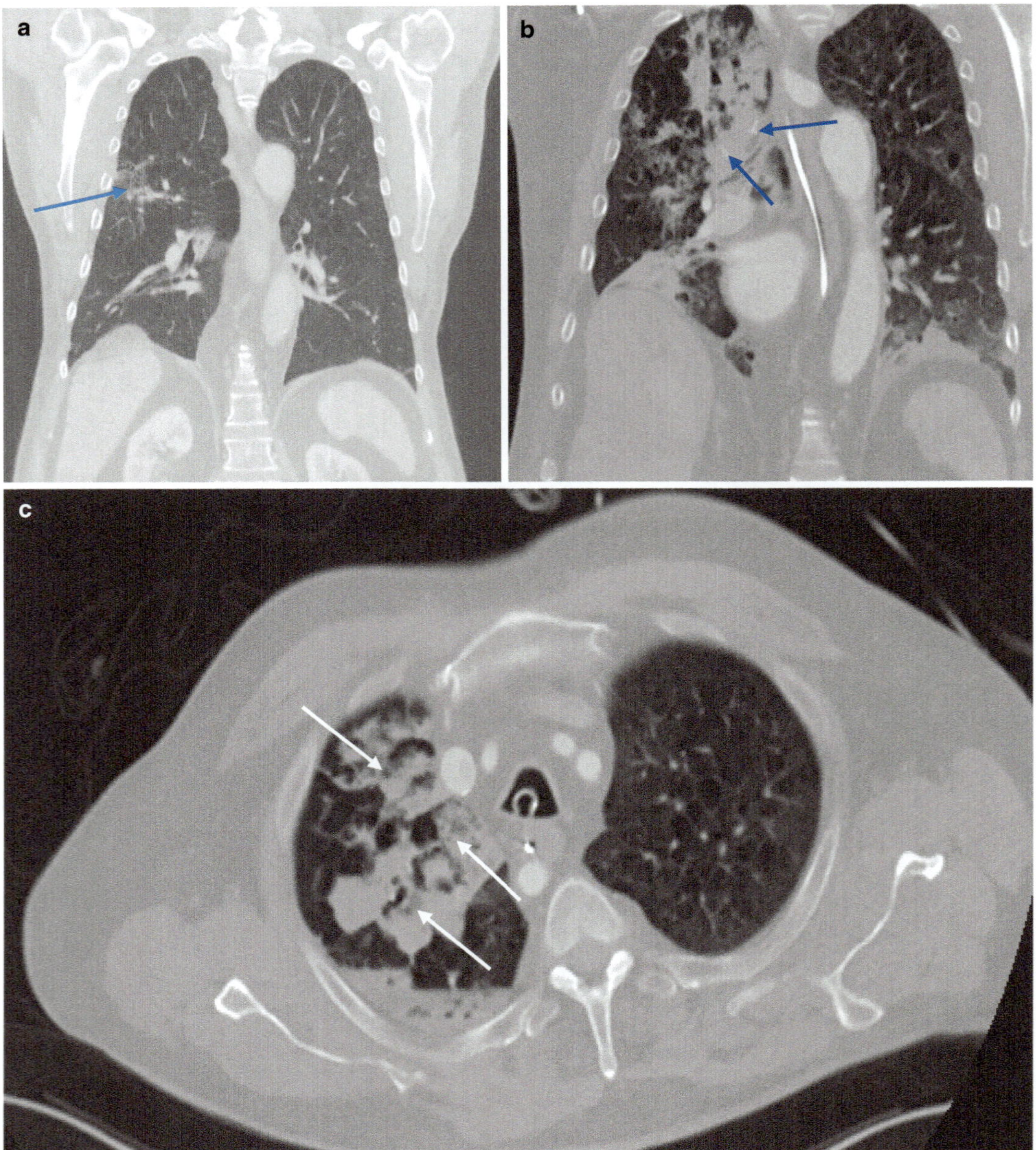

Fig. 3.100 (**a**) previous CT without interstitial infiltrates. NSCLC is present in the right upper lobe- (arrow). (**b**, **c**) CT after the patient experienced haemoptysis. Blue arrows indicate the right intercostal-bronchial artery as the bleeding source. White arrows indicate interstitial infiltrate bleeding

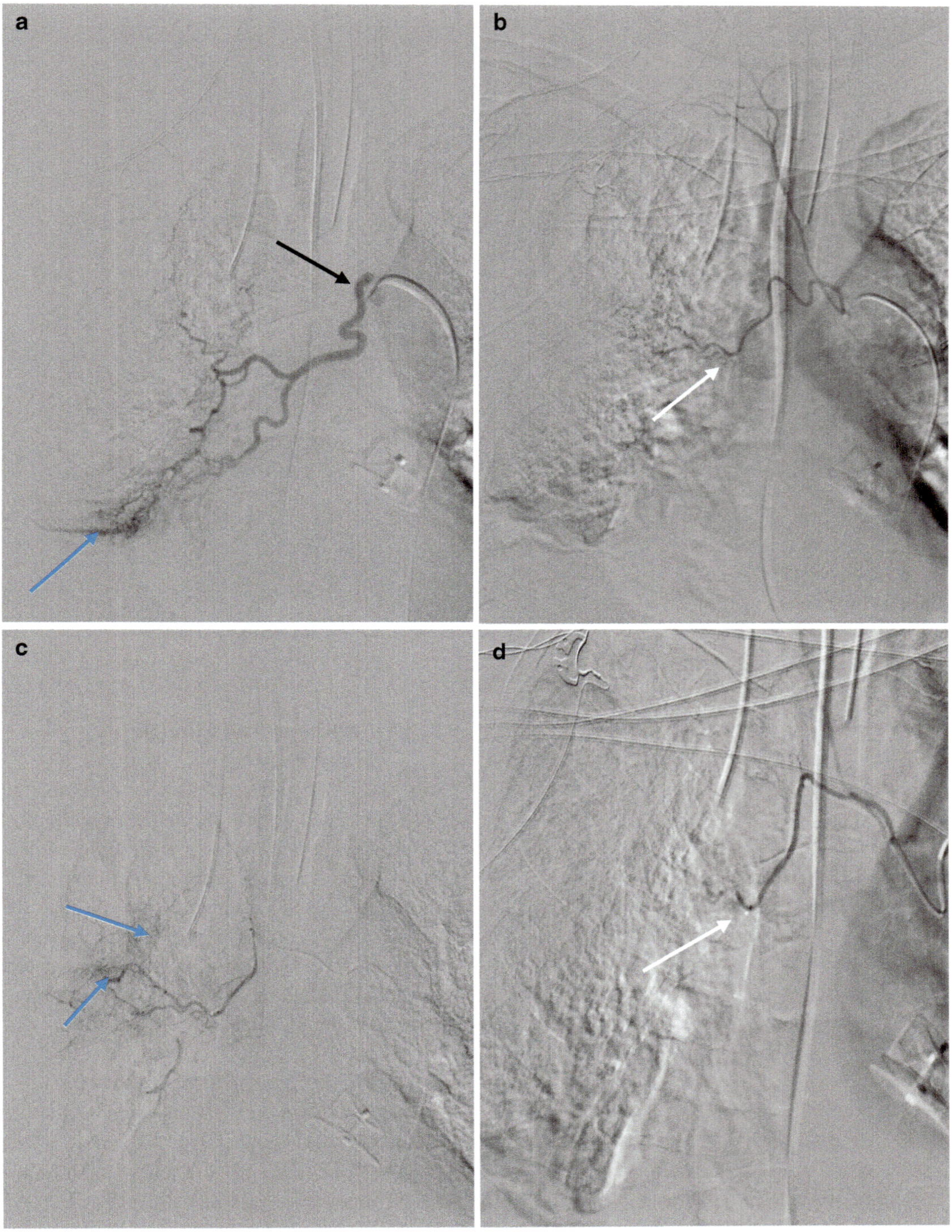

Fig. 3.101 Selective angiography of the right intercostal-bronchial trunk. Black arrow indicates a hypertrophic trunk (**a**). (**b**) white arrow indicates the tip of the micro-catheter advancing into one of the bleeding arteries. (**c**) blue arrows indicate contrast blush/hypervascularity and bleeding points. (**d**) white arrow shows arrested bleeding after embolization of one artery with 300–500 μm micro-spheres. (**e**) advancement of the microcatheter into another bleeding branch- (black arrow). The blue arrow indicates additional micro-coil embolization of one branch. (**f**) final control after embolization with a combination of micro-spheres and micro coils

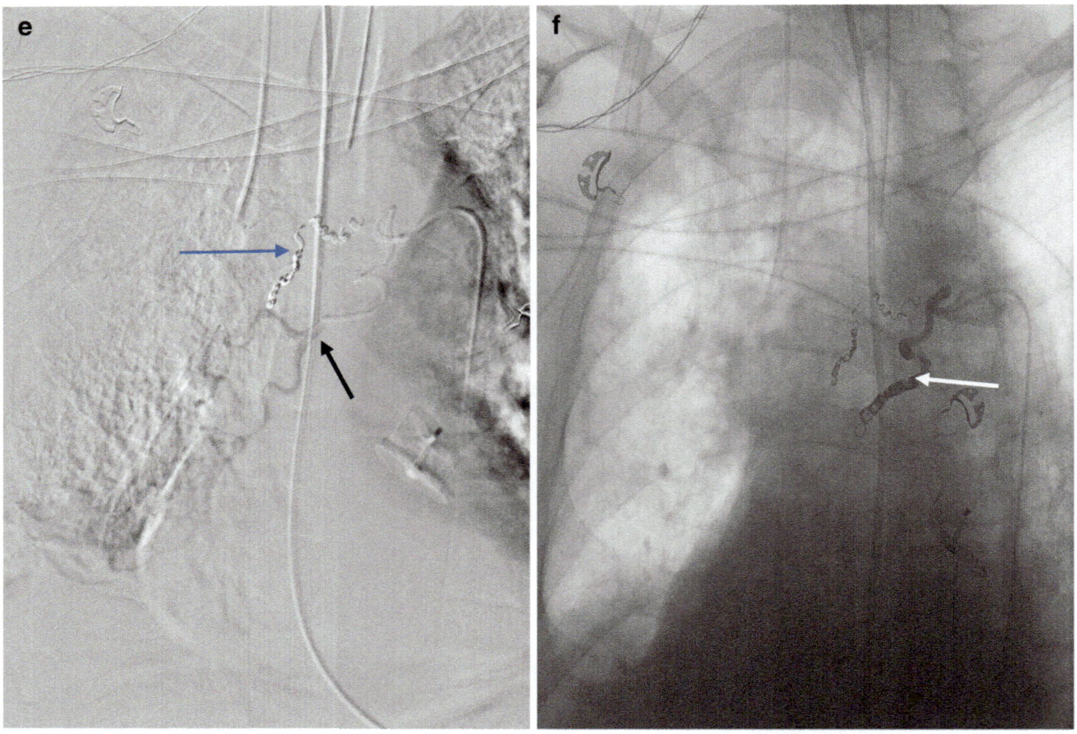

Fig. 3.101 (continued)

complete resorption of the infiltrate in the right lung (Fig. 3.102). The NSCLC remains stable in size.

3.7.2 Bleeding from the Bronchial Artery

Key Points

- The bronchial artery is the most frequent bleeding source in haemoptysis cases.
- Sometimes bleeding from the pulmonary artery can occur; therefore, it is important to exam the artery.
- Embolization is very useful and is the first-line treatment choice.
- Microspheres should never be used in cases involving arterio-venous fistulas.

3.7.2.1 Aetiology and Clinical Presentation

A-35-year-old patient experiences a number of episodes of haemoptysis in the last few months. The last episode was massive, and the patient was admitted to the emergency department. The patient was haemodynamically stable but the haemoptysis was ongoing. The patient had tuberculosis as a child. Testing revealed an active tuberculosis infection, and the patient was placed on antituberculosis treatment.

3.7.2.2 Pre-interventional Diagnosis

The contrast-enhanced CT lung window showed consolidation and ground glass opacities in the right lower lobe (Fig. 3.103). There were no visible vascular abnormalities in the pulmonary arteries.

3.7.2.3 Endovascular Treatment

Percutaneous insertions were performed through the right femoral vein and artery. First, a

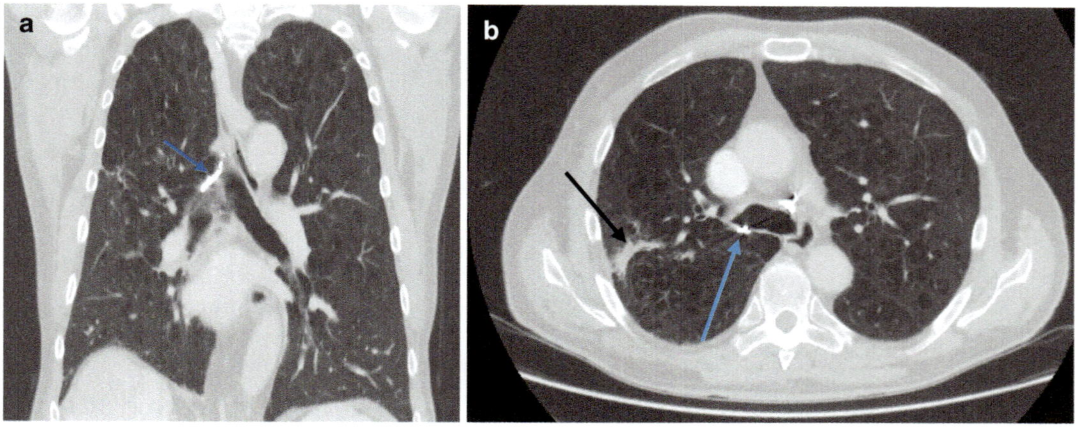

Fig. 3.102 Control contrast-enhanced CT 3 months after embolization. Blue arrows indicate micro-coils. Black arrow indicates right NSCLC. The infiltrate on the right side was completely resolved

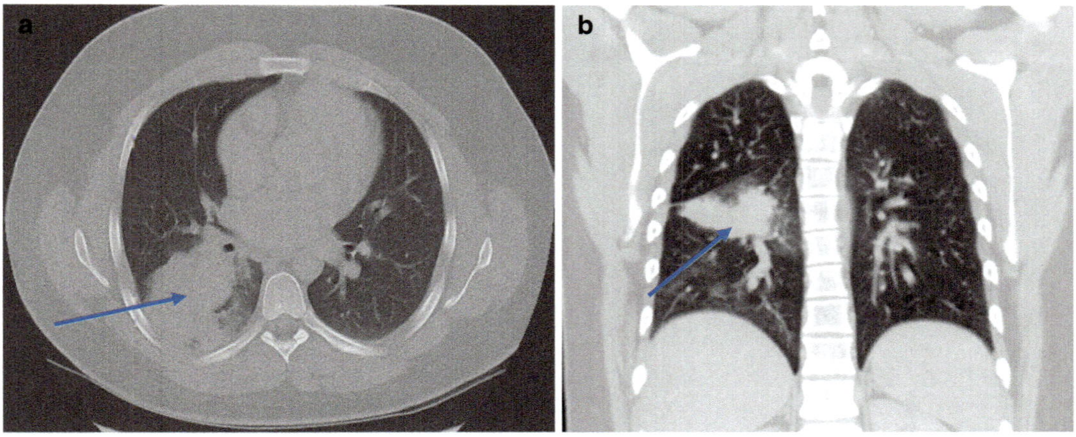

Fig. 3.103 Lung window CT scan with consolidation in the right lower lobe (arrows)

diagnostic catheter was advanced into the pulmonary artery, but angiography did not find a bleeding source or any other abnormality (Fig. 3.104a). After that, aortography was performed and showed a hypertrophic right intercostal-bronchial trunk and hypervascularity (Fig. 3.104b–d).

Selective angiography of the right intercostal trunk showed better hypervascularity and revealed a fistula in the right pulmonary vein (Fig. 3.105). The microcatheter was advanced further to approach the hypervascularity. The artery measured between 3.6 and 3.7 mm, and micro-coils with a diameter of 6 mm were deployed to avoid complications and migration into the heart. Control angiography after micro coil deployment showed still flow, and a micro plug with a diameter of 5 mm was finally advanced, achieving complete flow cessation.

3.7.2.4 Outcome

The patient was discharged from the hospital the next day without any complications. There was no new bleeding episode in the follow-up. It is vital to understand the anatomy and possible frequent communication of the intercostal bronchial artery with the subclavian, vertebral, internal thoracic, spinal and other arteries to avoid catastrophic complications during embolization with microspheres.

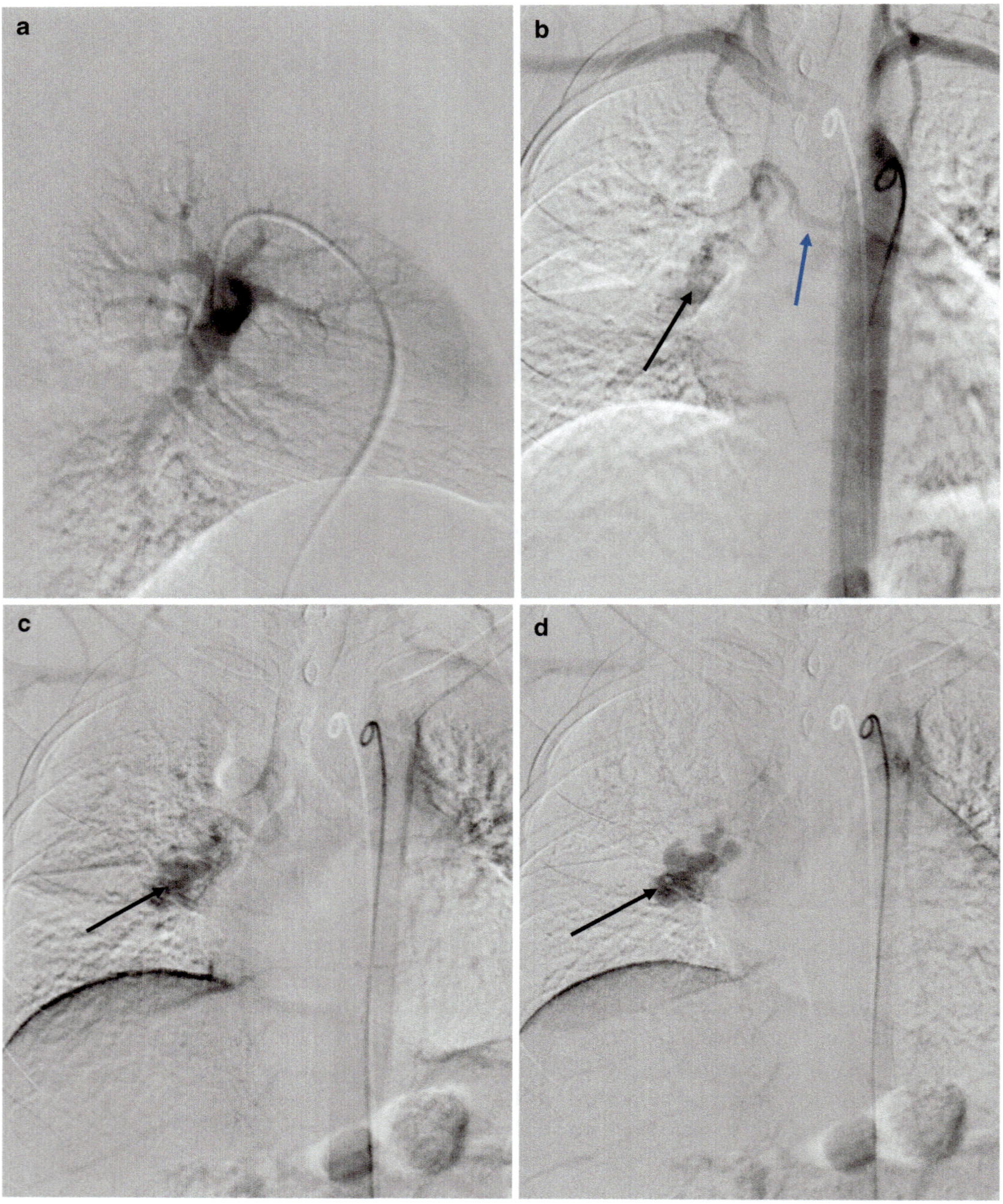

Fig. 3.104 Angiography of the right pulmonary artery, which was found to be normal (**a**). (**b**–**d**) aortography showing a hypertrophic right intercostal-bronchial trunk (blue arrows) and hypervascularity (black arrows)

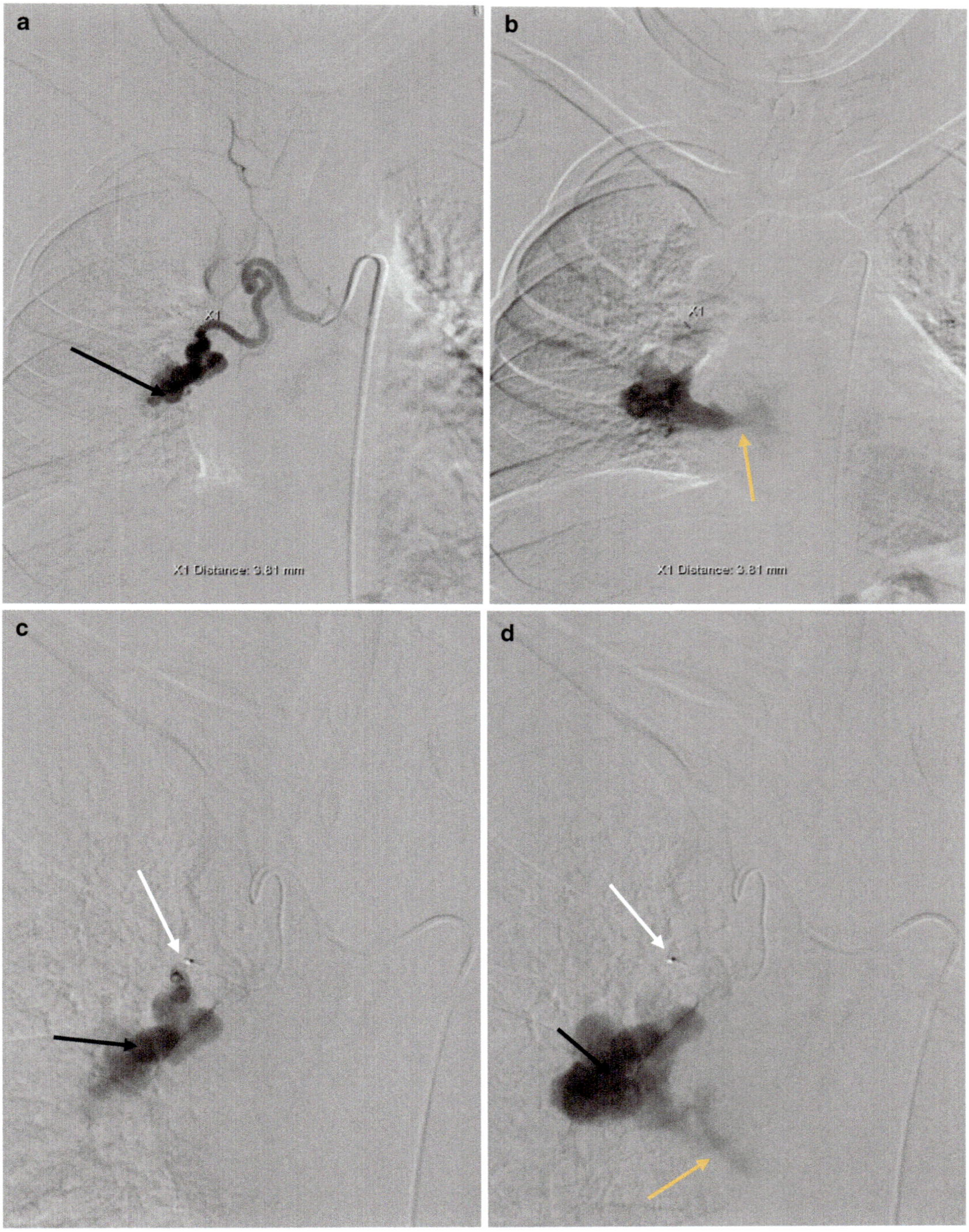

Fig. 3.105 Selective angiography of the hypertrophic right intercostal-bronchial trunk with hypervascularity-(black arrows). Yellow arrows indicate a fistula to the pulmonary vein. White arrows indicate the tip of the microcatheter, close to the hypervascularity. (**e–g**) embolization with micro-coils measuring 6 mm in diameter (blue arrows). Finally, the 5 mm diameter micro plug was advanced and deployed, achieving complete cessation of the flow (orange arrow)

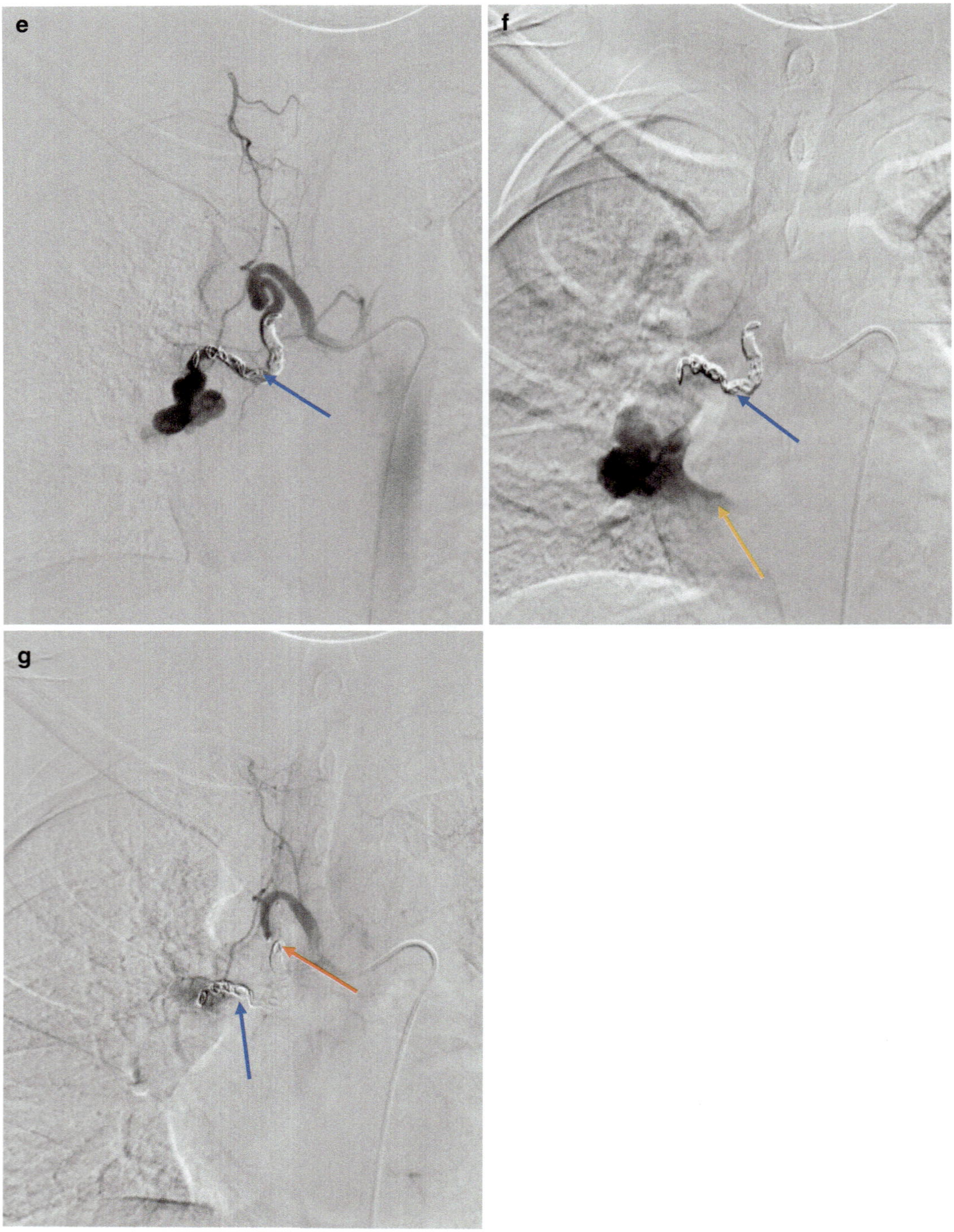

Fig. 3.105 (continued)

3.7.3 Bleeding from the Intercostal Artery

Key Points

- Chronic lung diseases and infections are the most frequent cause of intercostal-bronchial bleeding.
- Traumatic lesions of the intercostal-bronchial artery can occur
- Embolization is usually straightforward and safe. One level above and below the pseudoaneurysm should be examined.

3.7.3.1 Aetiology and Clinical Presentation

A 64-year-old patient with advanced non-small-cell lung cancer had been receiving palliative chemotherapy. In the last few weeks, the patient began experiencing haemoptysis, gradually increasing to almost 300–400 mL per day. The patient had a chronic cough and temperature of 37.8 °C.

3.7.3.2 Pre-interventional Diagnosis

Contrast-enhanced CT 4 months prior showed secondary changes in the tumour in the right lower lobe (Fig. 3.106a), and the current CT scan (Fig. 3.106b, c) showed tumour progression and

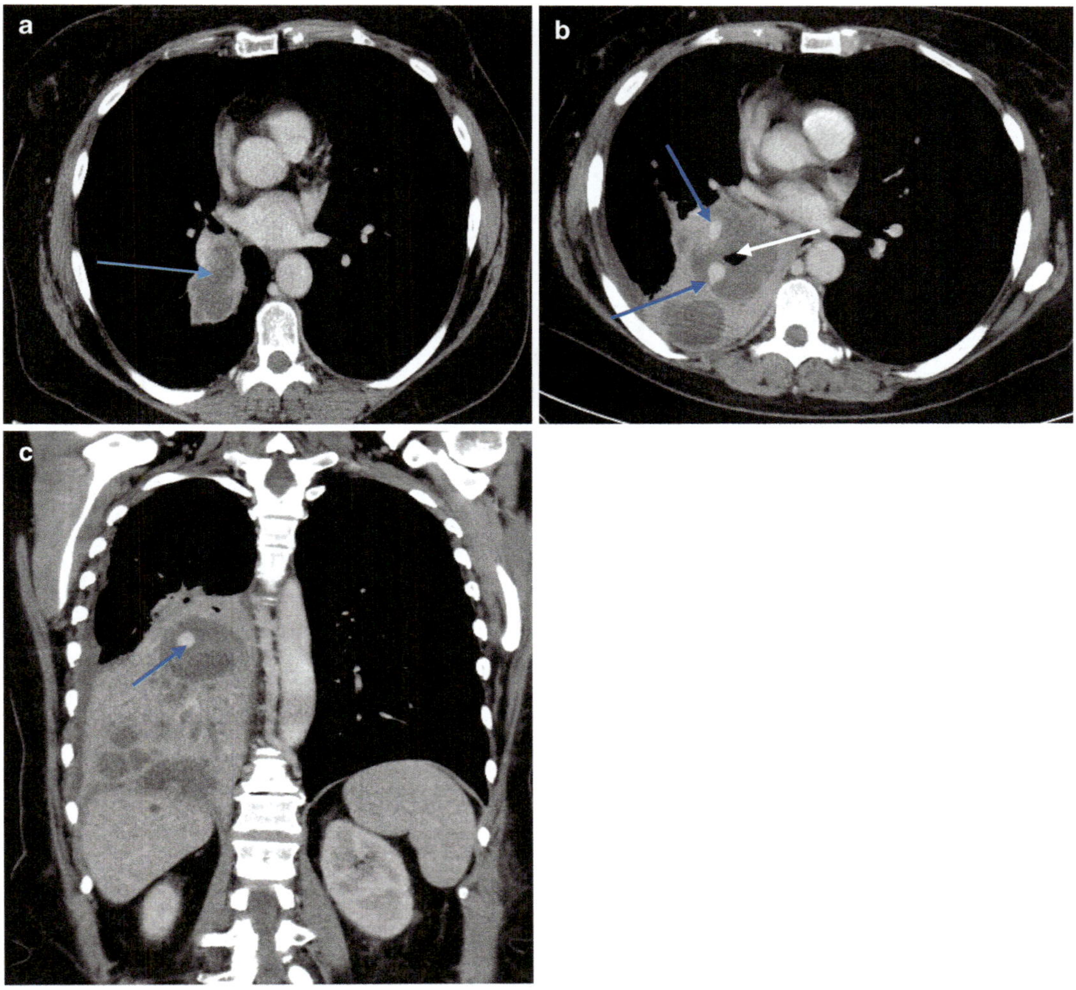

Fig. 3.106 (**a**) contrast-enhanced CT 4 months before the episode with haemoptysis; arrow indicates secondary changes in the tumour. (**b** and **c**) current CT shows tumour progress, abscess development (white arrow) and pseudoaneurysm (blue arrows)

abscess development with pseudoaneurysm. The eventual exclusion of bleeding from the pulmonary artery was challenging.

3.7.3.3 Endovascular Treatment

Percutaneous insertions were performed through the right femoral vein and artery. First, pulmonary angiography was performed and showed no bleeding or pseudoaneurysm (Fig. 3.107a). Next, selective angiography of the lower intercostal artery showed a pseudoaneurysm arising from the VI and VII intercostal arteries (Fig. 3.107). The microcatheter was advanced behind the pseudoaneurysm, and micro-coil embolization was performed. The same procedure was performed one level below the first intercostal artery.

3.7.3.4 Outcome

The patient had no new haemoptysis and did not experience complications during the embolization. The patient was placed on broad-spectrum antibiotic treatment. In such cases, pseudoaneurysm embolization with micro-coils is very safe and straightforward.

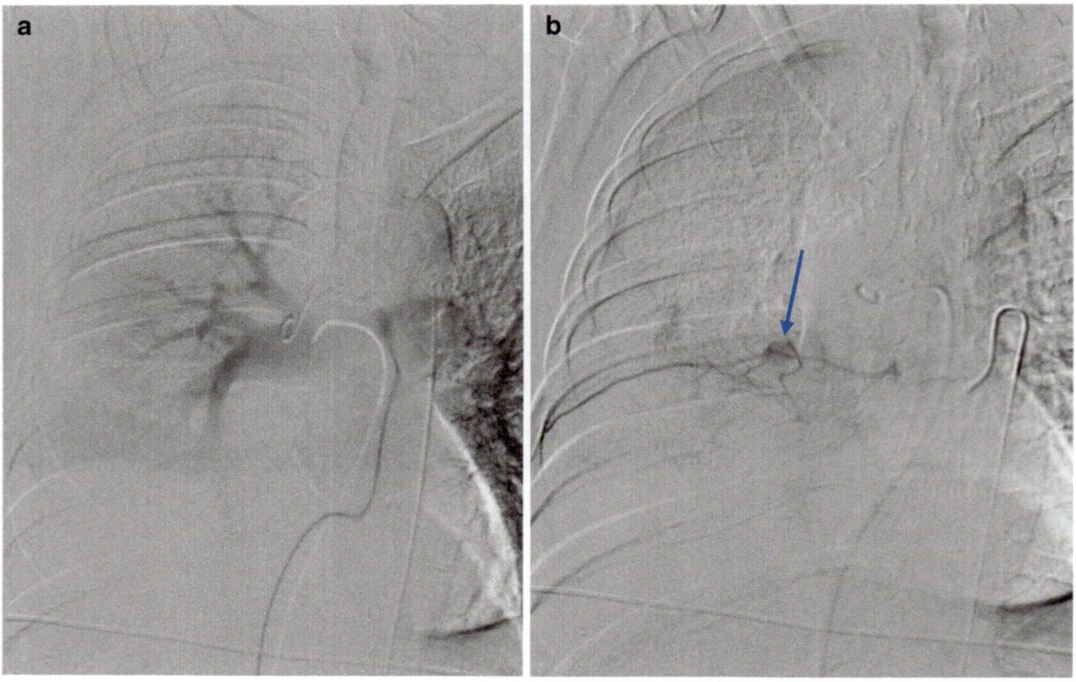

Fig. 3.107 (**a**) pulmonary angiography of the right pulmonary artery shows no pseudoaneurysm. (**b**, **c**) selective intercostal angiography revealed pseudoaneurysm (blue arrows). (**d**) advancement of the microcatheter behind the pseudoaneurysm and embolization with micro-coils (arrow). (**e** and **f**) the next intercostal artery below the first was occluded with micro-coils (arrow)

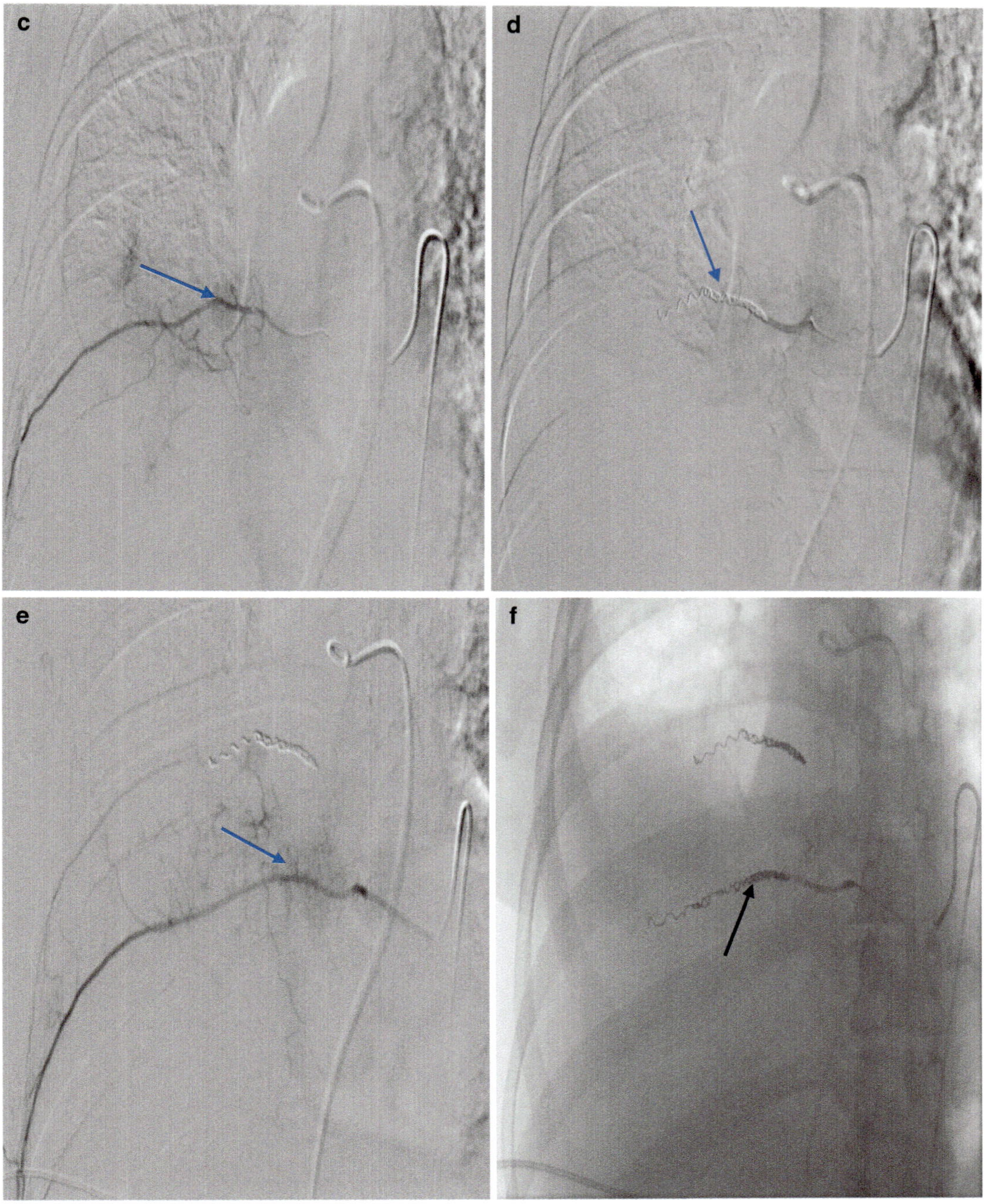

Fig. 3.107 (continued)

Abdominal Vascular Emergency

4

Contents

S. Duvnjak, *Endovascular Treatment of Arterial Emergencies*,
https://doi.org/10.1007/978-3-030-68832-5_4

4.1 Abdominal Aortic Emergencies

4.1.1 Abdominal Aortic Aneurysm-Symptomatic

Key Points

- An adequate infrarenal neck should be ensured to achieve a seal. No compromise should be made.
- Familiarity with adjunctive procedures such as renal stenting, the chimney technique, endoanchors, etc., is important.
- Local anaesthesia can be used as part of the protocol and as an "exercise" for the ruptured cases.

4.1.1.1 Aetiology and Clinical Presentation

A 65-year-old patient with aortic dissection type B and hypertension complained about chest and abdominal pain that had begun 4 days prior. The patient was haemodynamically stable, with a blood pressure of 180/120 mmHg and no other symptoms. Chest auscultation, ECG and coronary enzymes were within the standard limit, and the patient did not demonstrate coronary ischaemia. The white blood cell count was normal and CRP and the abdomen showed no signs of peritonitis, but pain could be provoked with aneurysm palpation. The patient had only one kidney (right), and renal function was impaired with an eGFR of 34 mL/min/1.73 m^2 and creatinine of 112 μmol/L (normal range 60–105 μmol/L).

4.1.1.2 Pre-interventional Diagnosis

Contrast-enhanced CT of the aorta showed type B aortic dissection, starting distally from the left subclavian artery. The aortic dissection had progressed relative to that on CT scanning 6 months prior, and the false lumen had expanded by approximately 1 cm. The patient had a 7 cm abdominal aortic and right iliac artery aneurysm measuring 24 mm, which had not been treated before according to the wishes of the patient (Fig. 4.1). Thoracic endovascular stent graft deployment was planned first, and abdominal aortic repair with EVAR stent grafts was eventually planned for later. The patient responded well to antihypertensive medicine and pain killers.

4.1.1.3 Endovascular Treatment

The TEVAR stent graft was deployed uneventfully via right femoral artery access under general anaesthesia. The stent graft was deployed distally from the left subclavian artery and extended distally around the diaphragm. There were no complications, and the patient showed no symptoms and was discharged 3 days after TEVAR. The need for AAA treatment was discussed once again, and the patient considered the treatment. Approximately 1 week after the patient was admitted to the hospital with abdominal pain and pain during aneurysm palpation, there were no signs of aneurysm rupture, and the patient was haemodynamically stable. The patient accepted the treatment, and due to the tortuous course of the iliac vessels and angulated aortic neck, an Aorfix stent graft was used and deployed as close to the right renal artery as possible (Fig. 4.2). The right internal iliac artery was occluded, and the distal landing zone was extended into the right external iliac artery. On the left side, the landing zone was in the common iliac artery, and the left internal iliac artery was open. Completion angiography showed severe stenosis of the right renal artery, and the stent graft likely partially occluded the right renal artery. Therefore, the renal stent was placed to preserve the right renal artery, with satisfactory results (Fig. 4.2).

4.1.1.4 Outcome

The patient did not have any complications, particularly spinal ischaemia, and had no deterioration of renal function. The patient was discharged 2 days after EVAR without symptoms or pain in the abdomen. Control contrast-enhanced CT 3 months later showed a well-deployed stent graft, no endoleak and an open right renal stent (Fig. 4.3).

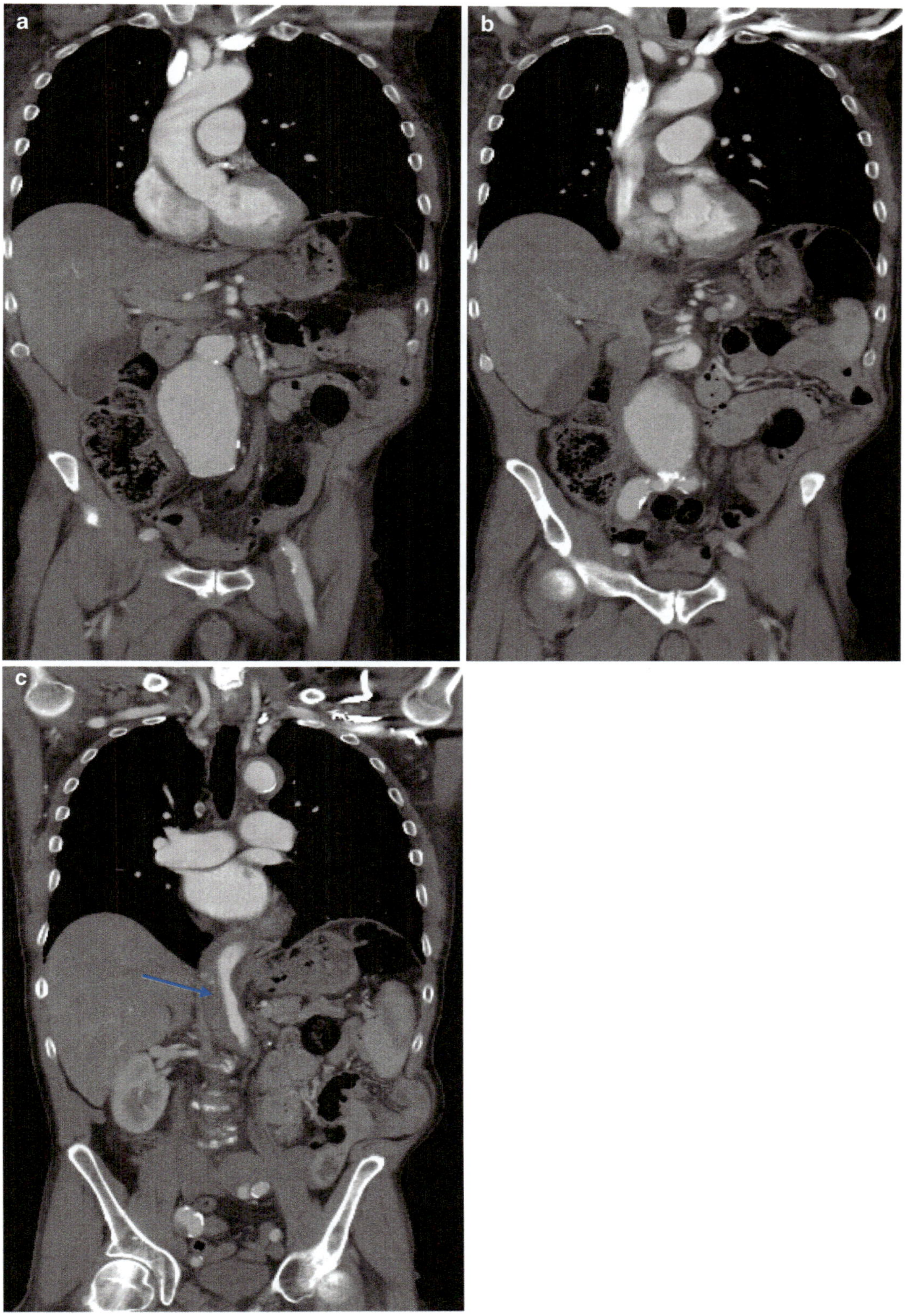

Fig. 4.1 Contrast-enhanced CT showing an aortic dissection (blue arrow) (**c**). Abdominal aortic aneurysm measuring 7 cm in the infrarenal aorta (**a, b**)

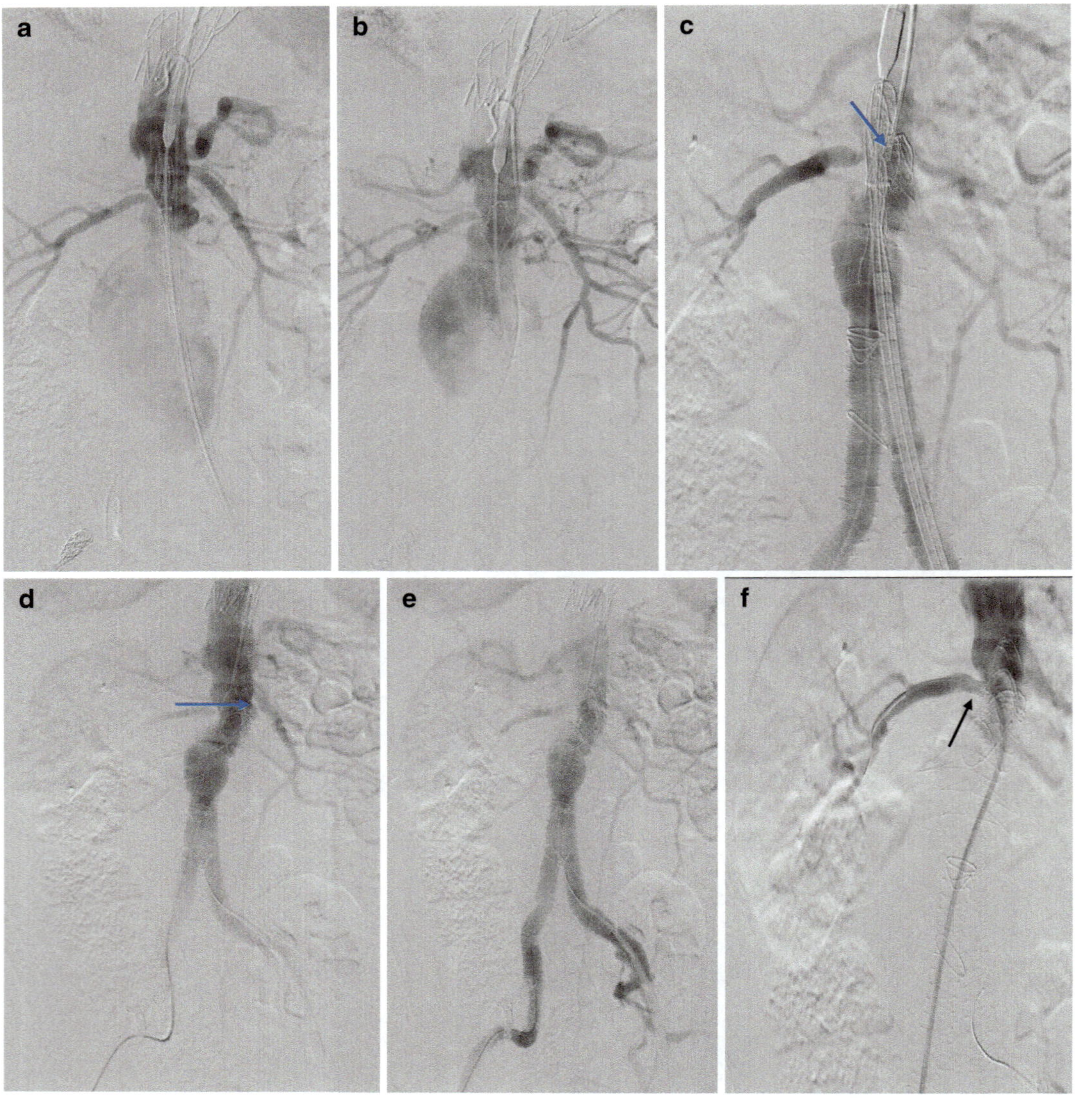

Fig. 4.2 Details from the EVAR intervention. (**a**–**c**) deployment of an Aorfix stent graft close to the right renal artery. (**d**) stenosis of the right renal artery-(blue arrows). (**e**) late-phase angiographic image showing no endoleak. (**f**) control image after renal stent placement showing a good result- (black arrow)

4.1.2 Abdominal Aortic Aneurysm-Ruptured

Key Points

- An adequate infrarenal neck should be ensured to achieve a seal in cases of ruptured. No compromise should be made.
- An occlusive aortic balloon can be used in unstable cases.
- Local anaesthesia is preferred in cases of rupture.

4.1.2.1 Aetiology and Clinical Presentation

A 71-year-old patient with a known abdominal aortic aneurysm was admitted to the emergency room due to acute sharp abdominal pain and hypotension. Blood pressure was 80/53 mmHg.

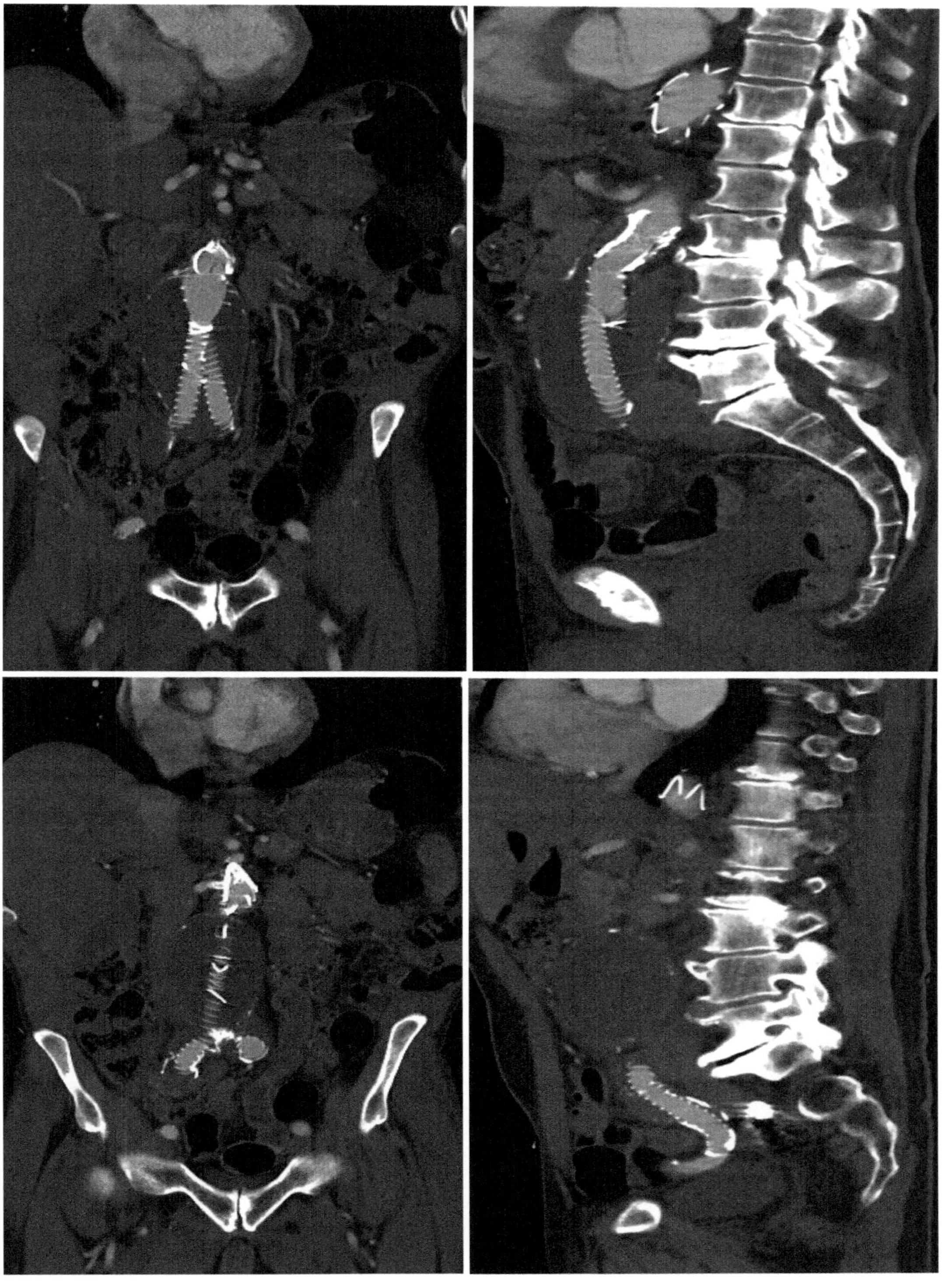

Fig. 4.3 Control contrast-enhanced CT 3 months after EVAR. No endoleak and an open right renal artery is observed

The patient had previous heart surgery and chronic pulmonary diseases. Bedside ultrasound revealed liquid in the abdomen and confirmed the clinical suspicion of ruptured AAA.

4.1.2.2 Pre-interventional Diagnosis

The patient was haemodynamically unstable and underwent a massive blood transfusion; therefore, emergency endovascular aneurysm repair (EVAR) was planned without CT scanning. Ultrasound revealed a potentially sound aneurysm neck.

4.1.2.3 Endovascular Treatment

Under local anaesthesia, percutaneous access was achieved through both femoral arteries. Angiography confirmed a sound aneurysm neck, and the EVAR stent graft was advanced (Fig. 4.4). The left femoral artery was easier to puncture. Therefore, the stent graft body was advanced through the left side. Immediately after stent graft deployment, the patient became unresponsive, and the blood pressure dropped precipitously. Fast advancement of the aortic occlusive balloon and infrarenal placement into the main body of the deployed stent graft were performed, and the blood pressure started to increase (Fig. 4.5). The contralateral leg was cannulated, and the occlusive balloon was inflated. The balloon was partially deflated, allowing the advancement of the stiff guidewire and fast deployment of the limb. Finally, angiography showed a good result with no endoleak. Both renal arteries were open and had improved calibre (Fig. 4.6).

4.1.2.4 Outcome

The patient recovered completely without complications and was discharged from the hospital 12 days after EVAR. A control CT scan 3 months later (Fig. 4.7) showed a satisfactory result without endoleak. The retroperitoneal haematoma was almost entirely resorbed.

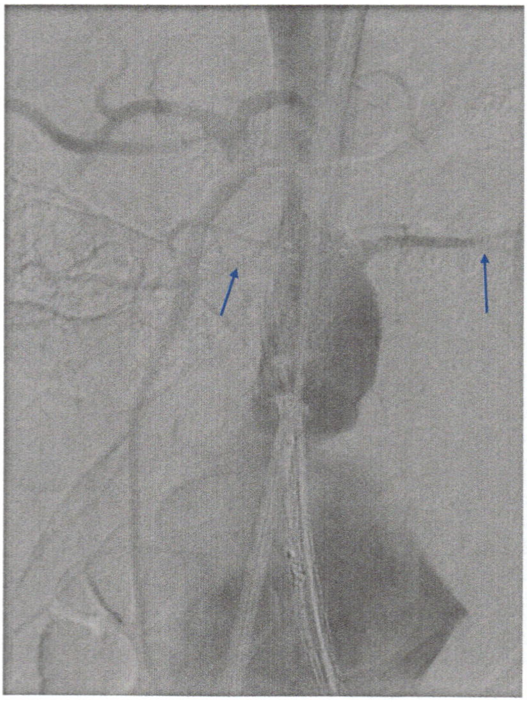

Fig. 4.4 Angiography and deployment of the stent graft. Note the spasming renal arteries-(arrows)

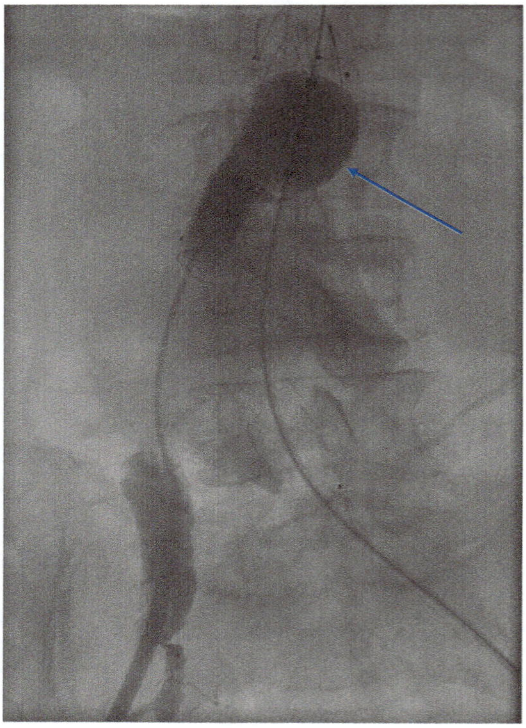

Fig. 4.5 The aortic occlusive balloon was advanced and placed infrarenally inside the main stent graft body (arrow)

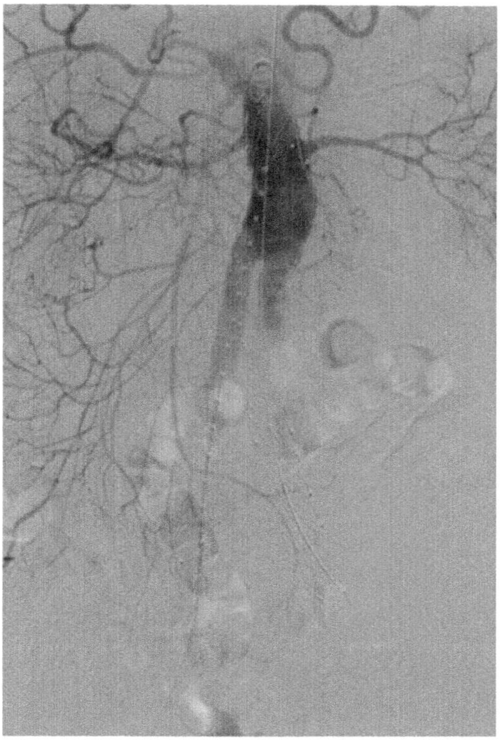

Fig. 4.6 Final angiography showed a well-deployed stent graft with no endoleak. Renal arteries now show an approximately standard calibre

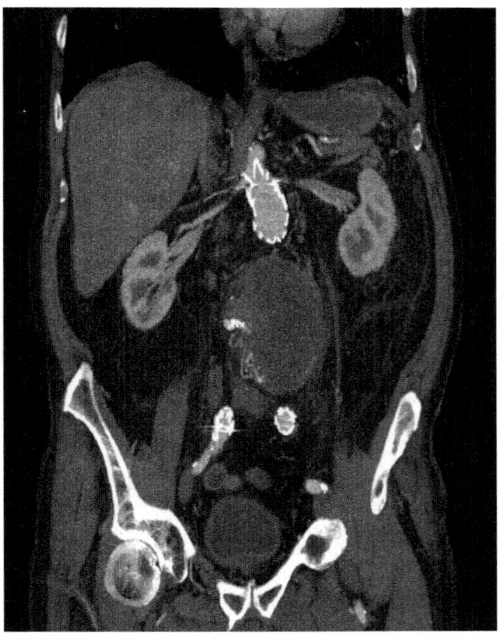

Fig. 4.7 Control contrast-enhanced CT 3 months after EVAR showing almost entirely retroperitoneal haematoma resorption and no endoleak

4.1.3 Iliac Artery Aneurysm-Ruptured

Key Points

- An adequate infrarenal neck should be ensured to achieve a seal. No compromise should be made.
- A bifurcated stent graft should be used in cases with inadequate landing zones.
- Local anaesthesia is preferred.

4.1.3.1 Aetiology and Clinical Presentation

A 65-year-old patient underwent aortic surgery with aorto-bi-iliac bypass grafts 10 years prior due to atherosclerotic diseases. There were no complaints after the surgery until recent pain in the abdomen. The patient did not visit the hospital after he experienced the pain the day before. The patient was brought to the emergency department in haemodynamic shock with a blood pressure of 90/62 mmHg and pulse rate of 122.

4.1.3.2 Pre-interventional Diagnosis

After the initial stabilization and resuscitation, emergency CT was performed and showed a ruptured 66 mm anastomotic pseudoaneurysm on the right side and retroperitoneal haematoma (Fig. 4.8). There was no sign of mycotic pseudoaneurysm paraclinically or clinically. There was a small pseudoaneurysm of the proximal anastomosis as well. The right internal iliac artery was open.

4.1.3.3 Endovascular Treatment

An occlusive balloon was percutaneously inserted in the distal aorta through the left femoral artery. Percutaneous access through the right femoral artery was not possible; therefore, it was surgically exposed. The right internal iliac artery was occluded with micro-coils afterwards through the right femoral artery. After that, a 7 Fr sheath was advanced, and the first stent graft, 8 mm in diameter and 59 mm in length, was advanced and deployed in the external iliac artery, followed by placement of a second stent graft with a diameter

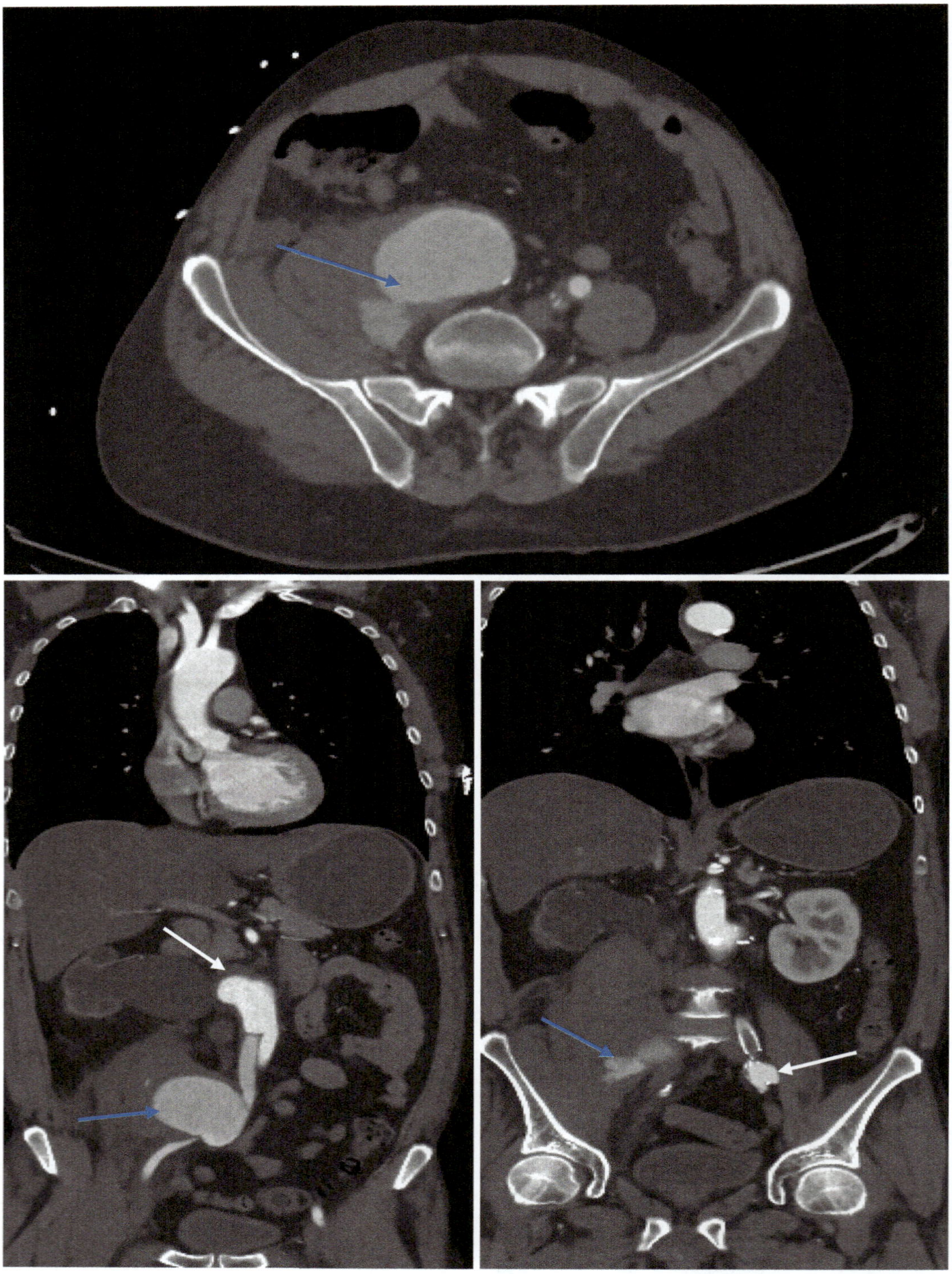

Fig. 4.8 Ruptured right 66 mm anastomotic pseudoaneurysm indicated by blue arrows. The proximal anastomosis and the left iliac anastomosis each presented with pseudoaneurysm (white arrows)

of 9 and 59 mm in length in the common iliac artery with good overlap with the first stent graft (Fig. 4.9). A 3000 IU heparin bolus was administered before stent graft deployment. Control angiography showed a well-deployed stent graft and no endoleak.

4.1.3.4 Outcome

The patient recovered completely without any complications. Elective treatment of the proximal anastomotic and left iliac anastomotic pseudoaneurysms with a bifurcated stent graft is scheduled. Control CT 3 months after the treatment showed a satisfactory result and no endoleak (Fig. 4.10).

4.1.4 Mycotic Abdominal Aortic Aneurysm

Key Points

- Mycotic aneurysms are complicated to treat.
- Stent graft deployment usually serves as a bridging procedure.
- Long-term antibiotics are required.

4.1.4.1 Aetiology and Clinical Presentation

A 71-year-old patient with arterial hypertension was admitted to the hospital with a 38 ° fever and diffuse abdominal (but not peritoneal) pain lasting between 2 and 3 weeks, without diarrhoea or blood in the stool. The white cell blood count was 23,000 mm^3, and the CRP was 105 mg/L. There were no other significant comorbidities and no history of vascular surgery. The blood culture was positive for *Salmonella enteritidis*, and intravenous antibiotics were administered.

4.1.4.2 Pre-interventional Diagnosis

Contrast-enhanced CT showed an unusually shaped abdominal aortic aneurysm, and a fluorodeoxyglucose positron emission tomography (FDG-PET) scan delineated the infection and mycotic infrarenal aortic aneurysm (Fig. 4.11). The patient was treated with broad-spectrum intravenous antibiotics during the first 2 weeks. After that, the aneurysm was surgically treated using deep femoral vein as an aortic tube graft. The patient continued with intravenous antibiotics for two additional weeks and was discharged and continued with oral antibiotic treatment. The surgery went well, and the patient did not experience any significant complications. A few weeks after the patient experienced abdominal, a new control CT scan revealed a pseudoaneurysm at the proximal anastomosis that showed evidence of rupture (Fig. 4.12).

4.1.4.3 Endovascular Treatment

There was enough length between the renal arteries and pseudoaneurysm to deploy the stent graft, and the intervention was planned. An aortic tube stent graft was deployed infrarenally without difficulties through the right femoral artery percutaneously, yielding satisfactory results (Fig. 4.13). The patient was discharged and continued on oral antibiotics, the white cell count fell to 9 /L × 10^9 /L, and the CRP was 25 mg/L.

4.1.4.4 Outcome

The patient was doing well the first month after the treatment, and 1 month control CT showed satisfactory results (Fig. 4.14). Two months after endovascular treatment, the patient was readmitted due to abdominal pain, and control CT showed a new rupture and pseudoaneurysm at the distal anastomosis (Fig. 4.15). The occurrence of rupture and pseudoaneurysm could probably be explained by the mechanical stiffness of the stent graft, its influence on the vein graft, and the still-active infections. The patient was treated surgically by removing the stent graft and vein graft, performing stump occlusion of the infrarenal aorta and creating an axillo-femoral bypass. A few weeks after surgery, the patient returned with signs of axillo-femoral bypass infection, and a PET scan revealed infections of the bypass and in both groins (Fig. 4.16). The patient underwent

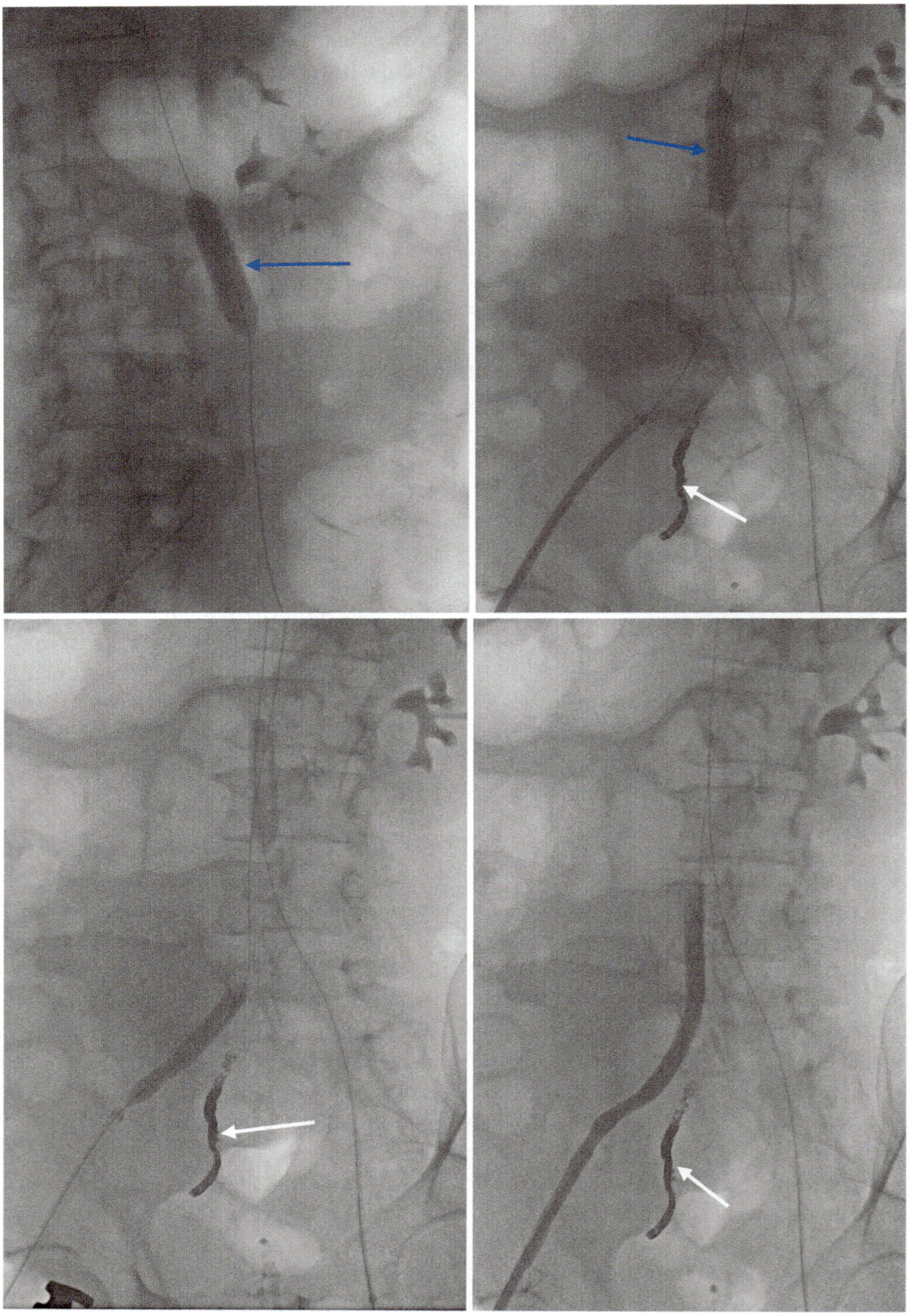

Fig. 4.9 Details from the emergency endovascular treatment. An occlusive balloon was placed via the left femoral artery (white arrows). The right femoral artery was used to perform embolization of the right internal iliac artery with microcoil occlusion of the "back door" (blue arrows). Advancement of the two stent grafts, the first, measuring 8 mm × 59 mm, placed distally in the external iliac artery, and the second, with a diameter of 9 mm × 59 mm, placed proximally with complete pseudoaneurysm exclusion

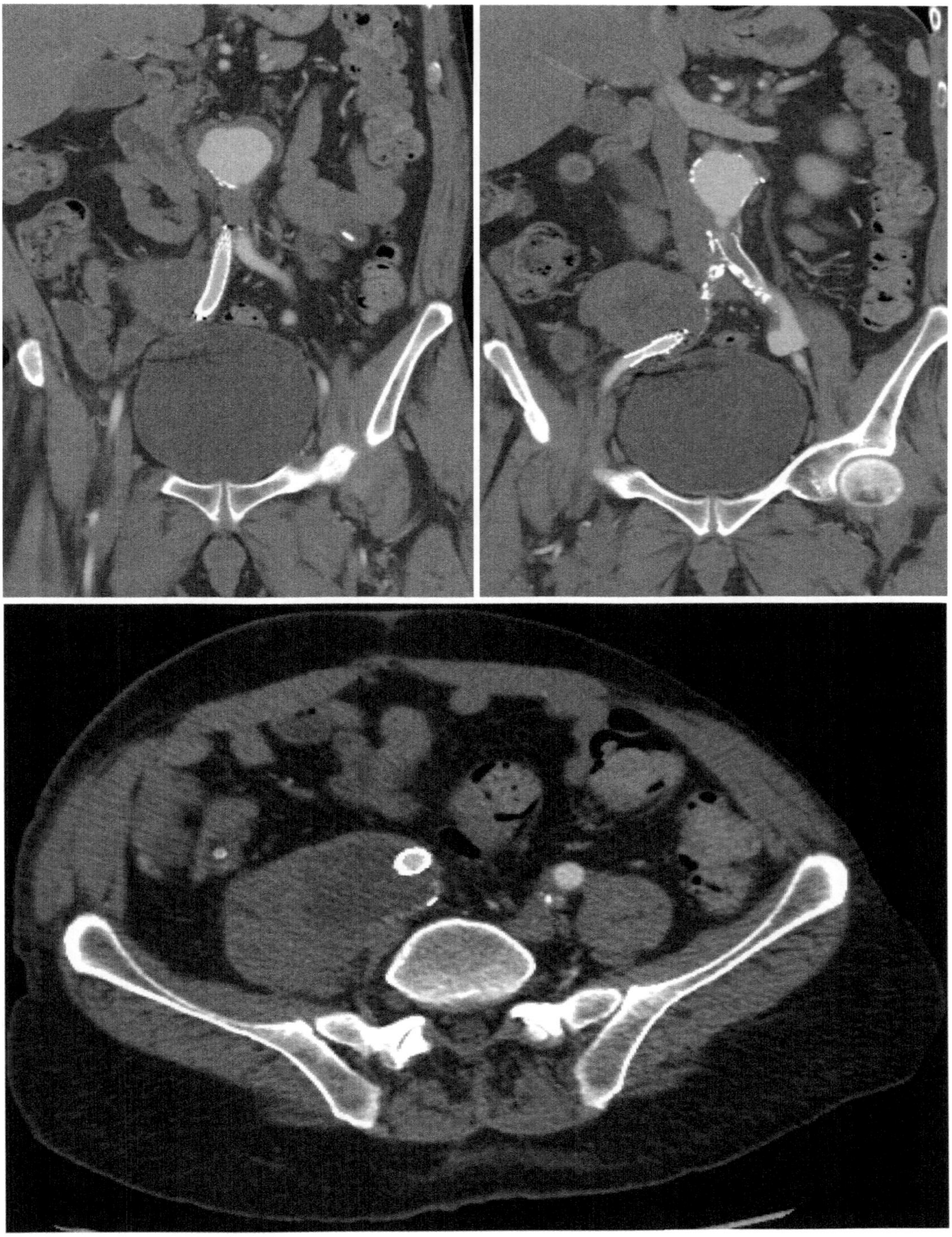

Fig. 4.10 Control contrast-enhanced CT 3 months after treatment. The –stent graft is open, and no endoleak is shown. The proximal pseudoaneurysm is scheduled for treatment at a later date. The pseudoaneurysm of the anastomosis on the left side will be treated together with the scheduled proximal anastomosis treatment

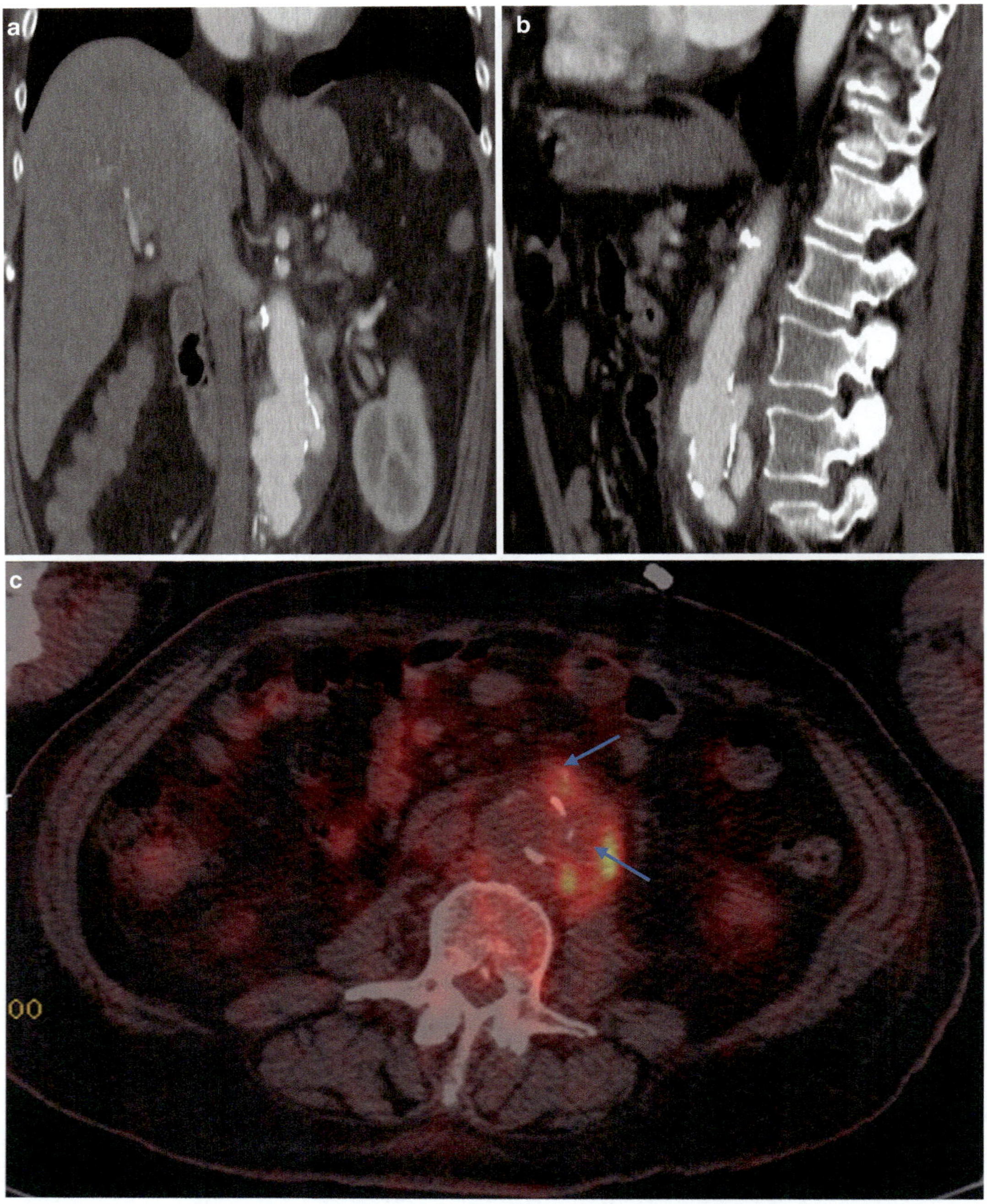

Fig. 4.11 Index CT scan (**a** and **b**) showing an "unusual" infrarenal aortic aneurysm. (**c**) FDG-PET scan showing infective aneurysm (arrows)

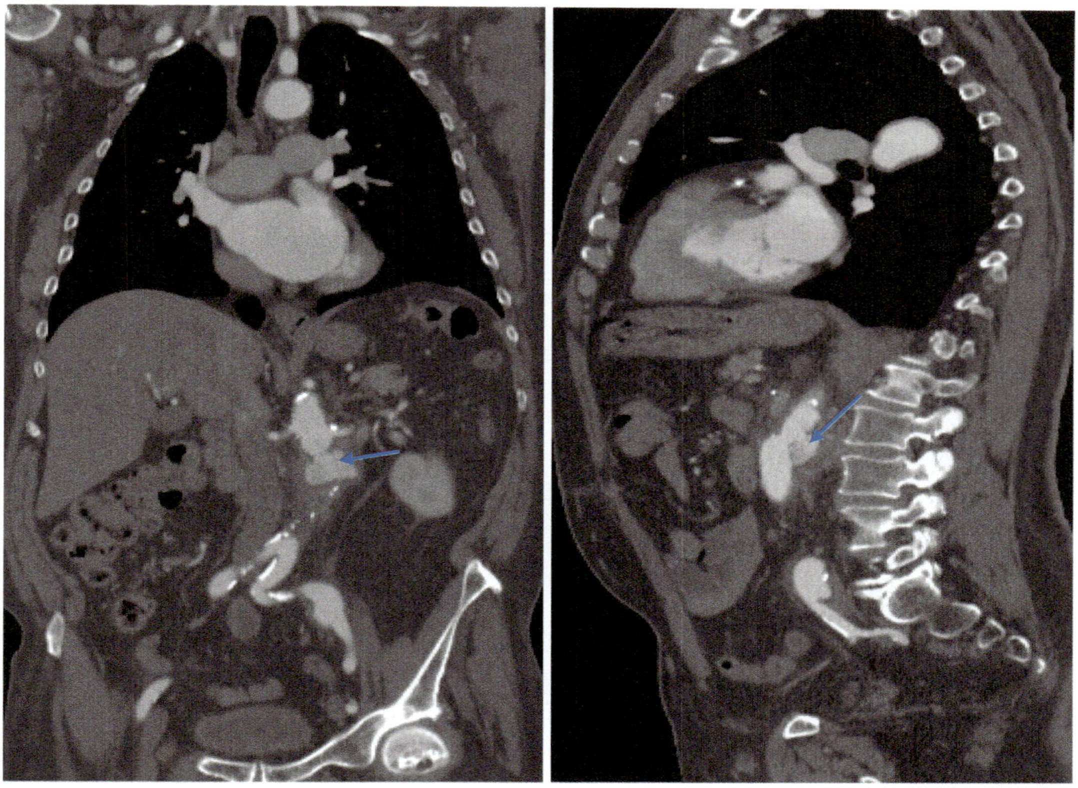

Fig. 4.12 Control contrast-enhanced CT showing a proximal anastomotic pseudoaneurysm and evidence of rupture (arrows)

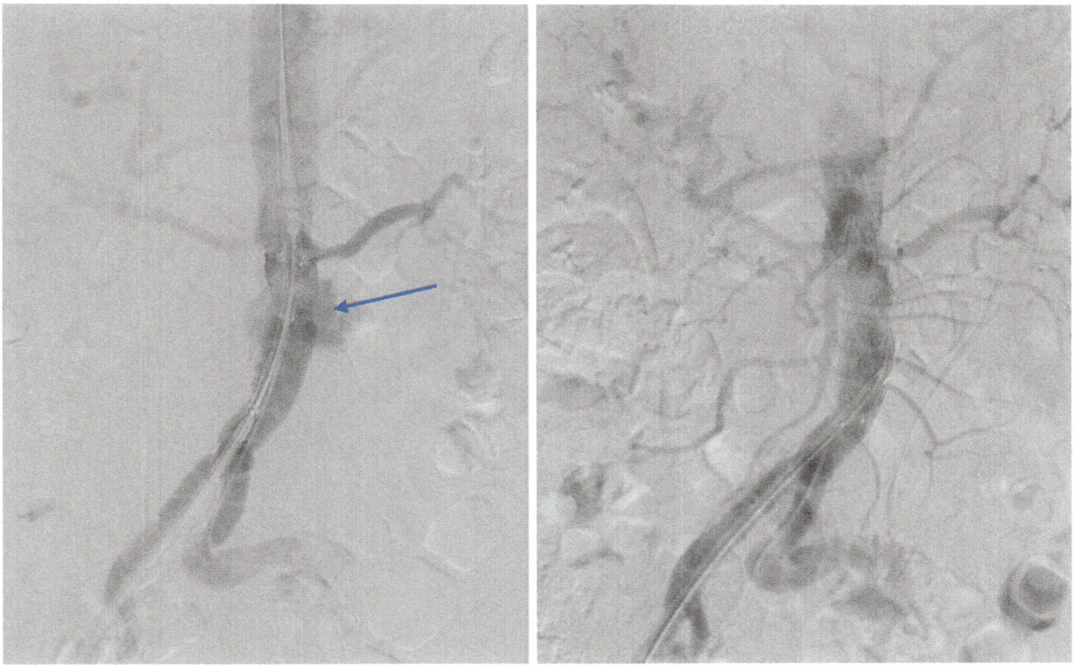

Fig. 4.13 An aortic stent tube graft was deployed infrarenally with an excellent outcome. The blue arrow indicates the proximal anastomotic pseudoaneurysm

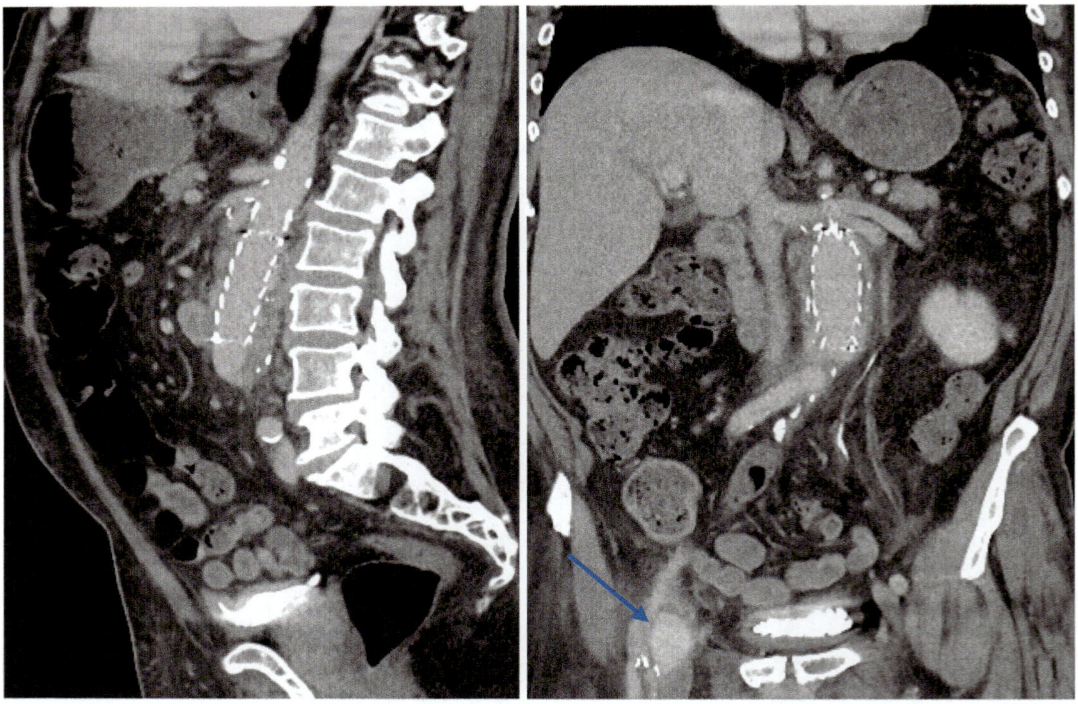

Fig. 4.14 Control contrast-enhanced CT 1 month after stent graft deployment shows a satisfactory result and no endoleak. The patient developed a pseudoaneurysm in the right groin (blue arrow)

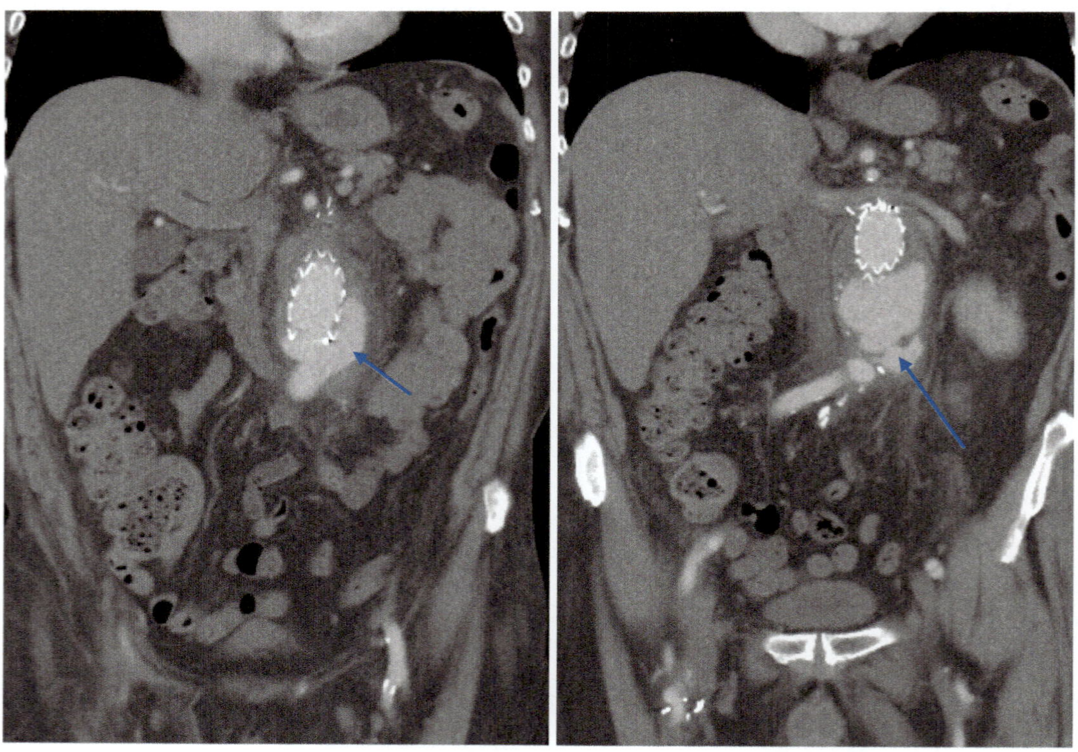

Fig. 4.15 Control CT 2 months after stent graft deployment showed a new rupture and pseudoaneurysm on the distal anastomosis (arrows), probably induced mechanically due to stiffness of the stent graft

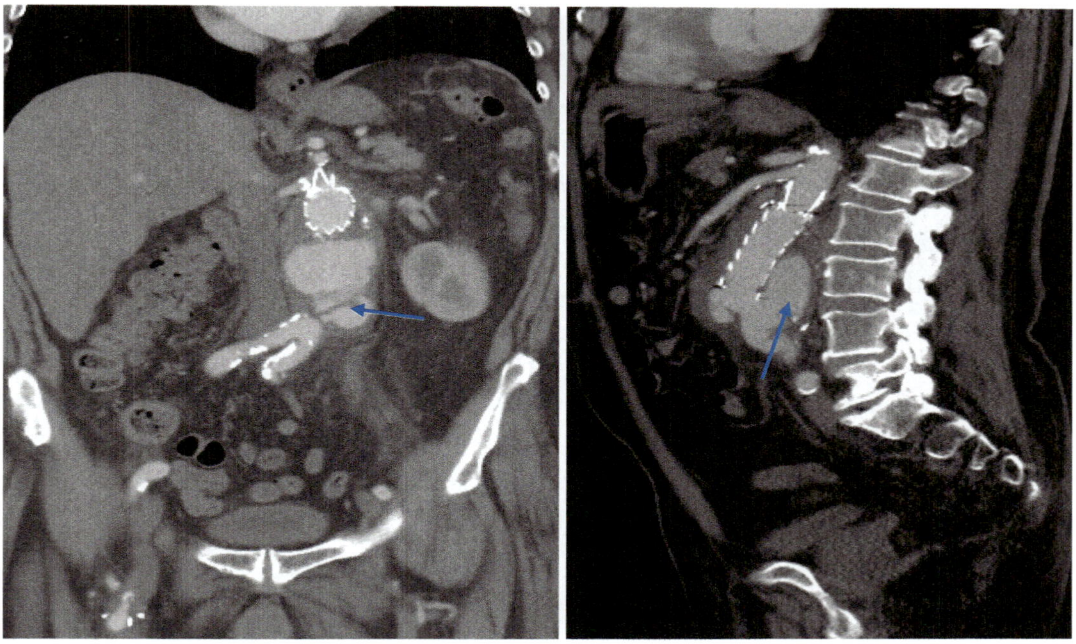

Fig. 4.15 (continued)

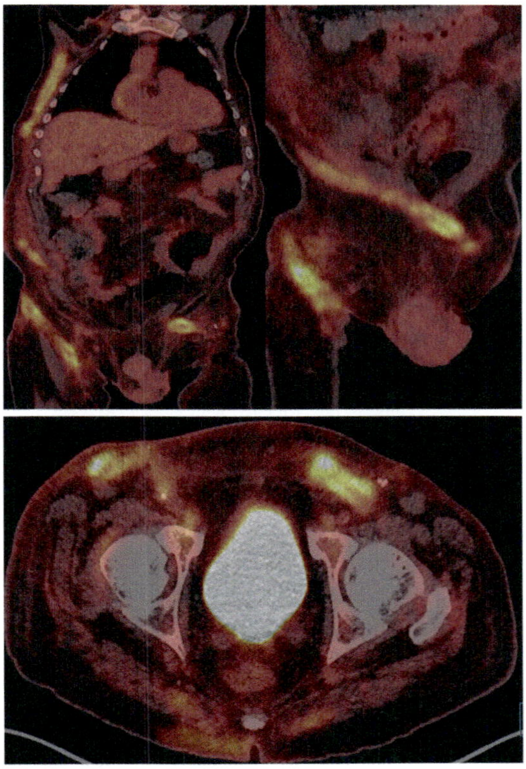

Fig. 4.16 FDG-PET scan showing infection of the right axillo-femoral bypass and in both groins

one more surgery for removal of the infected right axilla femoral bypass and creation of an axillo-femoral bypass on the left side (Fig. 4.17). A few weeks after the last surgery, the patient was readmitted again with abdominal pain, and CT showed blowout syndrome and aortic stump rupture (Fig. 4.18). There were no further surgical options for the patient.

4.1.5 Abdominal Aorto-Iliac Occlusion

Key Points

- Extensive aorto-iliac occlusive diseases can be treated with a covered stent with good patency.
- The percutaneous approach under local anaesthesia works for the majority of the patients.
- Familiarization with some re-entry devices is recommended.

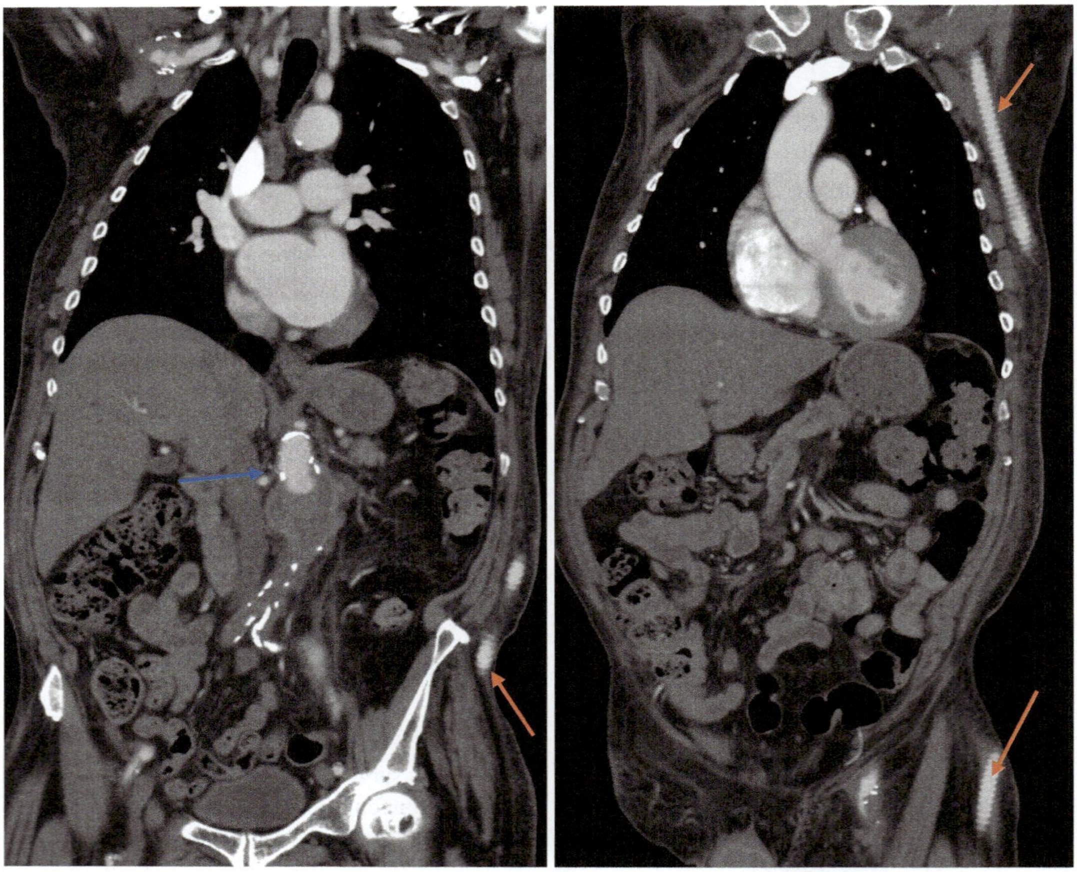

Fig. 4.17 Control CT after the creation of a left axillo-femoral bypass-(orange arrows). Blue arrow indicates an occluded intrarenal aortic stump

4.1.5.1 Aetiology and Clinical Presentation

A 67-year-old overweight patient with a long history of intermittent bilateral claudication was admitted. Recently, the patient experienced significant reduction and increasing pain during everyday work. The ankle-brachial index (ABI) was 50% on the right side and 55% on the left side. The patient was a heavy smoker and took antihypertensive medication.

4.1.5.2 Pre-interventional Diagnosis

Contrast-enhanced MRI showed occlusion of the infrarenal aorta and both common iliac arteries (Fig. 4.19). The external iliac arteries, femoral arteries, popliteal arteries and all three crural arteries were open bilaterally.

4.1.5.3 Endovascular Treatment

Percutaneous access was achieved via both femoral arteries under local anaesthesia, and a preclosure suture was deployed. After some time, it was possible to recanalize the occluded common iliac arteries and infrarenal aorta. Predilatation with 8 and 10 mm balloons was performed. After that, a covered aortic stent graft measuring 16 mm × 48 mm was deployed above the aortic bifurcation, followed by deployment of two covered stents measuring 9 mm × 59 mm in the common iliac arteries bilaterally (Fig. 4.20). Post-dilatation was performed with a balloon, and the final angiography showed good results and no distal embolization. There was no problem with haemostasis.

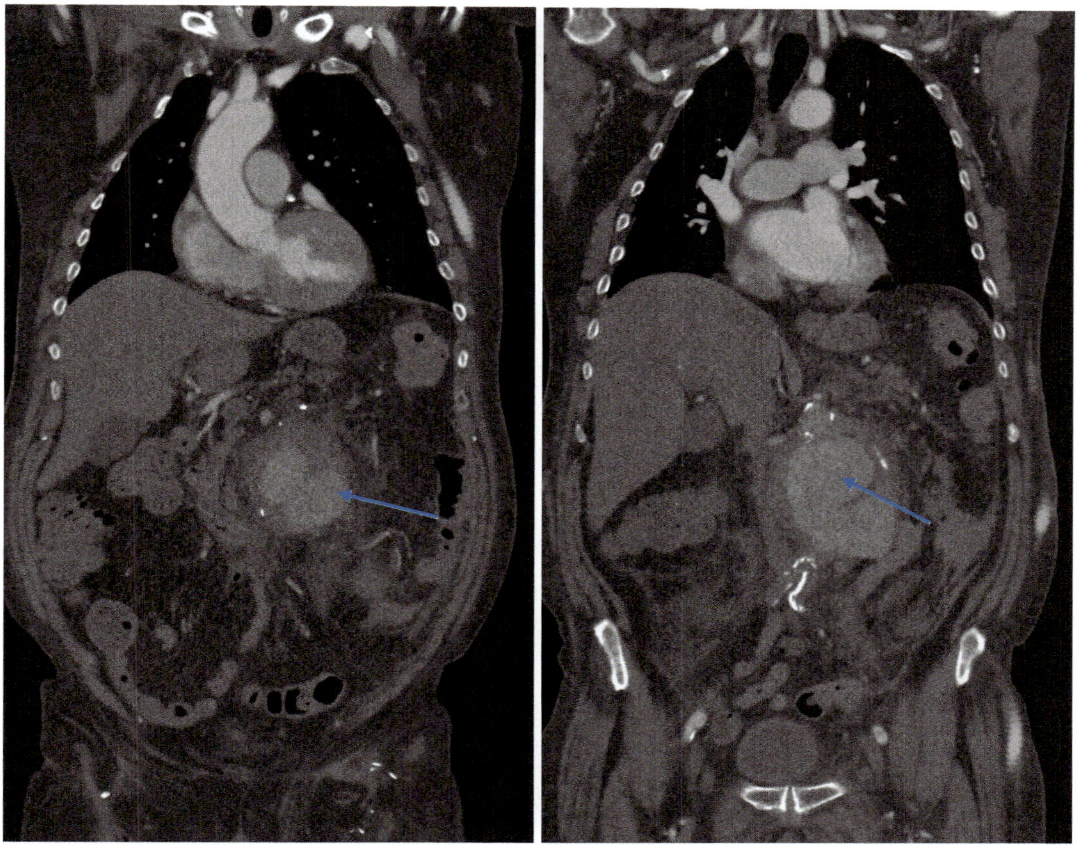

Fig. 4.18 Blowout syndrome and aortic stump rupture- (arrows)

4.1.5.4 Outcome

The patient was discharged from the hospital the next day and continued to be treated with acetylsalicylic medication. The ABI increased to 90% bilaterally.

4.2 Visceral Artery Aneurysms

4.2.1 Splenic Artery-I

Key Points

- A plan B and even a plan C must be considered.
- If the "back door" cannot be occluded, the aneurysm can be embolized.
- Ultrasound can be used during the follow-up in stable cases.

4.2.1.1 Aetiology and Clinical Presentation

A 59-year-old patient with arterial hypertension underwent contrast-enhanced CT due to unspecific abdominal pain lasting a few weeks after ultrasound of the abdomen that showed aneurysm in the visceral vessel. The patient did not experience vomiting, nausea, diarrhoea or blood in the stool and was afebrile. White blood cell count and other blood analyses were within normal limits. There was no anamnestic information on trauma or invasive vascular examination.

4.2.1.2 Pre-interventional Diagnosis

Contrast-enhanced CT of the abdomen showed an unruptured 59 mm splenic artery aneurysm (Fig. 4.21). The patient had not undergone any previous diagnostic examination. The strategy was to attempt to deploy a stent graft via the left brachial artery or, if not possible, to perform

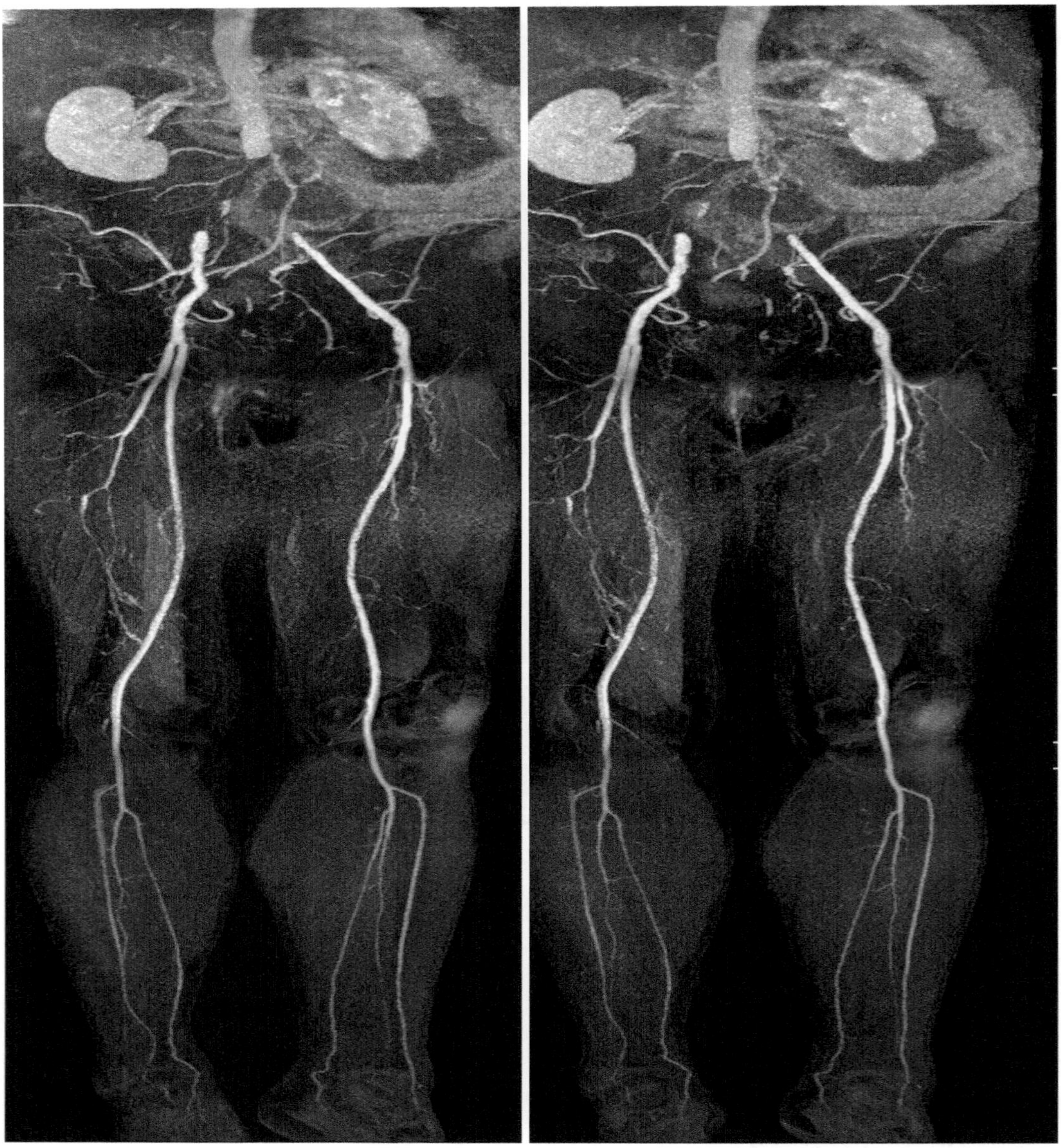

Fig. 4.19 Contrast-enhanced MRI of the lower extremities showing occlusion of the infrarenal aorta and common iliac arteries (arrow)

embolization and occlusion of the splenic artery with the stent graft.

4.2.1.3 Endovascular Treatment

A 6 Fr long sheath was advanced percutaneously into the descending aorta through the left brachial artery, and an attempt was made to navigate a diagnostic catheter and guidewire across the aneurysm and advance the stent graft. This attempt failed; therefore, the diagnostic catheter and later a microcatheter were advanced to embolized the "back and front doors" of the aneurysm. It was not possible to advance the microcatheter distally to occlude the "back door", and so the aneurysm itself was filled with micro-coils. Finally, the main splenic artery was occluded with 10 mm micro-coils distal to the dorsal pancreatic artery to allow vascular-

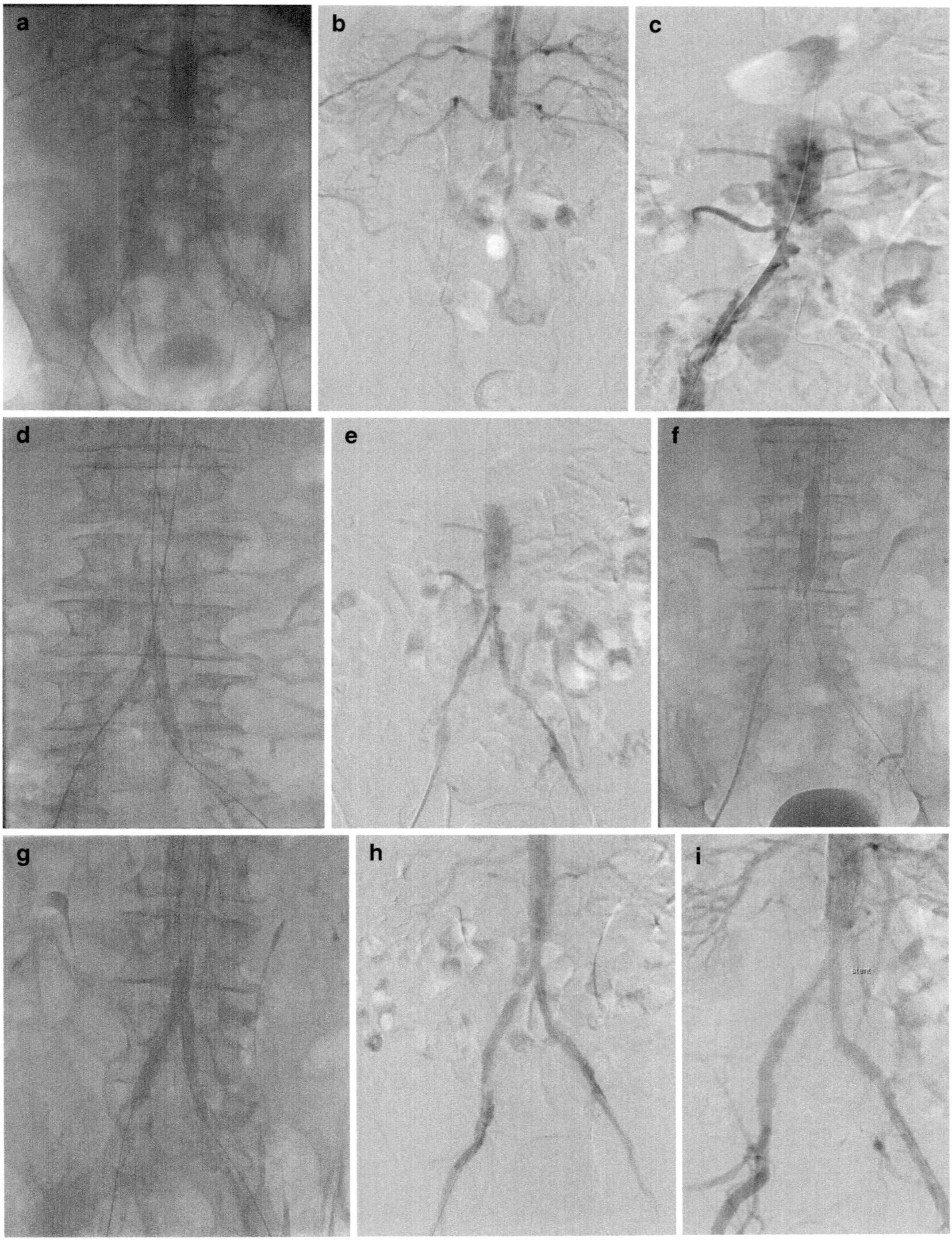

Fig. 4.20 (**a**, **b**) angiography after recanalization showing occluded distal abdominal aorta and iliac arteries bilaterally. (**c**–**e**) pre-dilatation with 8- and 10-mm balloons on both sides. (**f**, **g**) deployment of a covered stent in the aorta and both common iliac arteries and post-dilatation. (**h**, **i**) control angiography showing a satisfactory result

ization of the spleen collateral (Fig. 4.22). The intervention went well. The left brachial artery was manually compressed, and haemostasis was achieved. The patient was discharged the next day with anti-inflammatory medications and no complications.

4.2.1.4 Outcome

The patient is doing well and has had no complaints and no abdominal pain after a few days of expected pain after splenic artery embolization, splenic infarct and post-embolization syndrome. The patient did not experience any complications. One month control CT (Fig. 4.23a) showed a completely thrombosed splenic artery aneurysm and satisfactory contrast enhancement of the spleen through the collateral network. One-year control CT (Fig. 4.23b, c) showed shrinkage of the splenic artery aneurysm and adequate spleen vascularization.

4.2.2 Splenic Artery-II

Key Points

- In some ruptured splenic artery aneurysms, embolization can be performed very quickly to obtain haemostasis.
- If the "back door" cannot be occluded, aneurysm embolization can be performed.
- Non–contrast-enhanced CT and ultrasound can be used during follow-up in a patient with impaired renal function.

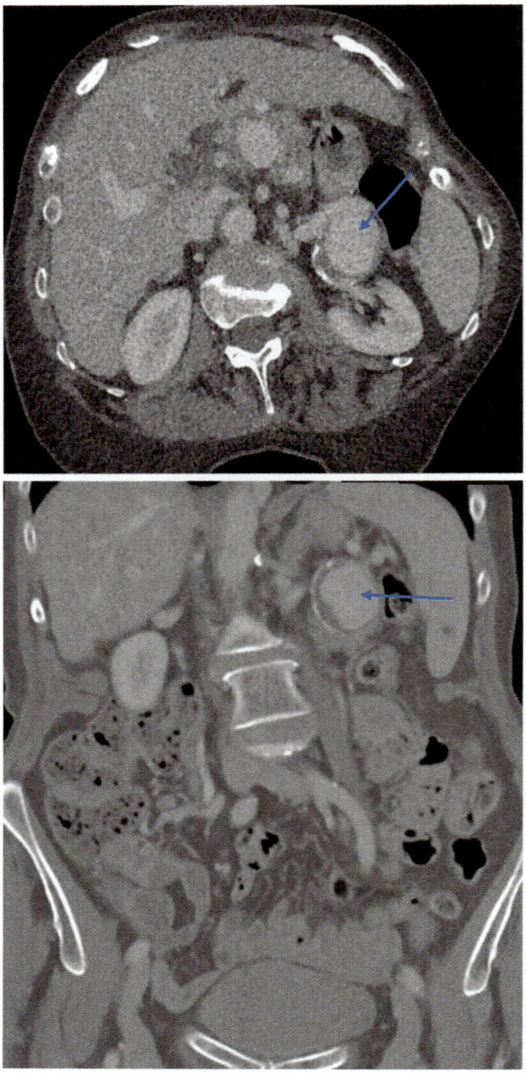

Fig. 4.21 Contrast-enhanced CT showing a 59 mm splenic artery aneurysm (arrows) and wall calcifications. There was no rupture

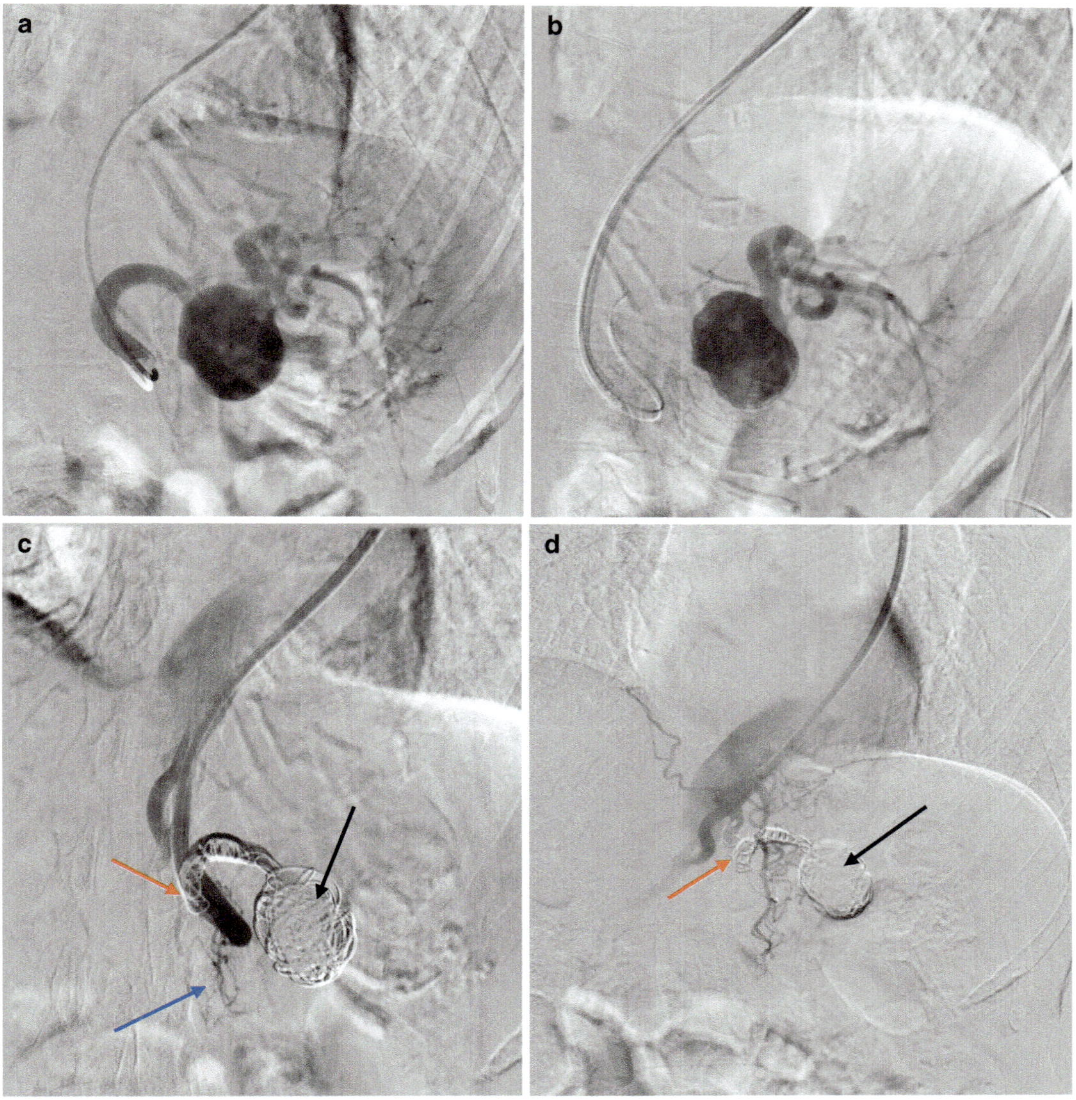

Fig. 4.22 (**a**, **b**) a 6 Fr sheath and 5 Fr diagnostic catheter have engaged the celiac trunk. It was not possible to advance the 6 Fr sheath further and secure a stable position to advance the stent graft. (**c**, **d**) embolization of the aneurysm itself(black arrows) and the "front door" with micro-coils (orange arrows) with a satisfactory result. The blue arrow indicates the dorsal pancreatic artery that provides collateral splenic vascularization

4.2.2.1 Aetiology and Clinical Presentation

A 61-year-old patient with known arterial hypertension for over a decade was treated with two drugs. The patient was admitted to the emergency room in hypotensive shock with blood pressure 80/50 mmHg and pulse 120/min. The patient experienced sharp severe pain in the left abdominal quadrant before becoming hypotensive. The patient had not undergone any diagnostic examinations previously. After the initial resuscitation, including blood transfusion due to a haemoglobin level of 4.1 mmol/L, ultrasound revealed a haematoma in the abdomen. However, it was

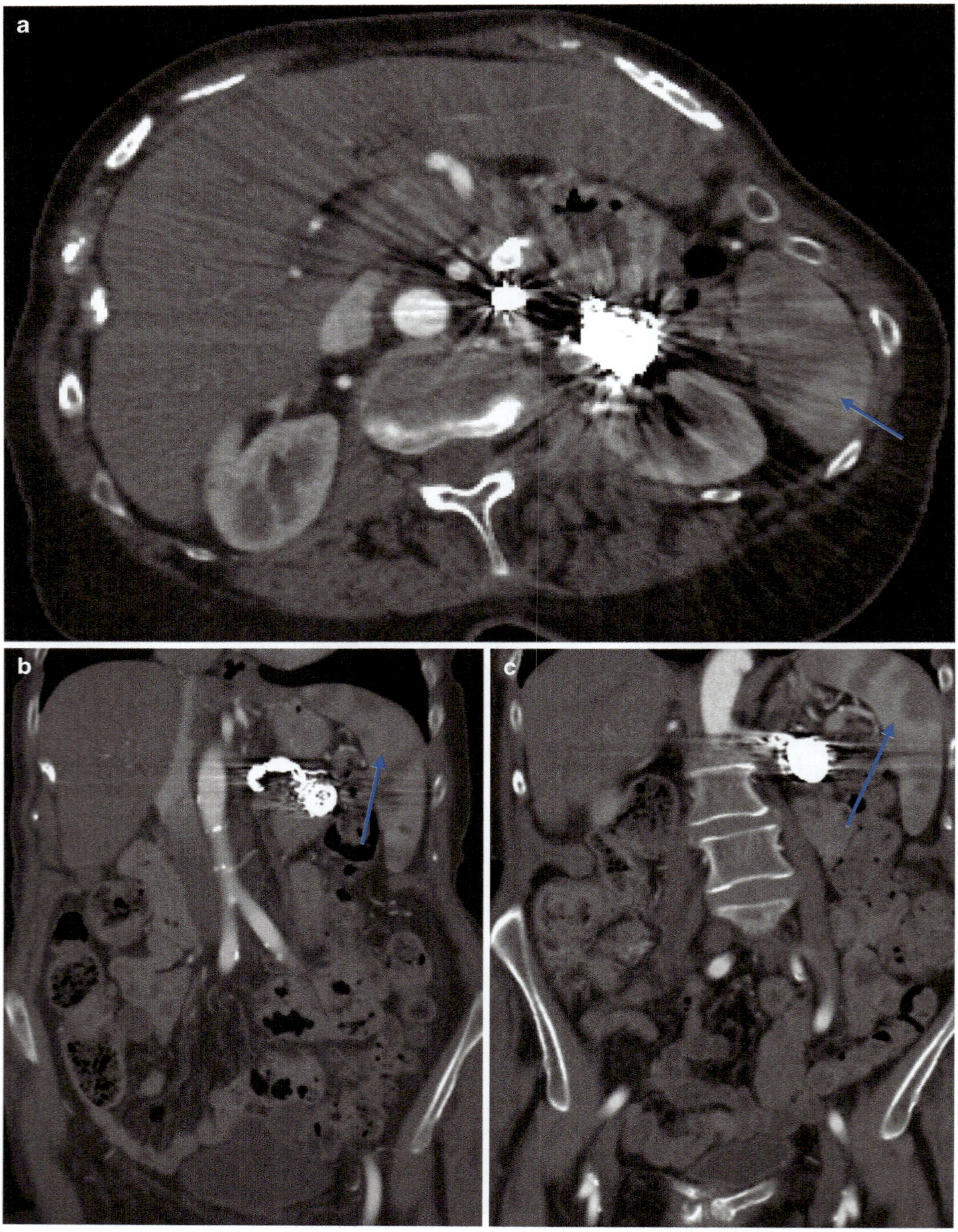

Fig. 4.23 (**a**) one month control CT after embolization with a completely thrombosed aneurysm; arrow indicates splenic contrast enhancement through the collateral network. One-year control CT with shrinkage of the aneurysm to 36 mm; arrows indicate splenic contrast enhancement (**b**, **c**)

impossible to precisely determine the source of the bleeding. Contrast-enhanced CT was performed to plan further treatment due to the temporary nature of the patient's stabilization and a blood pressure of 100/75 mmHg.

4.2.2.2 Pre-interventional Diagnosis

Contrast-enhanced CT showed a ruptured 65 mm splenic artery aneurysm and retroperitoneal haematoma (Fig. 4.24). Emergency embolization and, in case of deterioration of patient's status, emergency laparotomy were planned.

4.2.2.3 Endovascular Treatment

Under local anaesthesia, a 5 Fr sidewinder-shaped catheter was inserted percutaneously into the right femoral artery, engaging the celiac trunk, and subsequently, a microcatheter was advanced. It was not possible to advance the microcatheter beyond the aneurysm and embolize the "back door" of the aneurysm. Therefore, multiple micro-coils with diameters from 20 mm down to 10 mm were deployed into the aneurysm itself. The main splenic artery proximal to the aneurysm was occluded with 10 mm-diameter micro-coils

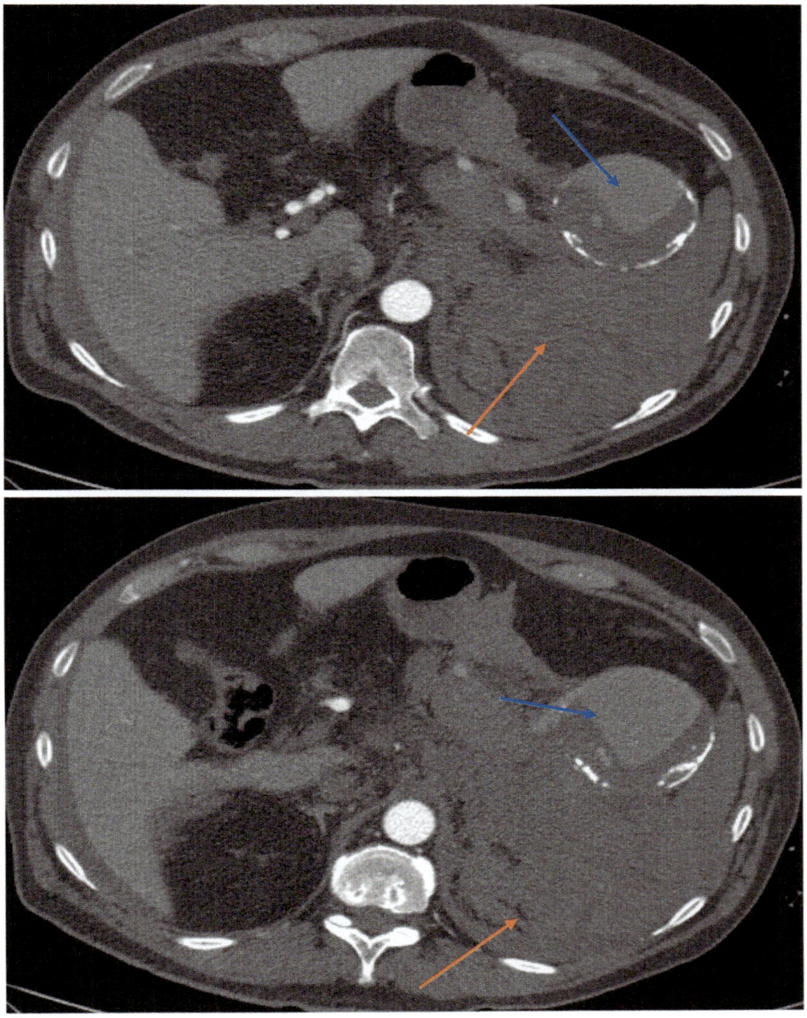

Fig. 4.24 The ruptured 65 mm splenic artery aneurysm. Blue arrows indicate the aneurysm. Orange arrows indicate a retroperitoneal haematoma. There was no aortic aneurysm, and both femoral and iliac arteries were open without stenosis

(Fig. 4.25). It is crucial to note that if the patient had become unstable, it would have been essential to occlude the main splenic artery without spending time occluding the aneurysm. The intervention went well, and the patient did not experience worsening of haemodynamic status. One complication that can occur in situations such as these is compartment syndrome, and laparotomy may be

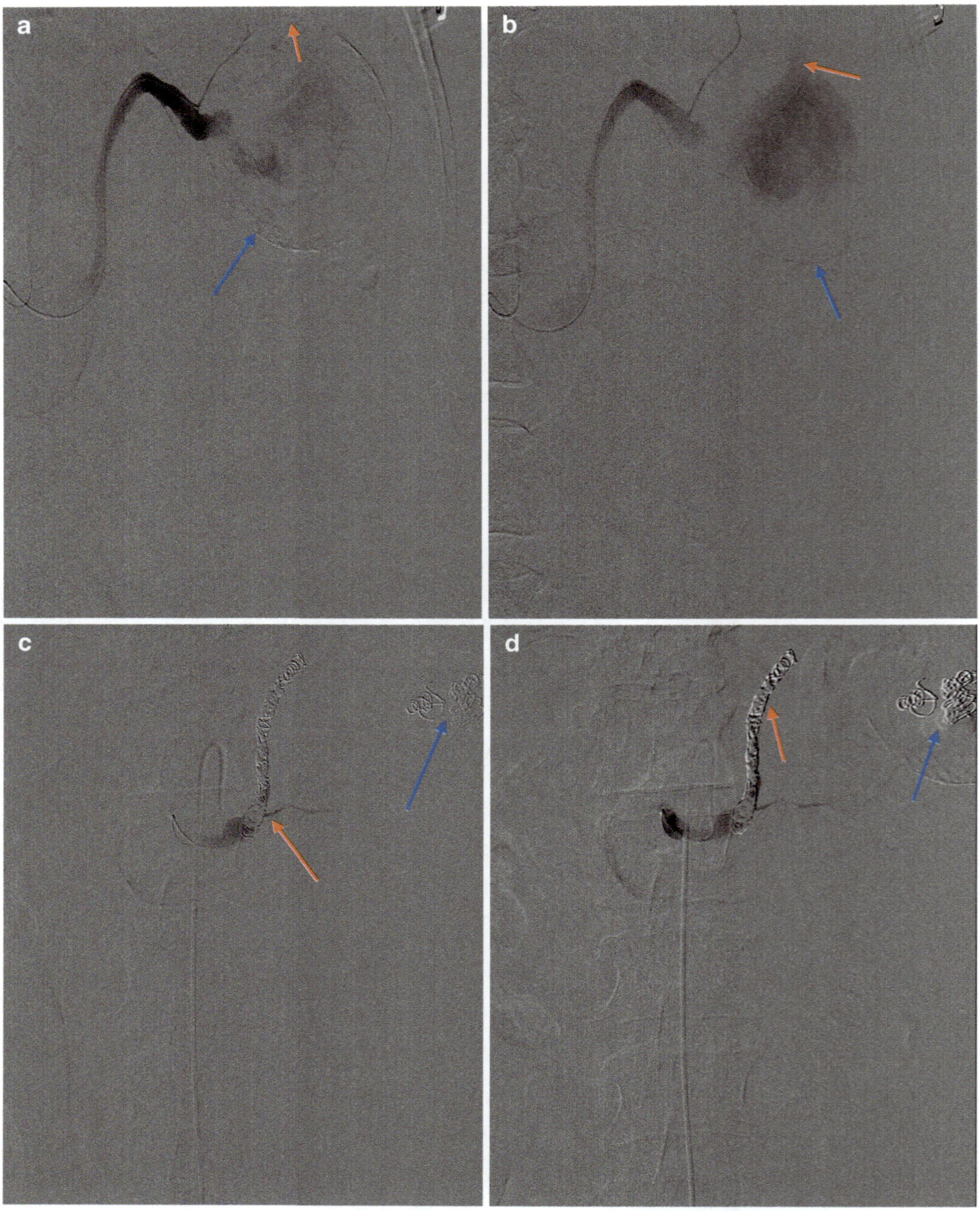

Fig. 4.25 Selective angiography of the splenic artery (**a**, **b**) blue arrows indicate calcification in the aneurysm wall. Orange arrows indicate breaks in the aneurysm calcification wall and probably the rupture point. (**c**, **d**) blue arrows indicate micro-coils inside the aneurysm. Orange arrows indicate micro-coils in the main splenic artery proximal to the aneurysm

required in case of multiorgan failure. The patient was discharged 2 weeks after the embolization and developed renal failure with decreasing eGFR and increased creatinine, but the situation stabilized, and no dialysis was required.

4.2.2.4 Outcome

The patient did not experience any complications during the follow-up, but the renal function remained impaired. One month control non-contrast-enhanced CT (Fig. 4.26) showed a stable

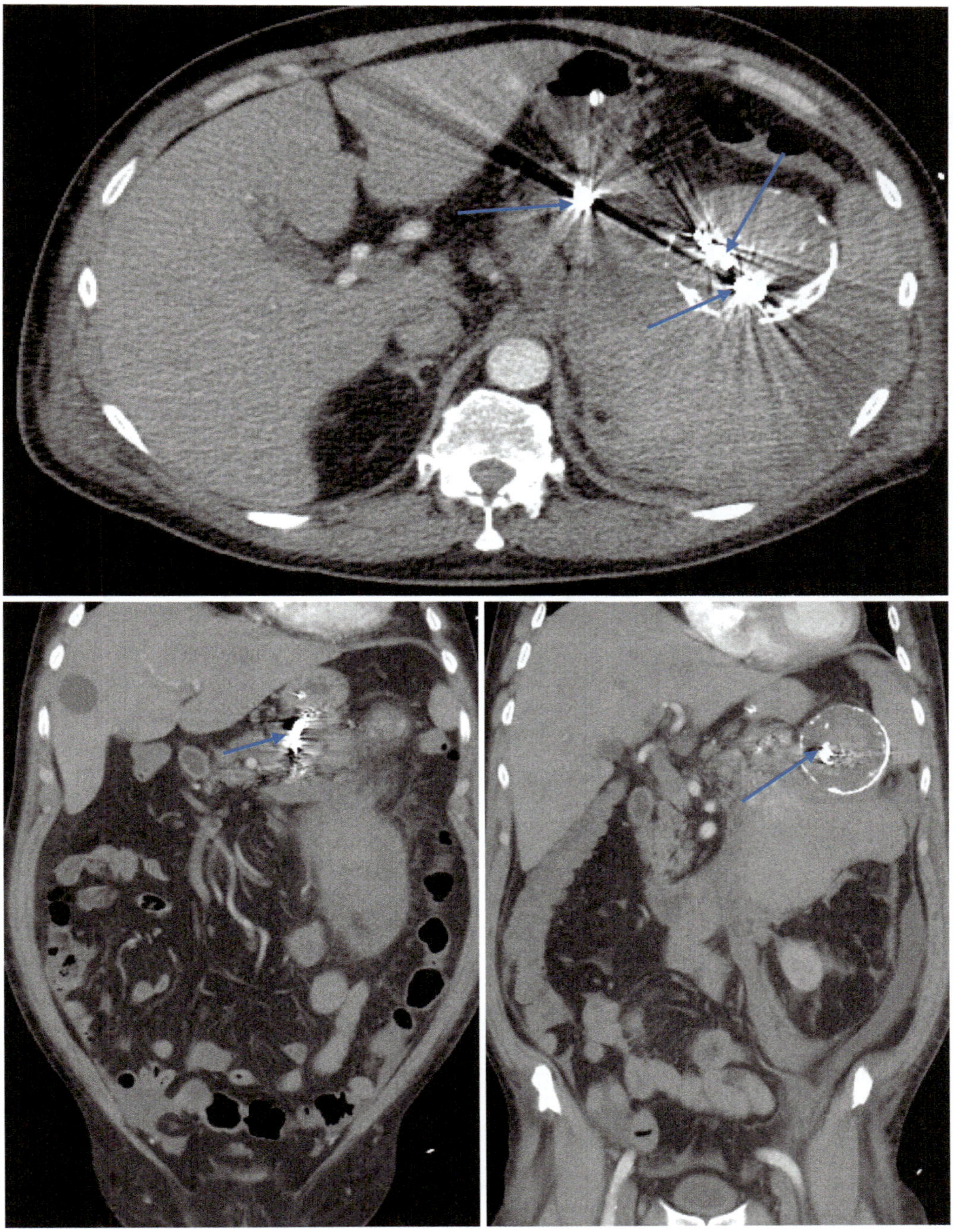

Fig. 4.26 Non–contrast-enhanced CT one-month after embolization. The size of the splenic artery aneurysm had stabilized. Arrows indicate micro-coils

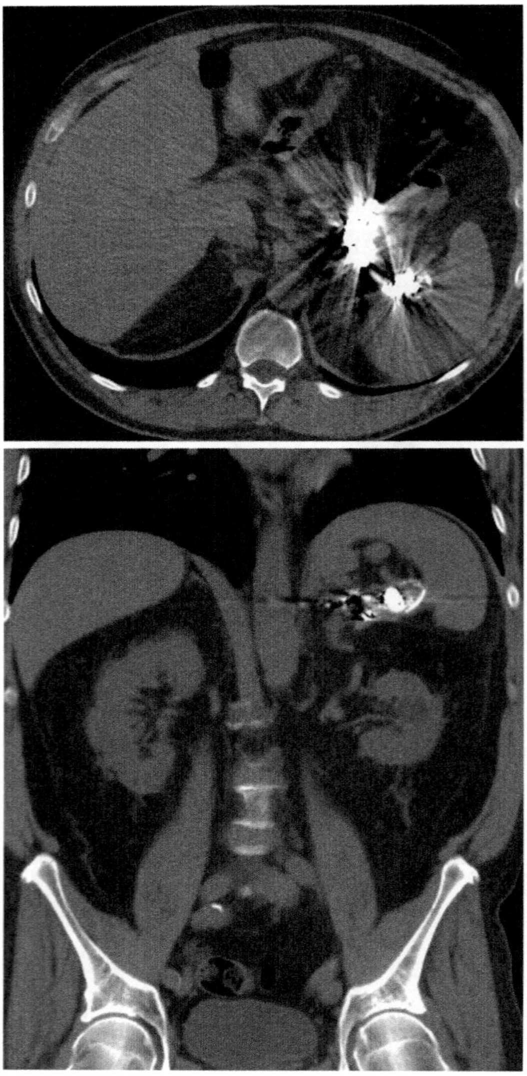

Fig. 4.27 Non–contrast-enhanced CT 1 year after embolization showing splenic artery aneurysm shrinkage

splenic aneurysm and retroperitoneal haematoma. The patient remained haemodynamically stable and had a stable haemoglobin level without the need for blood transfusion. A non-contrast-enhanced CT scan 1 year later showed shrinkage of the splenic aneurysm and resorption of the retroperitoneal haematoma (Fig. 4.27).

4.2.3 Hepatic Artery–I

Key Points
- Left trans-brachial access provides a stable position for stent graft deployment.
- Today, the steerable sheath is of excellent help and can provide a stable position for stent graft deployment.
- For large aneurysms coil embolization can facilitate thrombosis.

4.2.3.1 Aetiology and Clinical Presentation

A 67-year-old patient with advanced-stage chronic obstructive pulmonary disease complained of mild pain in the right upper abdominal quadrant. The pain was not constant and had become more intense in the previous few months. Ultrasound revealed a giant hepatic artery aneurysm, and contrast-enhanced CT was performed to confirm the diagnosis and to plan treatment.

4.2.3.2 Pre-interventional Diagnosis

Contrast-enhanced CT showed a 55 mm proper hepatic artery aneurysm with calcification (Fig. 4.28). There were no signs of rupture. The celiac trunk showed no stenosis, as did the femoral and pelvic arteries. Percutaneous stent graft deployment was planned, aiming to preserve arterial flow to the liver. The diameter of the artery anterior to the aneurysm was 5 mm, and that posterior to the aneurysm was 4.5 mm.

4.2.3.3 Endovascular Treatment

Under local anaesthesia, a 5 Fr multipurpose catheter was percutaneously inserted via the left brachial artery, engaging the celiac trunk, and a 0.035-in. guidewire was advanced into the hepatic artery. A 6 Fr sheath was then advanced into the celiac trunk, through which a diagnostic

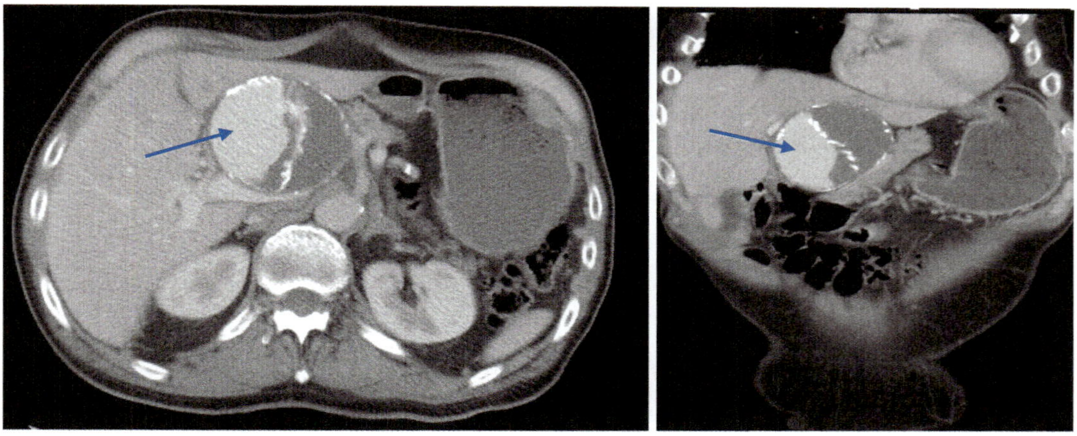

Fig. 4.28 A 55 mm proper hepatic artery aneurysm (arrows)

microcatheter was coaxially advanced into the aneurysm. After that, micro-coils with diameters from 20 mm down to 15 mm were deployed into the aneurysm itself. Two stent grafts with a diameter of 6 mm and a length of 28 mm were advanced and deployed into the proper and common hepatic arteries, and control angiography showed complete aneurysm exclusion (Fig. 4.29). The micro-coils were deployed into the aneurysm to facilitate thrombosis. However, stent grafts alone can be used in such cases as well.

4.2.3.4 Outcome

The patient was discharged from the hospital the next day without complications or pain. Two months after the embolization, the patient complained of pain in the right abdominal quadrant and had a fever of 38 degrees Celsius. The white blood count was 13 /L × 10^9 /L. The patient was suspected of having developed an infection of the stent graft, and an FDG-PET scan showed no infection of the stent graft or aneurysm (Fig. 4.30). No other sources of infection were found during the examination. The patient has recovered from the fever with a white blood cell count within the normal range after 1 week shows no symptoms.

4.2.4 Hepatic Artery-II

Key Points

- Today, the steerable sheath is of excellent help and can provide a stable position for stent graft deployment.
- The portal circulation should be assessed before deciding to occlude the hepatic artery.

4.2.4.1 Aetiology and Clinical Presentation

A 55-year-old patient presented with liver cirrhosis, portal hypertension, ascites and chronic pancreatitis. The patient had previously undergone numerous procedures for ascites and pancreatic cyst drainage, which were complicated with liver and gallbladder cyst collection treated with drainage (Fig. 4.31). The patient complained of mild pain in the right upper abdominal quadrant, which had become more intense in the last month. Contrast-enhanced CT was performed and revealed a 20 mm pseudoaneurysm arising from the cystic artery (Fig. 4.32). The patient did not want to be treated, and control imaging was scheduled.

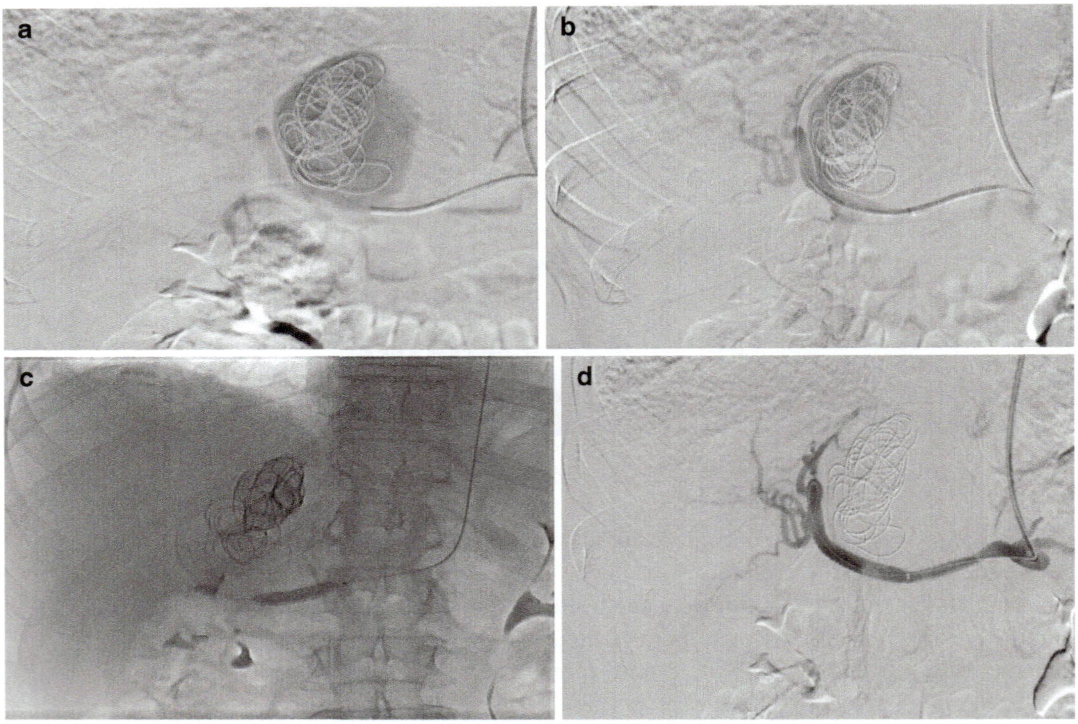

Fig. 4.29 (**a**, **b**) deployment of a number of 20 mm-diameter micro-coils through a microcatheter advanced coaxially into the aneurysm. (**c**, **d**) deployment of the two 6 mm-diameter stent grafts and post-dilatation with a satisfactory result and complete aneurysm exclusion

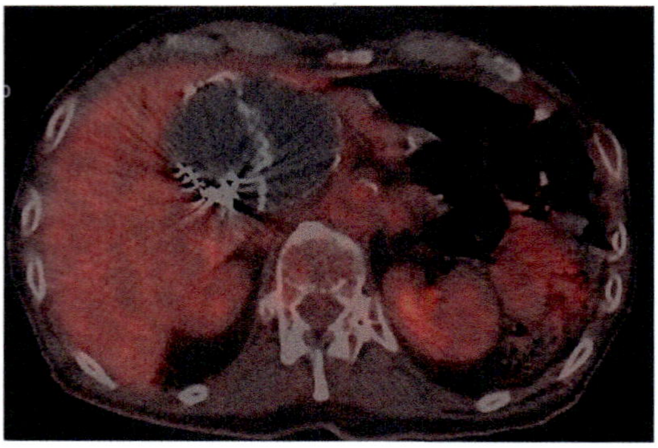

Fig. 4.30 FDG-PET scan showing no aneurysm infection and unchanged aneurysm size

4.2.4.2 Pre-interventional Diagnosis

Approximately 2 months later, the patient experienced severe constant pain but remained haemodynamically stable. Contrast-enhanced CT was performed and showed rapid enlargement of the cystic artery pseudoaneurysm to 50 mm (Fig. 4.33). The desirable option was to preserve flow to the right hepatic artery and deploy a stent graft. If it would not be possible, embolization was another option.

4.2.4.3 Endovascular Treatment

Under local anaesthesia, a 5 Fr sidewinder-shaped catheter was percutaneously inserted through the right femoral artery into the celiac trunk, and a 0.035-in. guidewire was further advanced into the right hepatic artery. After that, a 6 Fr, 90 cm-long sheath was advanced into the proper hepatic artery, and two stent grafts with diameters of 6 mm and lengths of 28 mm were deployed (Fig. 4.34). Control angiography showed a well-deployed stent graft and complete exclusion of the pseudoaneurysm.

The cystic artery was injured during percutaneous drainage, and a pseudoaneurysm developed. In such cases, it is relatively easy to treat either with stent grafts or embolization.

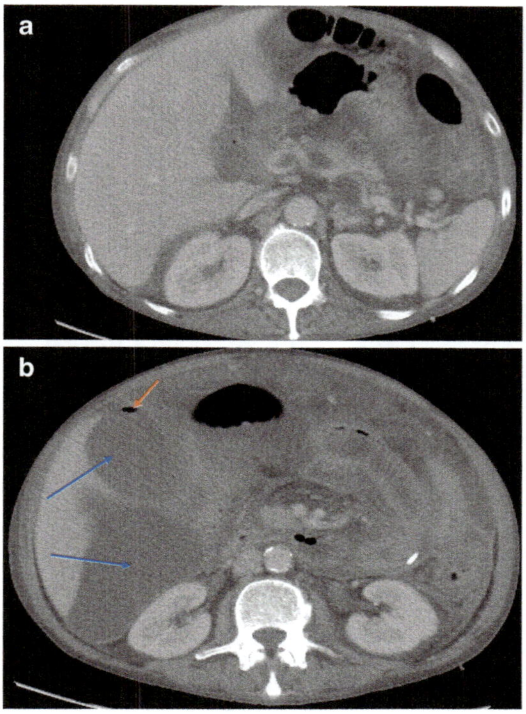

Fig. 4.31 Index CT scan showing ascites and post-pancreatitis cysts (**a**). (**b**) CT scan obtained after a number of ascites and pancreatic cyst drainages showing two new instances of cystic collection- (blue arrows) in the liver and gallbladder, with some air inside one collection (orange arrow) after recent ascites drainage

4.2.4.4 Outcome

The patient did not have ischaemic complications after occlusion of the cystic artery. Three month control CT (Fig. 4.35) showed a satisfactory result and complete resolution of the pseudoaneurysm.

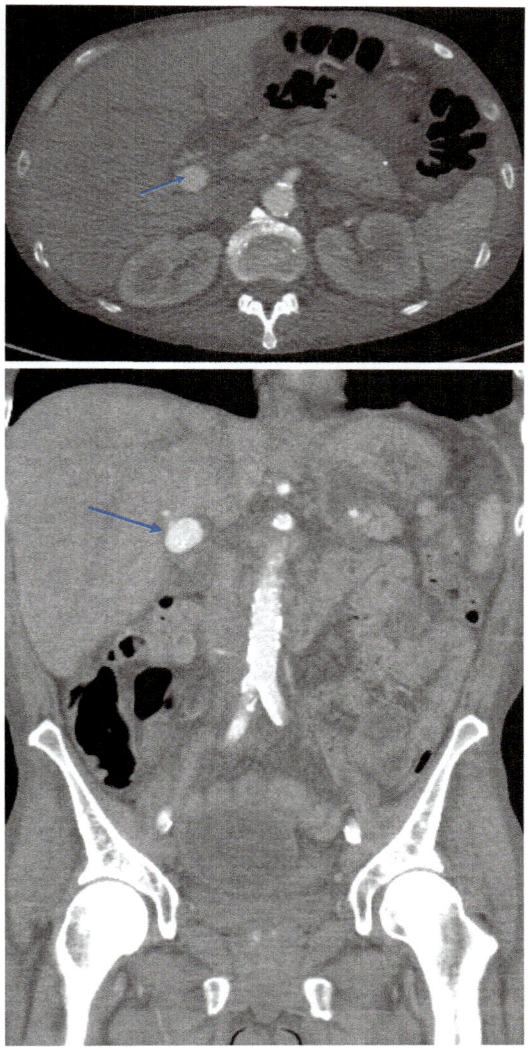

Fig. 4.32 Control contrast-enhanced CT 1 month after the last drainage showing a 20 mm cystic artery pseudoaneurysm (arrows)

4.2.5 Left Gastric Artery

> **Key Points**
> - If it is not possible to achieve a stable catheter position via transfemoral access, liberal left brachial access should be used.
> - A microcatheter should always be used.
> - Usually, 2 or 3 mm-diameter micro-coils are recommended. Today, micro-plugs are available as well.

4.2.5.1 Aetiology and Clinical Presentation

A 68-year-old patient with an implantable cardioverter-defibrillator (ICD) and heart insufficiency with an ejection fraction (EF) of 30% had complained of abdominal pain in the previous 5 days. The patient experienced a drop in blood pressure when the pain began but did not seek help. The blood pressure during the examination was 90/70 mmHg, and haemoglobin was 5.5 mmol/L. Ultrasound of the abdomen showed free fluid, and contrast-enhanced CT was planned.

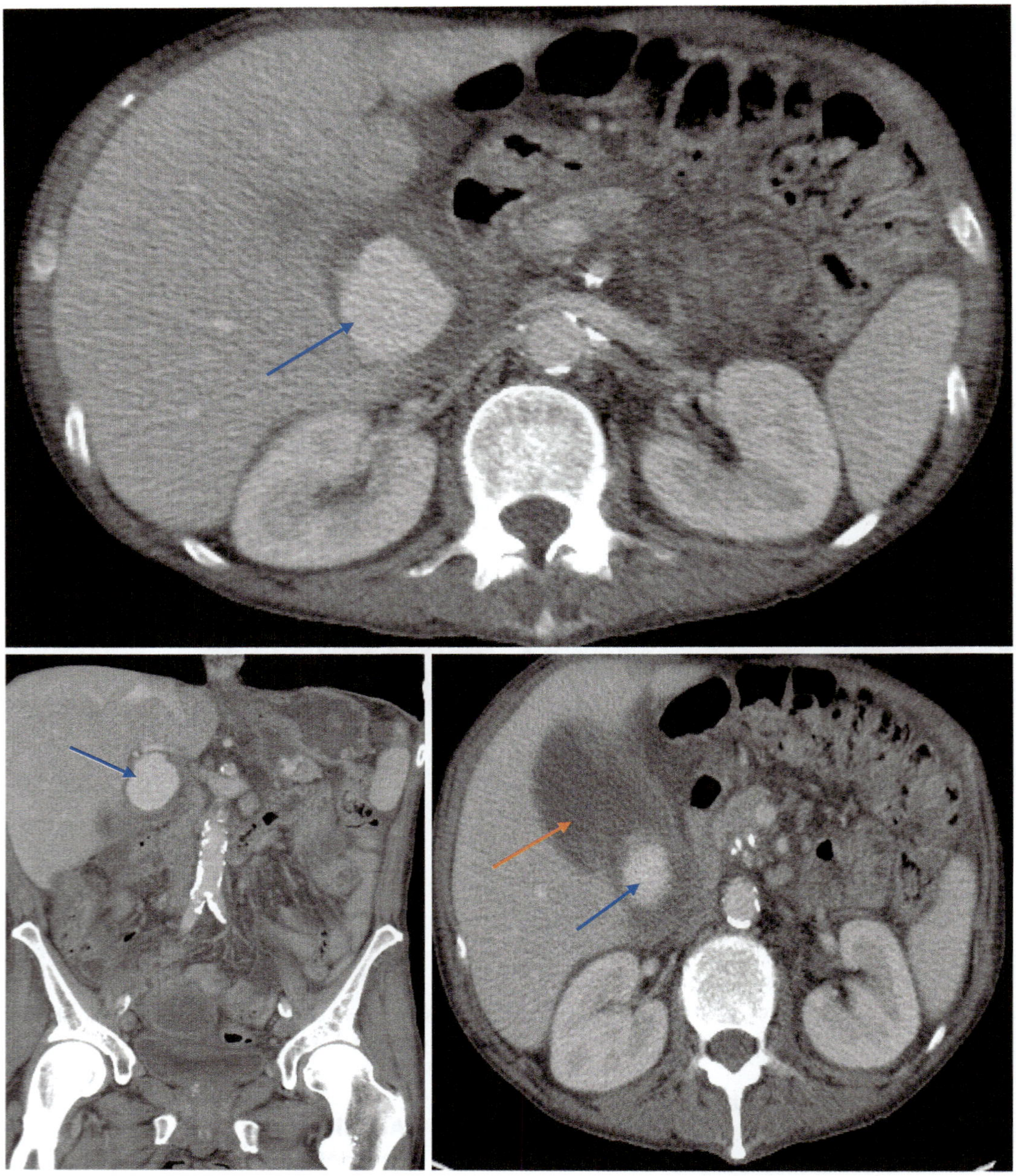

Fig. 4.33 Two months later, CT showed rapid enlargement of the 50 mm gastroduodenal pseudoaneurysm (arrows). The gallbladder was compressed and enlarged (orange arrow)

4.2.5.2 Pre-interventional Diagnosis

Contrast-enhanced CT showed an aneurysm arising from the left gastric artery and intraperitoneal and retroperitoneal haematomas (Fig. 4.36). It was decided to proceed with embolization of the left gastric artery.

4.2.5.3 Endovascular Treatment

Under local anaesthesia, a 5 Fr multipurpose catheter was inserted percutaneously through the left brachial artery for selective catheterization of the celiac trunk and further super-selective angiography of the left gastric artery. Angiography showed

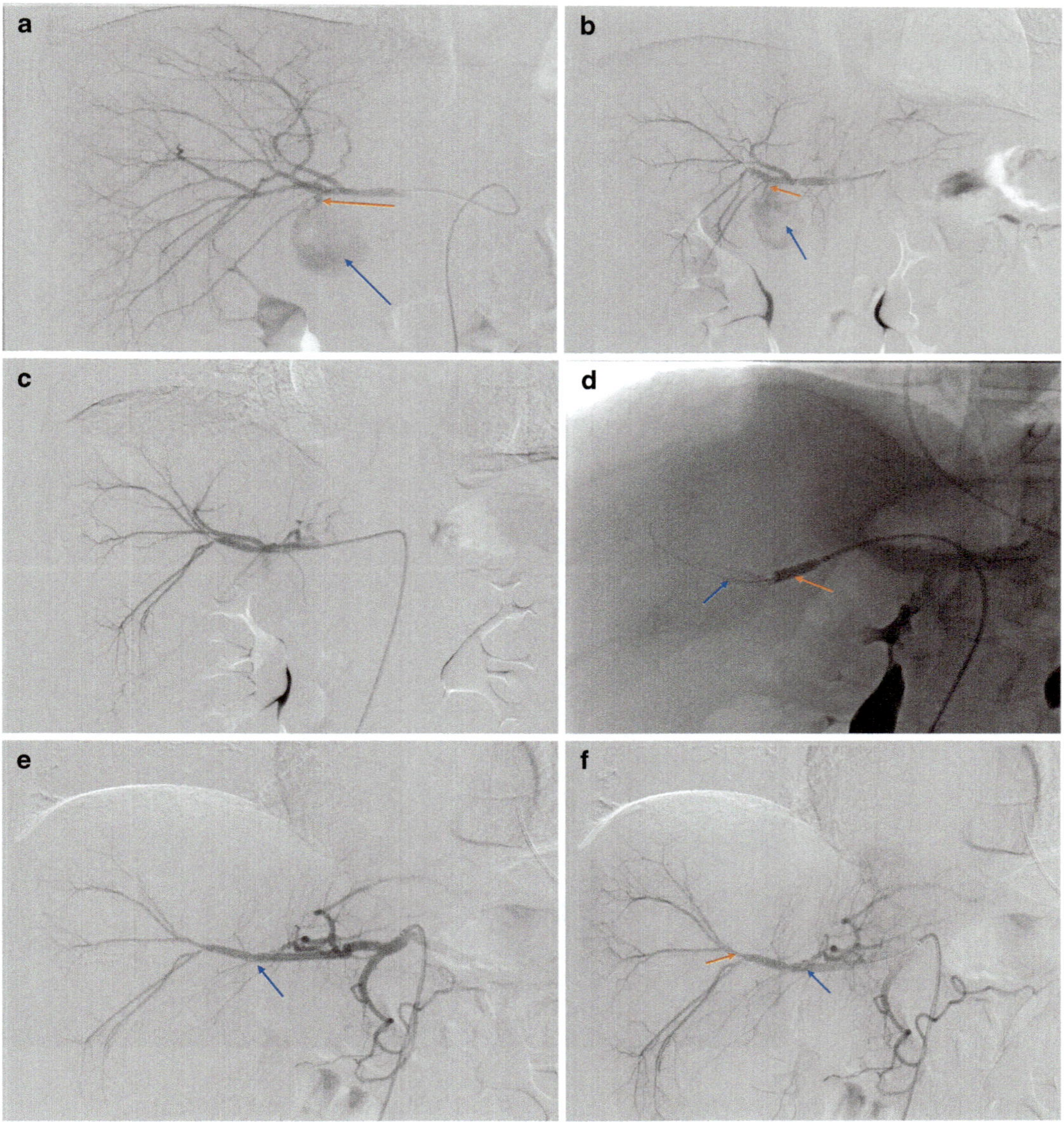

Fig. 4.34 Angiography showed a cystic artery pseudoaneurysm (blue arrow). Orange arrow indicates the origin of the cystic artery (**a**, **b**). (**c**, **d**) deployment of two 6 mm-diameter stents grafts. Blue arrow indicates the first stent graft. Orange arrow indicates the second stent graft. Control angiography shows well-deployed stent graft- (blue arrows). Orange arrow indicates spastic vessels after withdrawal of the guidewire (**e**, **f**)

aneurysms of the left gastric artery and discrete contrast extravasation (Fig. 4.37). A 0.021 in. micro-catheter was further advanced coaxially into the left gastric artery, and embolization was performed with 2 and 3 mm-diameter micro-coils. Final control imaging showed satisfactory results and arrested bleeding. The other branches of the coeliac trunk were patent (Fig. 4.37).

4.2.5.4 Outcome

The patient did not experience any complications during the follow-up. Three month control contrast-enhanced CT (Fig. 4.38) showed a thrombosed left gastric aneurysm and complete resorption of the retroperitoneal haematoma. The patient was haemodynamically stable and had a stable haemoglobin level.

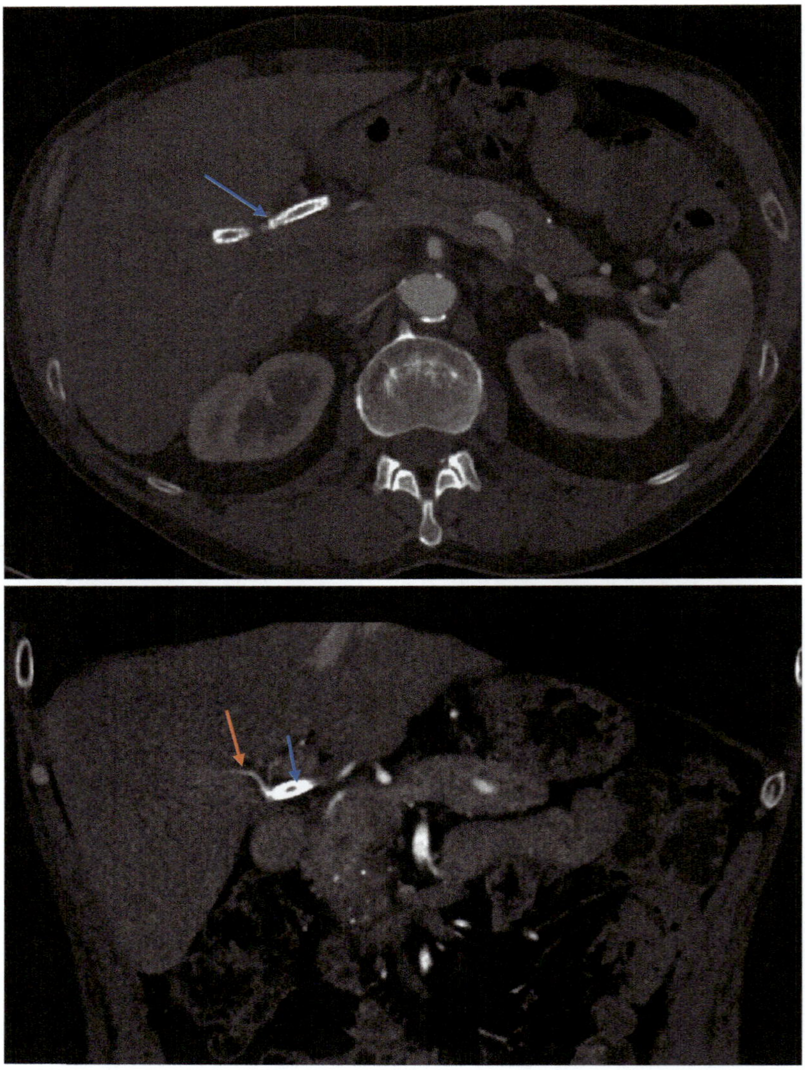

Fig. 4.35 Control contrast-enhanced CT showing complete resolution of the pseudoaneurysm. It is difficult to assess the flow in the stent (blue arrows), but there is flow behind the stent graft (orange arrow)

4.2.6 Gastroduodenal Artery I

Key Points

- The "front and back door" should always be embolized.
- Compression on the celiac trunk by the crus diaphragm has been described as the cause of gastroduodenal artery arcade aneurysm development.
- Microcatheters should always be used in such cases to perform a safe embolization.

4.2.6.1 Aetiology and Clinical Presentation

A 39-year-old healthy patient was admitted to the emergency department in hypovolemic shock after an acute onset of sharp abdominal pain approximately 6 h prior. The blood pressure was 80/50 mmHg, and there was no trauma in the anamnesis. Acute blood control revealed a drop in haemoglobin to 4.7 mmol/L. Abdominal ultrasound revealed free fluid in the abdomen, and haemoperitoneum was suspected. Emergency CT was scheduled. The patient responded well to resuscitation and blood transfusion, with blood pressure increasing to 110/70 mmHg, and remained stable.

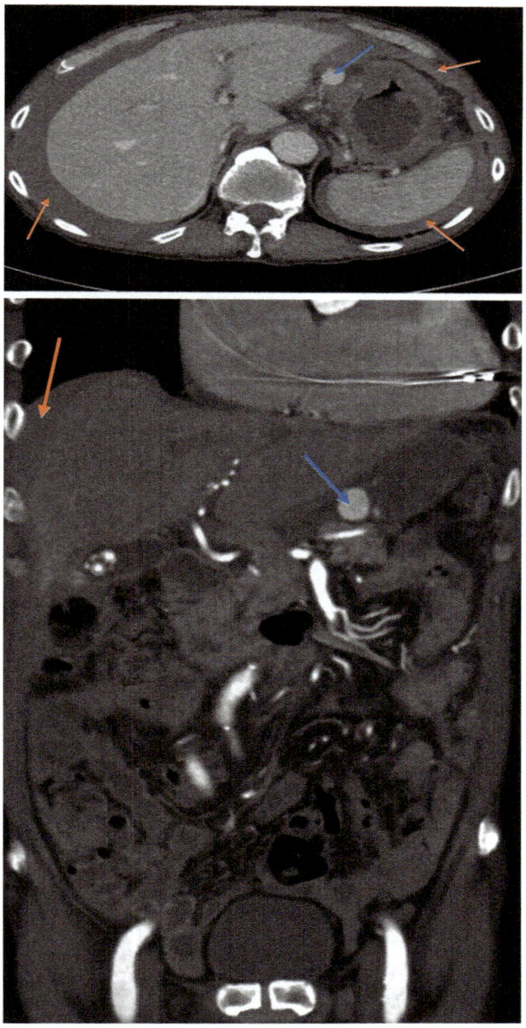

Fig. 4.36 Contrast-enhanced CT showing a 22 mm left gastric artery aneurysm (blue arrows) and haematoma around the liver and spleen (orange arrows)

4.2.6.2 Pre-interventional Diagnosis

Contrast-enhanced CT showed a ruptured pancreaticoduodenal arterial arcade aneurysm with intraperitoneal haematoma (Fig. 4.39). The celiac trunk was slightly compressed with the diaphragmatic ligament, and no other abnormalities were seen on CT. Emergency embolization was scheduled.

4.2.6.3 Endovascular Treatment

Under local anaesthesia, a 5 Fr cobra-shaped catheter was percutaneously inserted through the right femoral artery for selective catheterization of the superior mesenteric artery. The same catheter was also used to perform selective angiography through the inferior pancreaticoduodenal artery, which confirmed a pancreaticoduodenal arterial arcade aneurysm (Fig. 4.40). The 0.021 in. microcatheter was further advanced into the inferior pancreaticoduodenal artery, and embolization with 3 mm-diameter micro-coils was performed. After that, selective catheterization of the celiac trunk and super-selective catheterization of the gastroduodenal artery to embolize the "front door" were performed with the same microcatheter. Micro-coils with diameters of 3 and 5 mm were used, and control imaging showed a satisfactory result and no complications. One complication that can occur in such a situation is compartment syndrome, and laparotomy can be required in a case of multiorgan failure.

4.2.6.4 Outcome

The patient complained the next day of abdominal pain but remained haemodynamically stable. Control CT was performed to exclude residual bleeding and showed a satisfactory result without bleeding (Fig. 4.41). The patient recovered very well and did not develop any complications. Three-month control CT showed complete resolution of the intraperitoneal haematoma (Fig. 4.42). The aneurysm in this patient remains with an unknown aetiology. Compression of the celiac trunk can cause hyperdynamic flow through the pancreaticoduodenal artery and, consequently, aneurysm development.

4.2.7 Gastroduodenal Artery II

Key Points

- Post-pancreatitis pseudoaneurysms usually involve the splenic and gastroduodenal arteries.
- Both the gastroduodenal and pancreaticoduodenal arteries or the aneurysm itself should be occluded in such cases.
- A microcatheter should always be used.

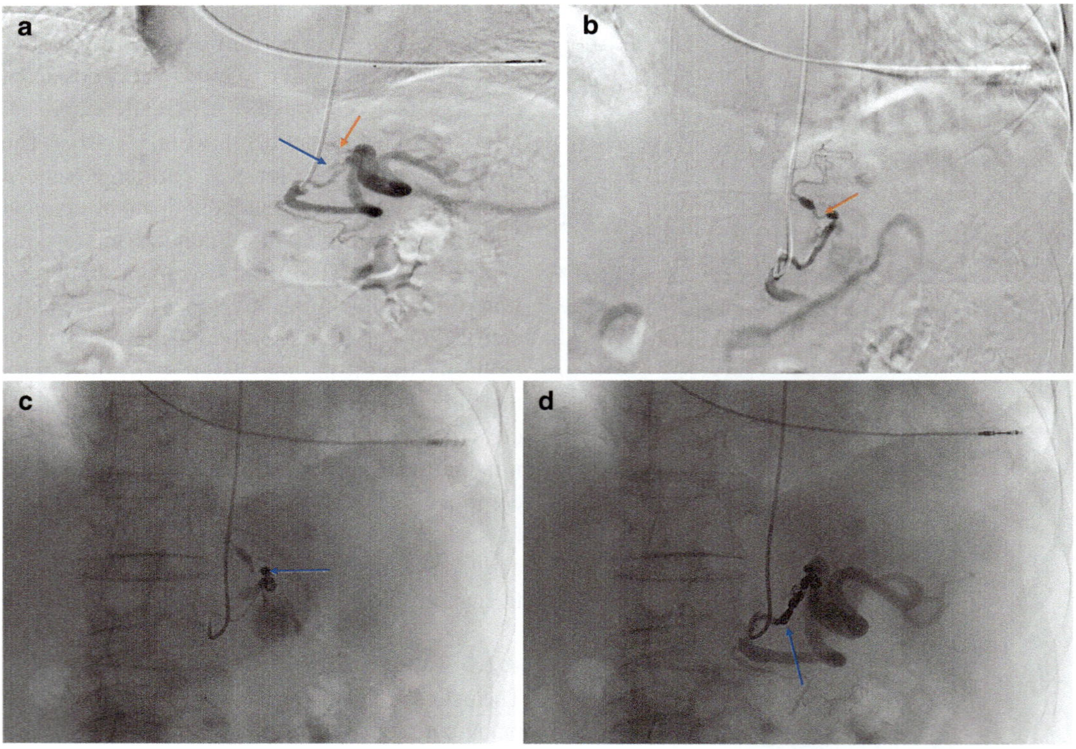

Fig. 4.37 Selective angiography of the left gastric artery, (**a**) blue arrow indicates discrete bleeding. Orange arrow indicates the spastic artery distal to the bleeding point (**b**). (**c**) blue arrow indicates the initially deployed 2 mm-diameter micro-coils. (**d**) blue arrow indicates finally deployed 3 mm-diameter micro-coils

4.2.7.1 Aetiology and Clinical Presentation

A 59-year-old patient with liver cirrhosis, portal hypertension and post-pancreatitis was admitted to the emergency department with abdominal pain. The patient previously experienced bleeding from oesophageal varices that were treated endoscopically and with medications. There was no bleeding at the time of admission, but the pain in the abdomen was constant. Control blood test did not show signs of acute pancreatitis. Abdominal ultrasound showed a visceral artery aneurysm, and contrast-enhanced CT was scheduled.

4.2.7.2 Pre-interventional Diagnosis

Contrast-enhanced CT showed a 67 mm gastroduodenal aneurysm/pseudoaneurysm with partial thrombosis. There was no active contrast extravasation (Fig. 4.43). The plan was to preserve the flow through the hepatic artery and to treat the aneurysm/pseudoaneurysm with a stent graft.

4.2.7.3 Endovascular Treatment

Under local anaesthesia, a 5 Fr sidewinder-shaped catheter was percutaneously inserted through the right femoral artery into the celiac trunk. A 0.035 inch guidewire and a 6 Fr sheath were advanced into the right hepatic artery. It was not possible to either secure a stable position for the sheath or to advance the stent graft via the femoral artery. Therefore, advancement of the stent graft through the left brachial artery was attempted, but this, too, failed. It was

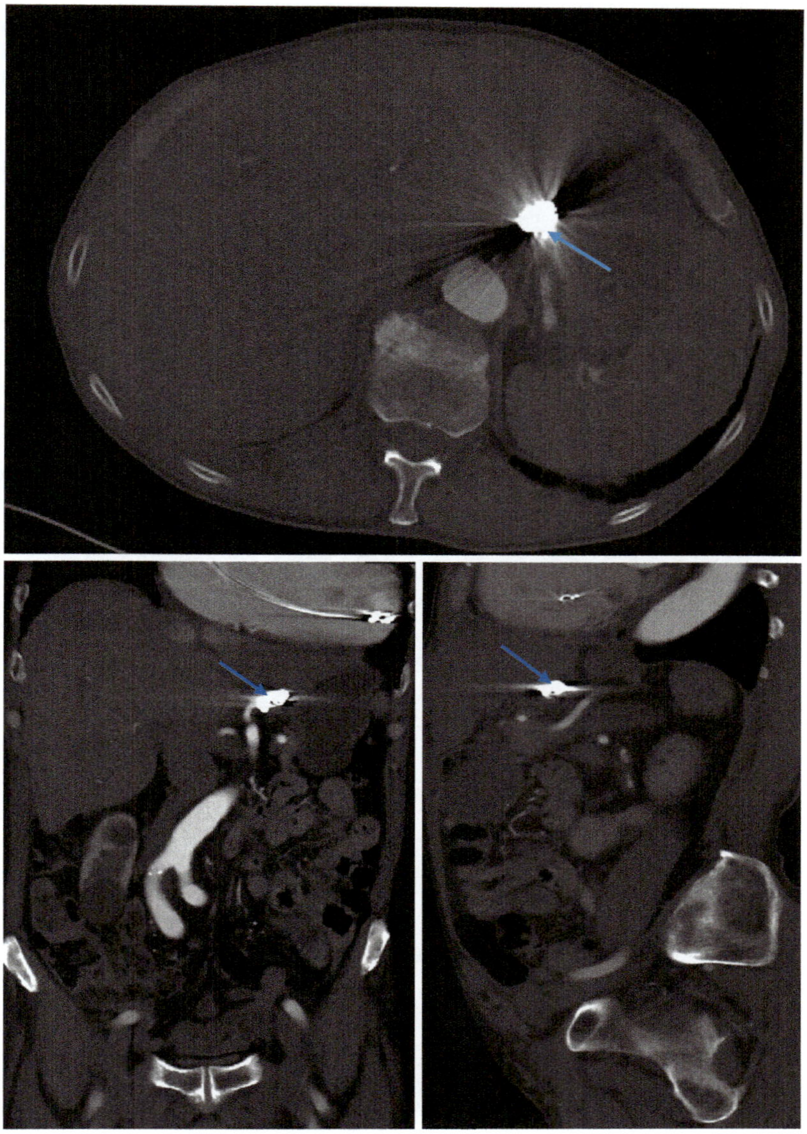

Fig. 4.38 Contrast-enhanced CT 3 months after embolization, showing resorptions of the intraabdominal haematoma and completely thrombosed left gastric artery aneurysms. Blue arrows indicate micro-coils

decided to perform embolization of the aneurysm itself with multiple micro-coils deployed through the microcatheter to preserve the hepatic artery flow. Finally, the origin of the gastroduodenal artery was occluded with a 6 mm Amplatz plug deployed through the 5 Fr diagnostic catheter, securing complete aneurysm exclusion (Fig. 4.44). Spasm of the hepatic artery resolved spontaneously after withdrawal of the different materials.

4.2.7.4 Outcome

The patient did not experience any complications and was discharged without pain. Three months later, control CT showed a completely thrombosed gastroduodenal artery aneurysm (Fig. 4.45).

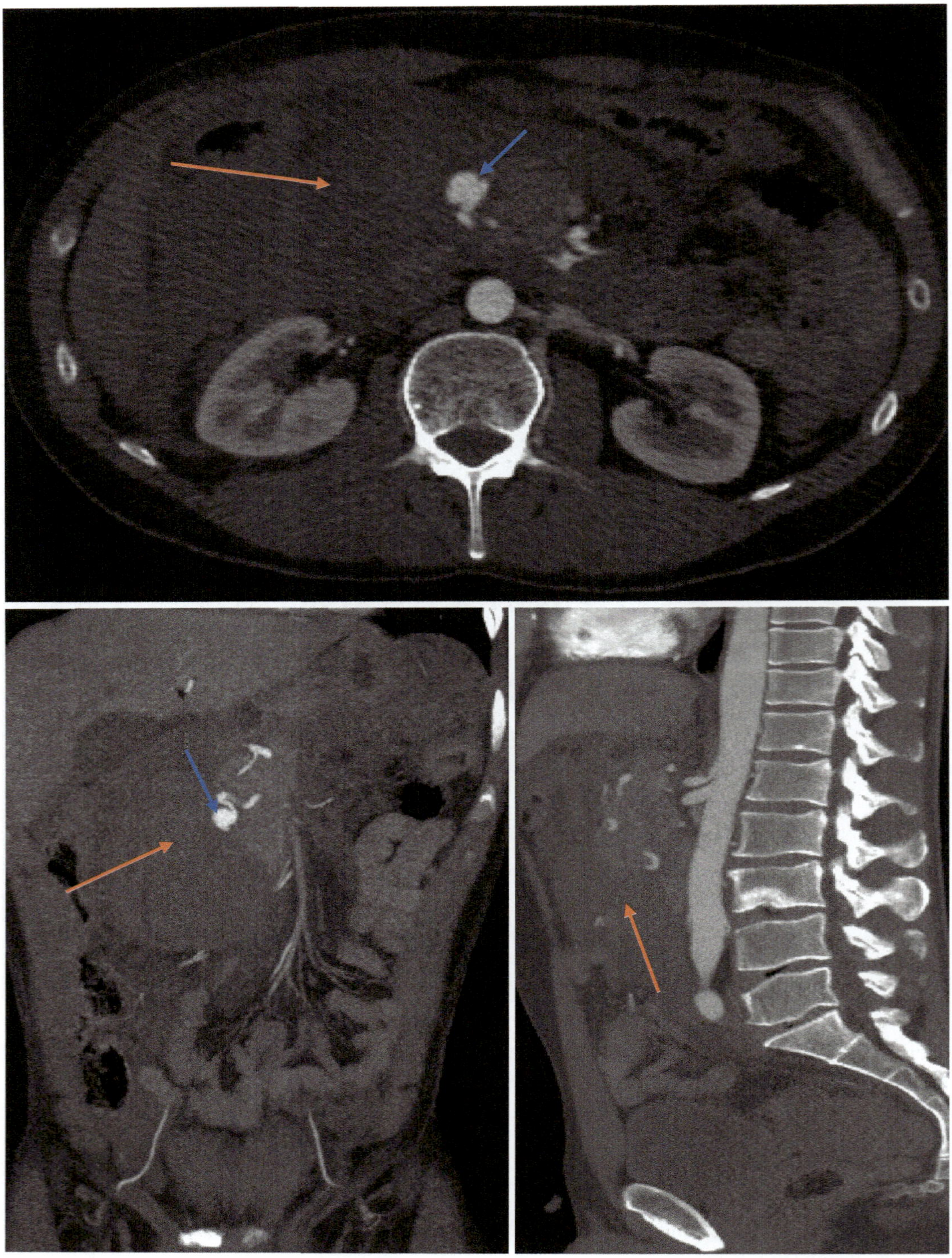

Fig. 4.39 Ruptured pancreaticoduodenal arterial arcade aneurysm (blue arrows). Orange arrows indicate intraperitoneal haematoma

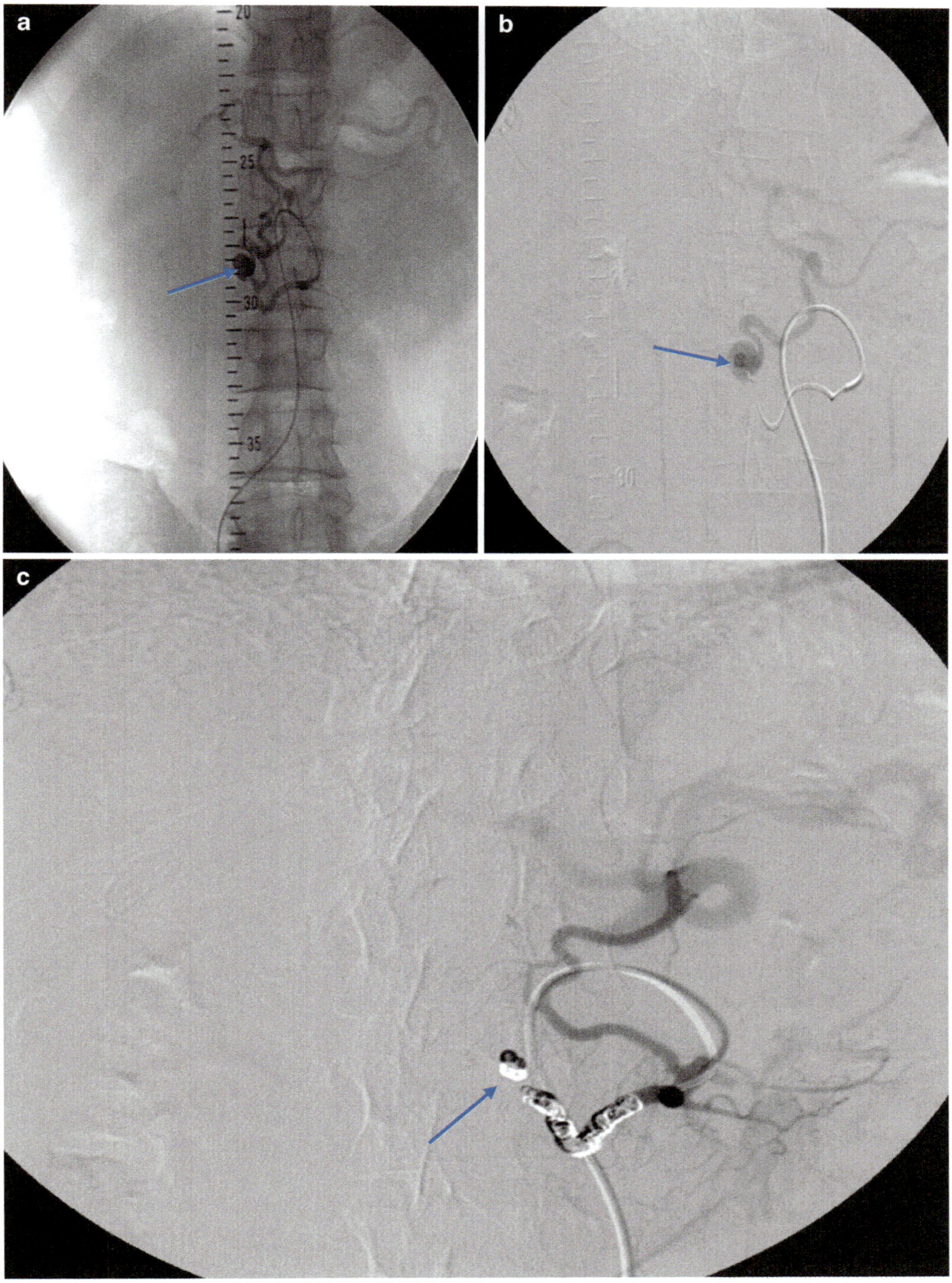

Fig. 4.40 Selective angiography of the inferior pancreaticoduodenal artery arising from the superior mesenteric artery shows a pancreaticoduodenal arterial arcade aneurysm (blue arrows) (**a**, **b**). (**c**) embolization of the "back door" with 3 mm-diameter micro-coils deployed through a microcatheter. (**d**) advancement of the microcatheter into the celiac trunk and further into the gastroduodenal artery to occlude the "front door". The blue arrow indicates that the tip of the microcatheter has advanced into the gastroduodenal artery. (**e**) final control image after occlusion of the "front door" (orange arrow) and "back door" (blue arrow). The micro-coils had diameters of 3 or 5 mm

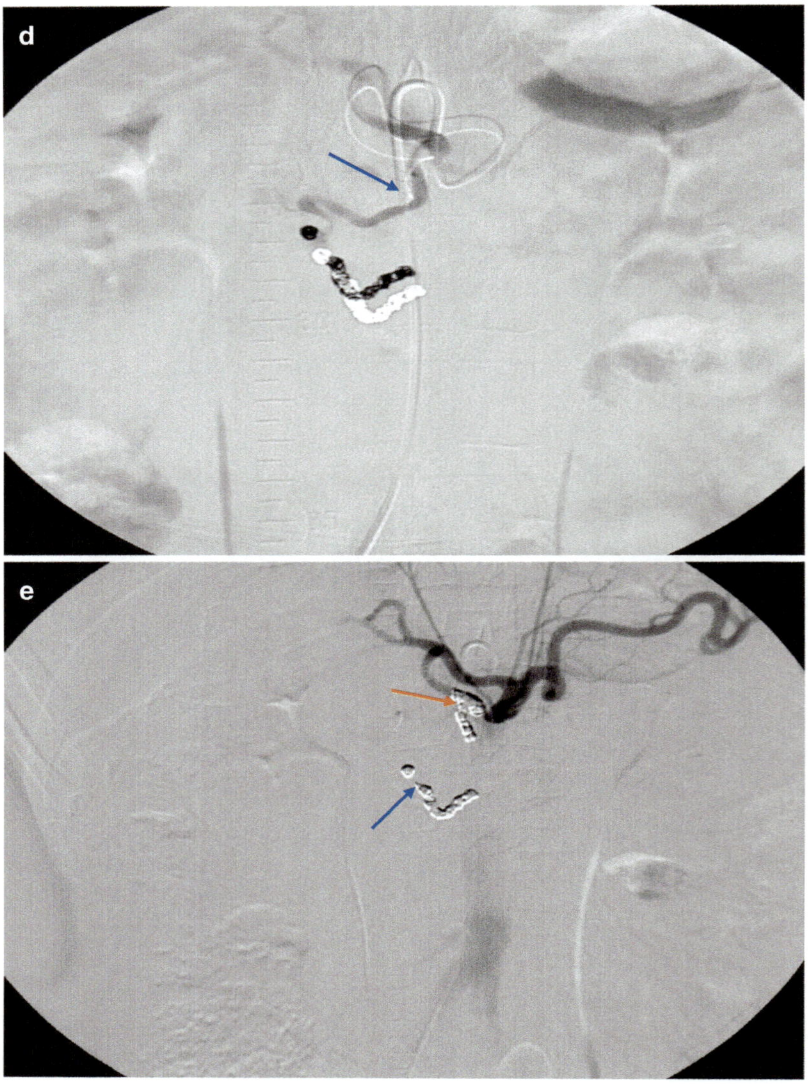

Fig. 4.40 (continued)

4.2.8 Superior Mesenteric Artery

> **Key Points**
> - Patients with impaired coagulation status can be treated with micro-plugs or hydro micro-coils.
> - CT imaging should be available before treatment decisions are made.
> - Microcatheters should always be used.
> - Glue is a potent embolic agent, but experience is essential.

4.2.8.1 Aetiology and Clinical Presentation

A 62-year-old patient with arterial hypertension was admitted to the emergency department with signs of hypovolemia after a sudden onset of sharp abdominal pain. No other comorbidities were present. Abdominal ultrasound confirmed free fluid in the abdomen, and an urgent CT scan was performed. The haemodynamic status deteriorated as blood pressure fell to 50/40 mmHg. Acute explorative laparotomy was performed, but the bleeding site could not be found. Abdominal packing was

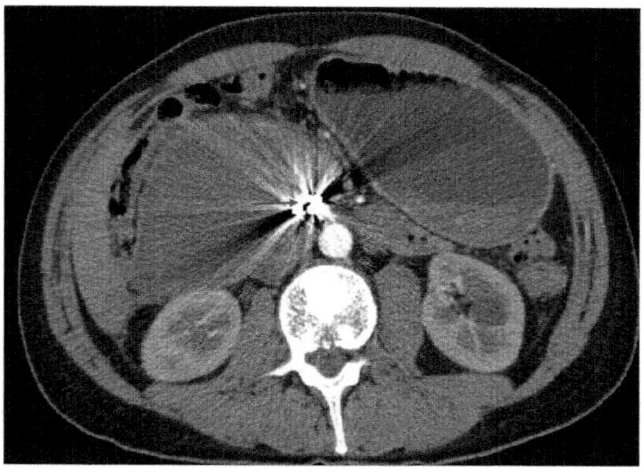

Fig. 4.41 Control CT performed the next day showing a satisfactory result. No expansion of the haematoma was observed, and the patient remained haemodynamically stable. Arrow indicates micro-coils in the gastroduodenal artery

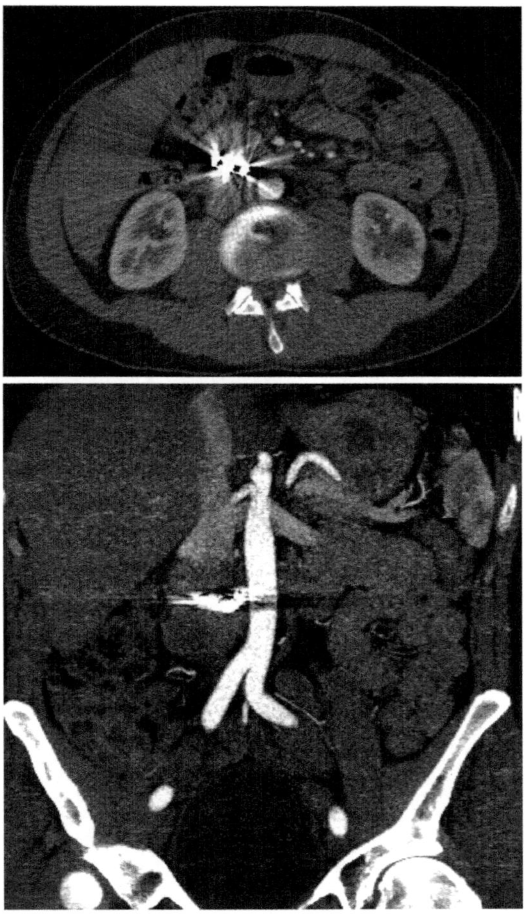

Fig. 4.42 Control contrast-enhanced CT 3 months after embolization showing complete resorption of the intraperitoneal haematoma

performed, and the haemodynamic status improved. The patient responded to resuscitation therapy.

4.2.8.2 Pre-interventional Diagnosis

Acute contrast-enhanced CT showed intraperitoneal haematoma and minimal contrast extravasation around the duodenum/jejunum (Fig. 4.46). After the CT scan, the patient underwent acute laparotomy. The next day, the patient's haemodynamic status deteriorated with ongoing bleeding. Control CT was performed and showed active bleeding from the superior mesenteric artery branch (Fig. 4.47).

4.2.8.3 Endovascular Treatment

A 5 Fr sidewinder-shaped catheter was inserted percutaneously through the right femoral artery for selective angiography of the superior mesenteric artery, which showed bleeding from the jejunal branch (Fig. 4.48). After that, a microcatheter was further advanced into the jejunal branch. The bleeding jejunal artery had a diameter of 1.9 mm, and the intention was to attempt to occlude only the bleeding artery. If the bleeding could not be arrested, the plan was to sacrifice an additional jejunal artery, followed by eventual bowel resection. The microcatheter was advanced into the bleeding artery as far as possible. Small micro-coils with a diameter of 2 mm were deployed very carefully. Control angiography showed arrested bleeding, and only the bleeding vessels were occluded. All other jejunal branches were open. The intervention went well, and the patient recovered gradually. There was no need for bowel resection, and the patient did not develop compartment syndrome.

4.2.8.4 Outcome

The patient did not experience any complications during the recovery period. There were no new bleeding episodes, and the patient remains haemodynamically stable. We believe that a small visceral aneurysm ruptured in a healthy patient and caused hypovolemic shock and intraabdominal bleeding. No other visceral aneurysms were observed.

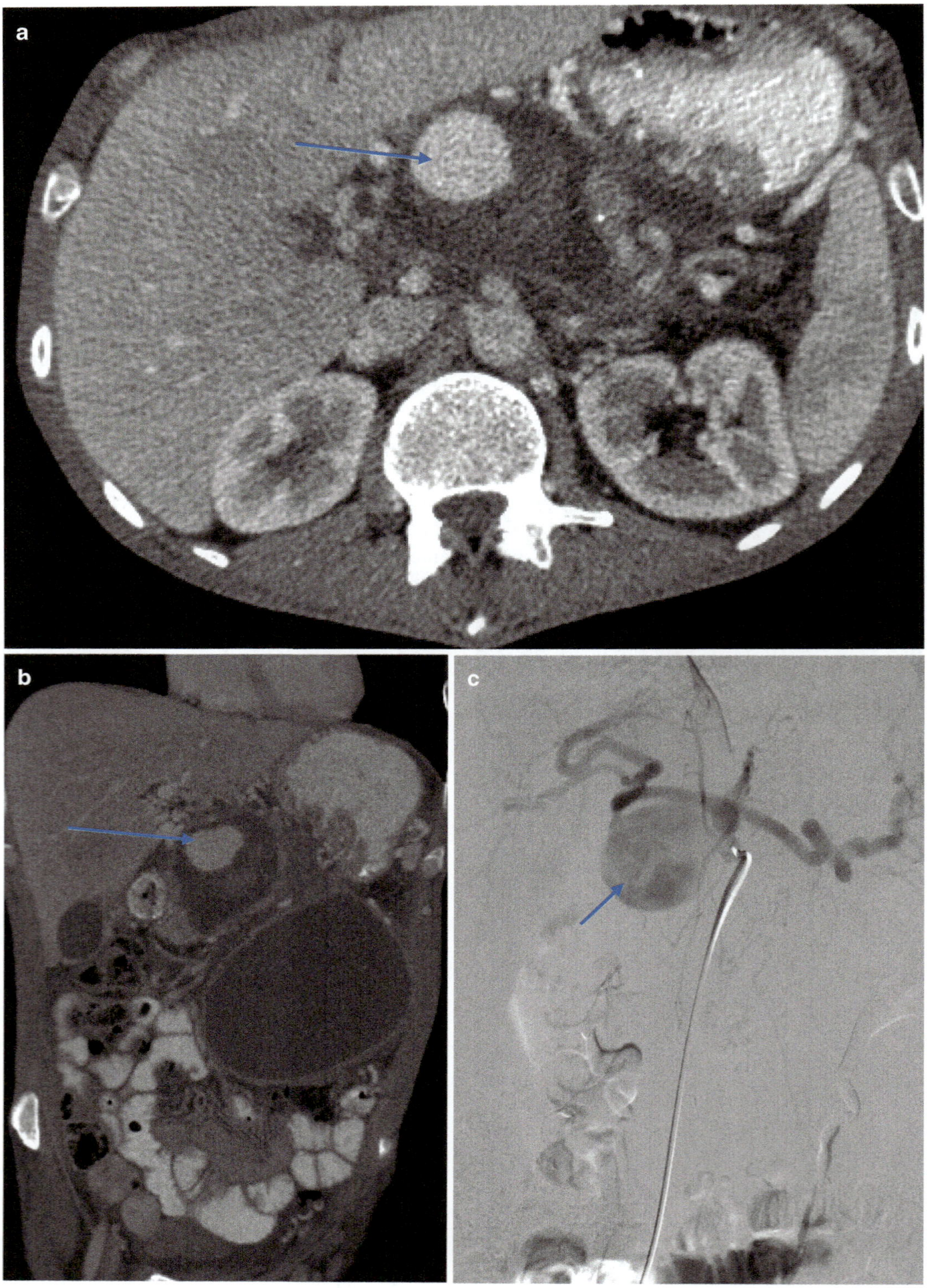

Fig. 4.43 (**a**, **b**) CT showing a vast gastroduodenal aneurysm (blue arrows). (**c**) angiography obtained through femoral access; arrow indicates the aneurysm. It was not possible to advance the stent graft, and thus left brachial access was prepared

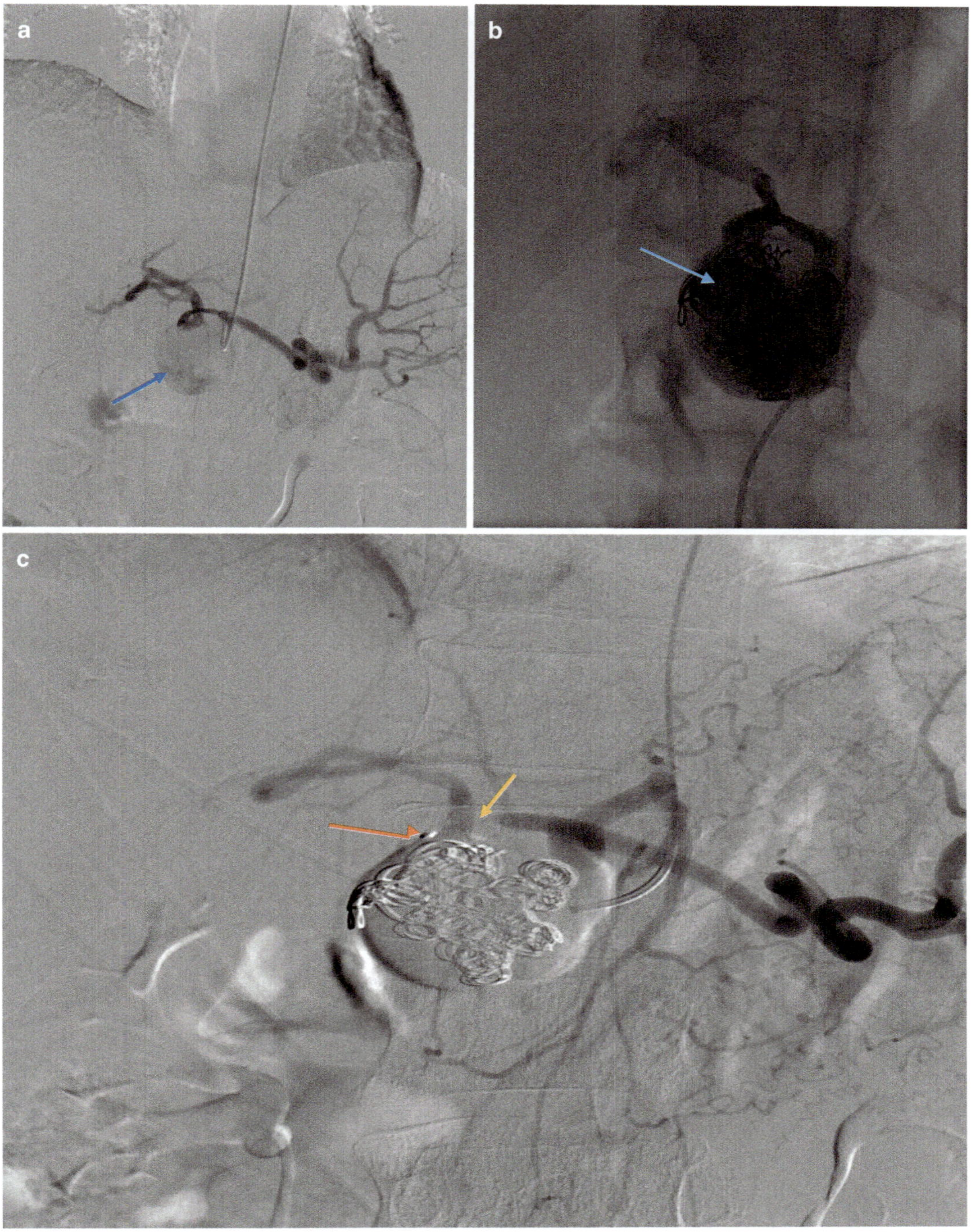

Fig. 4.44 Angiography via left brachial access. It was not possible to advance the stent graft; therefore, the aneurysm was embolized at the origin of the gastroduodenal artery. Blue arrows indicate the aneurysm (**a**, **b**). (**c**) orange arrow indicates the tip of the 6 mm Amplatz Plug used to occlude the origin of the gastroduodenal artery. Yellow arrow indicates the spastic hepatic artery after manipulation with different materials

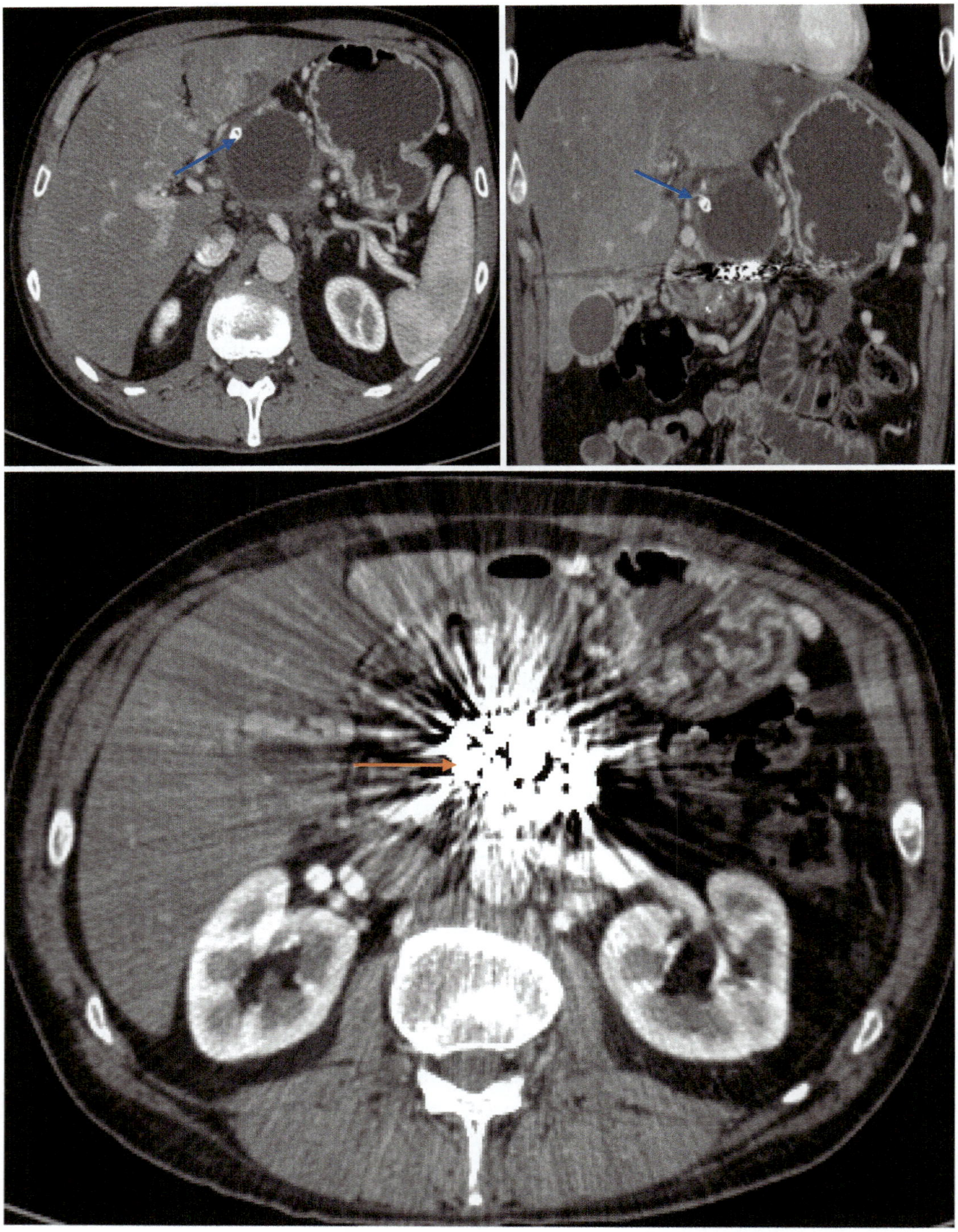

Fig. 4.45 Three months later, control CT showing a completely thrombosed gastroduodenal artery- Blue arrows indicate the tip of the Amplatz plug. Orange arrow indicates the micro-coils inside the aneurysm

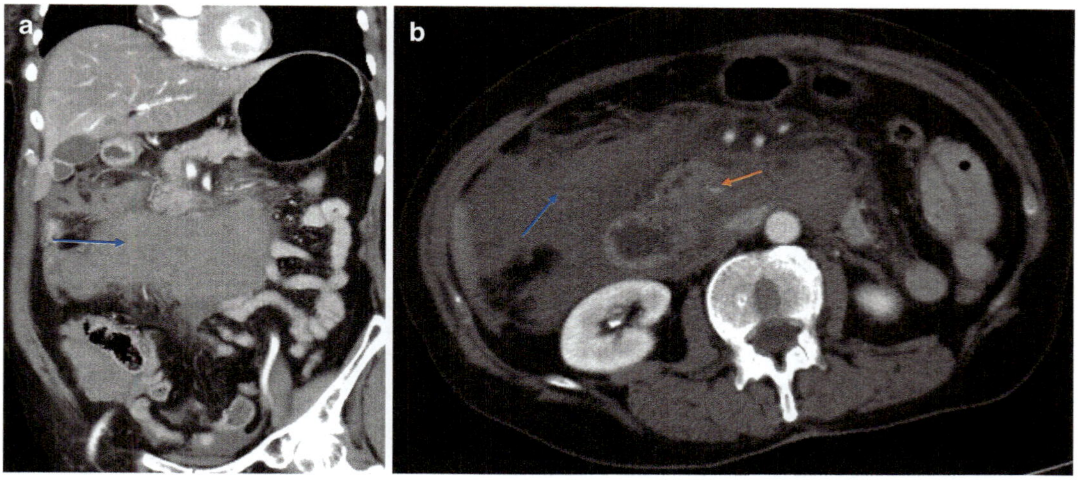

Fig. 4.46 Index contrast-enhanced CT showing intraperitoneal haematoma (**a** and **b**) (blue arrows). (**b**) orange arrow indicates a small focus with active bleeding

4.2.9 Inferior Mesenteric Artery

Key Points

- CT imaging should be carefully assessed before treatment decisions are made.
- Microcatheters should always be used, and super-selective embolization should always be performed.
- Liquid embolic agents should never be used for arteriovenous fistulas.

4.2.9.1 Aetiology and Clinical Presentation

A 67-year-old patient underwent aortic surgery due to a 6 cm abdominal aortic aneurysm 7 years prior. The patient was not controlled after the surgery. In the last few months, the patient complained of constant pain in the lower abdomen. There were no other symptoms or abnormalities. Abdominal ultrasound showed an enlarged inferior mesenteric artery, and a CT scan was scheduled.

4.2.9.2 Pre-interventional Diagnosis

Contrast-enhanced CT showed an enlarged, dilated inferior mesenteric artery, an aneurysm at the distal part and an arteriovenous fistula (Fig. 4.49). The inferior mesenteric vein was dilated as well. Embolization of the arteriovenous fistula and aneurysm was planned.

4.2.9.3 Endovascular Treatment

Under local anaesthesia, a 5 Fr pigtail catheter was percutaneously inserted through the right femoral artery for abdominal aortography, and a sidewinder catheter was used for selective angiography of the inferior mesenteric artery (Fig. 4.50). The microcatheter was coaxially advanced close to the aneurysm, and micro-coils with diameters of 10 mm were used for embolization with a satisfactory outcome. The diameter of the artery proximal to the aneurysm and fistula was 6–6.5 mm, and 10 mm micro-coils were used to avoid potential migration due to high flow through the fistula.

4.2.9.4 Outcome

The patient did not experience any complications during the follow-up, and the pain disappeared. Contrast-enhanced CT 3 months after embolization showed a thrombosed aneurysm and an occluded arteriovenous fistula (Fig. 4.51).

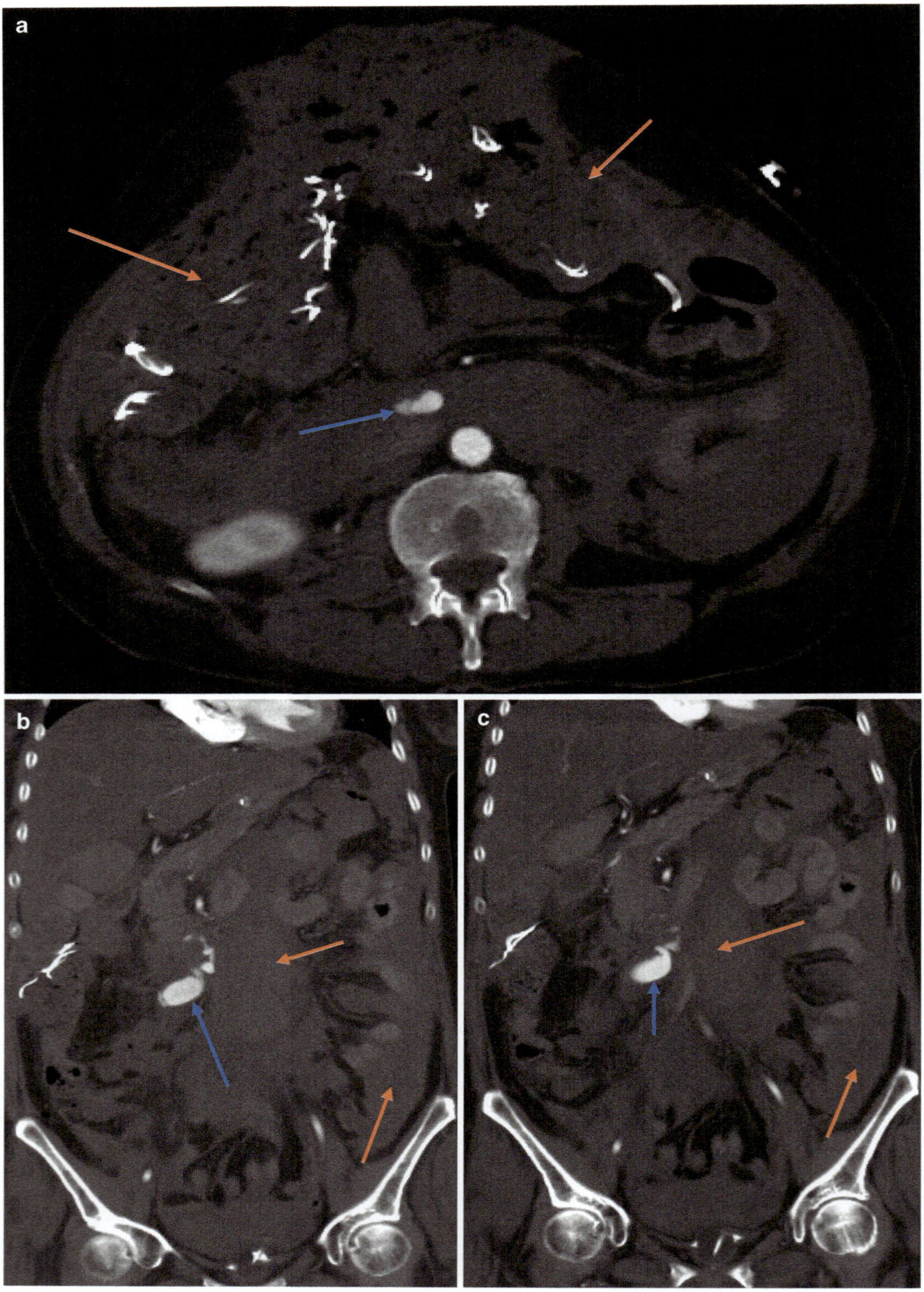

Fig. 4.47 Control contrast-enhanced CT after explorative laparotomy and packing. The patient was haemodynamically unstable with clinical signs of ongoing bleeding. Active bleeding was observed from the superior mesenteric artery branch (blue arrows). Orange arrow indicates gauze (**a**). (**b**, **c**) orange arrows indicate haemoperitoneum

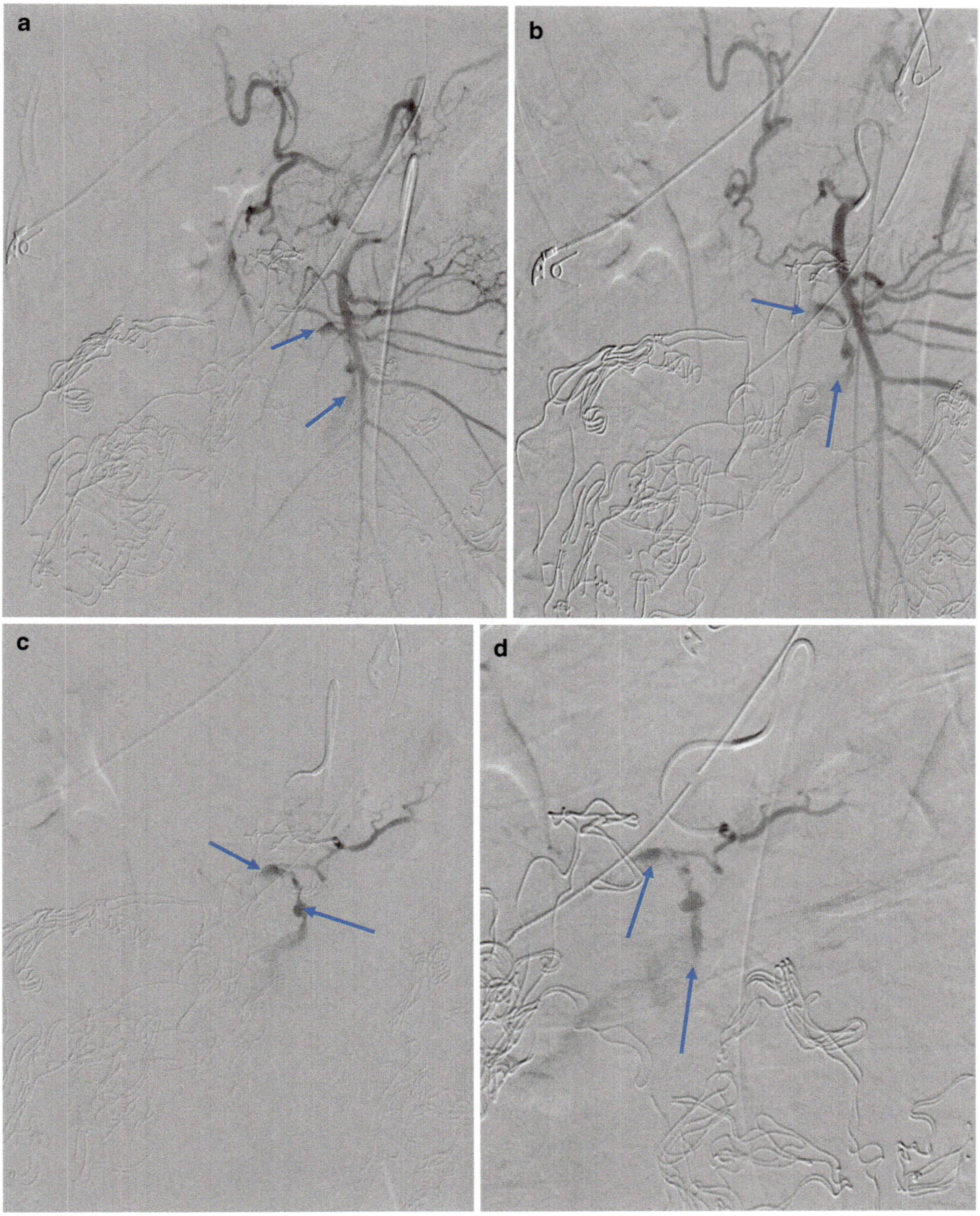

Fig. 4.48 Selective superior mesenteric artery angiography showing active bleeding from the jejunal branches (arrows) (**a**, **b**). (**c**, **d**) images; super-selective angiography advanced through a microcatheter of the jejunal artery with active bleeding (arrows). (**e**) the diameter of the bleeding artery was 1.93 mm. (**f**, **g**) control imaging after successful embolization with 2 mm micro-coils –(arrows)

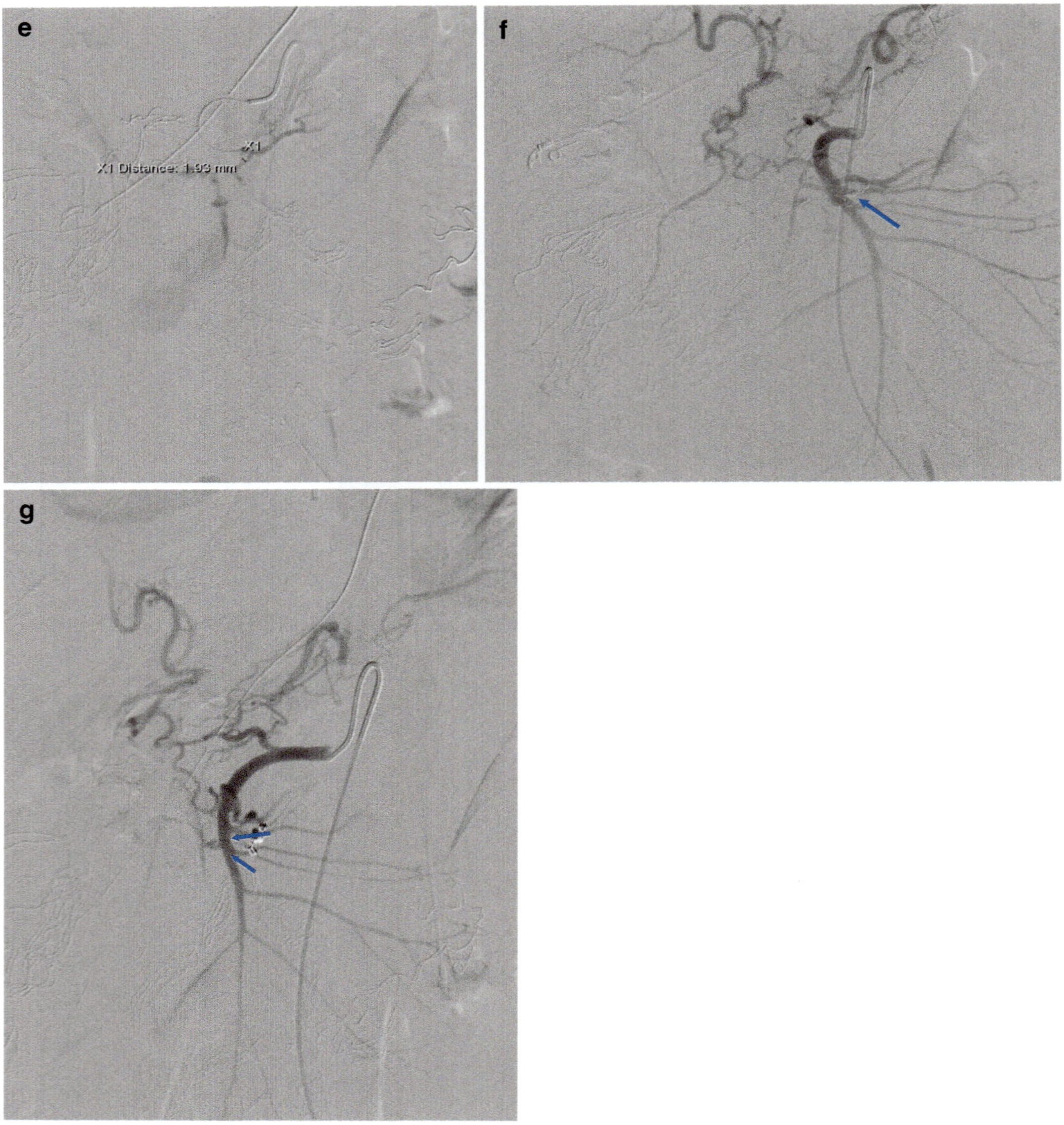

Fig. 4.48 (continued)

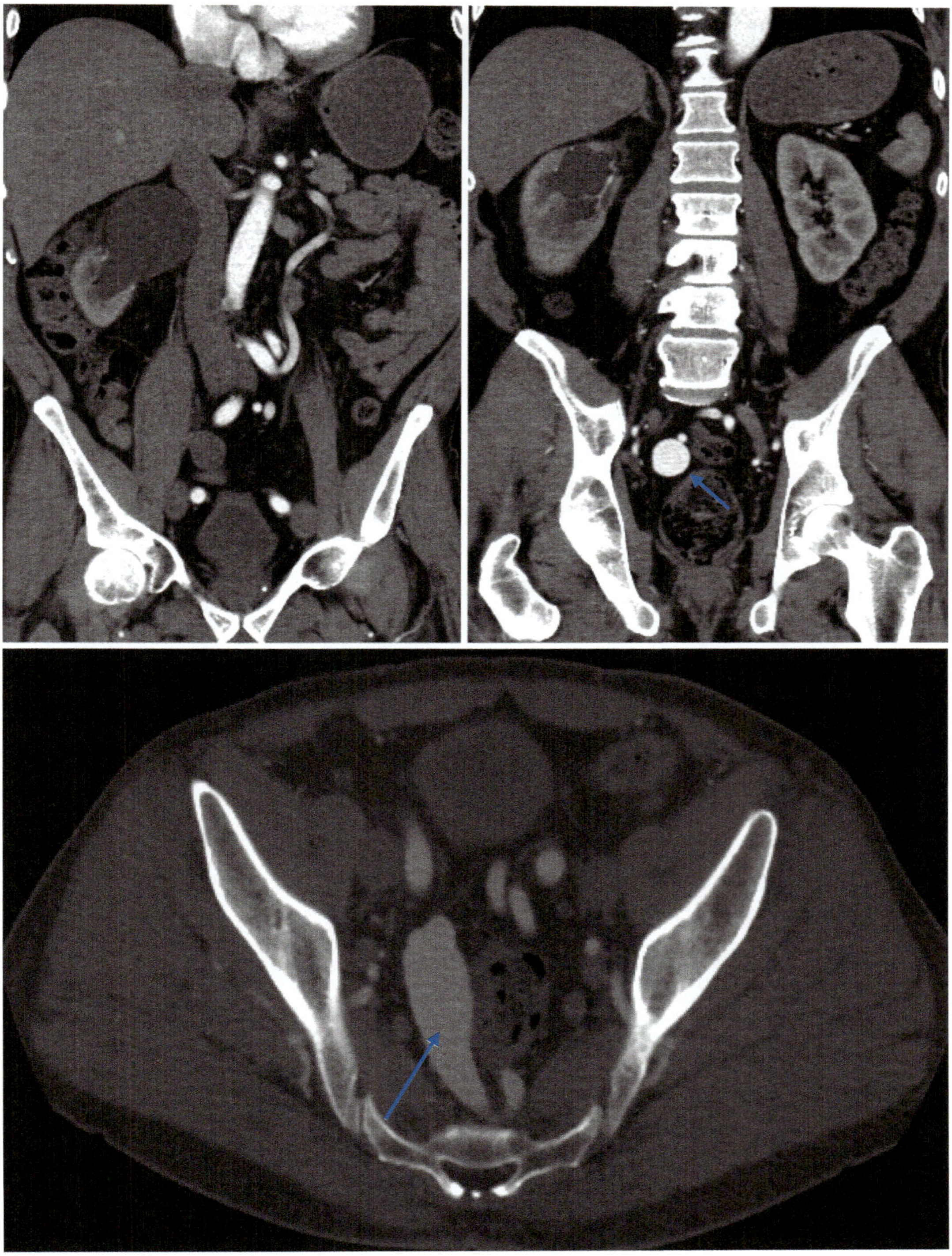

Fig. 4.49 Contrast-enhanced CT showed an enlarged inferior mesenteric artery and an aneurysm at the distal part (blue arrows)

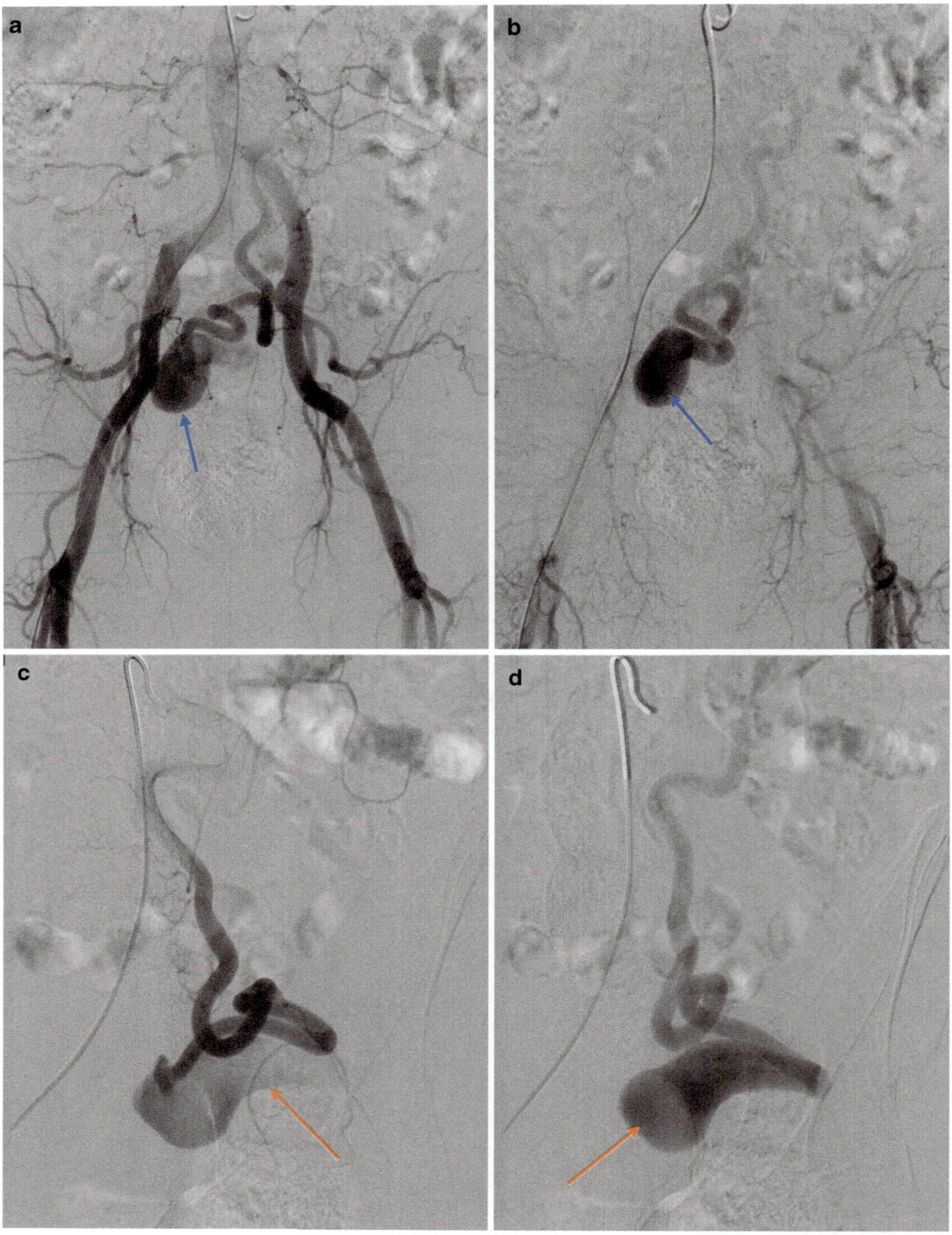

Fig. 4.50 (**a**, **b**) Abdominal aortography showed enlarged an inferior mesenteric artery and an aneurysm-(blue arrows). (**c**, **d**) Selective angiography of the inferior mesenteric artery showed arteriovenous fistula-(orange arrows). (**e**, **f**) Embolization of the aneurysm and fistula; blue arrows indicate micro-coils and arrested flow

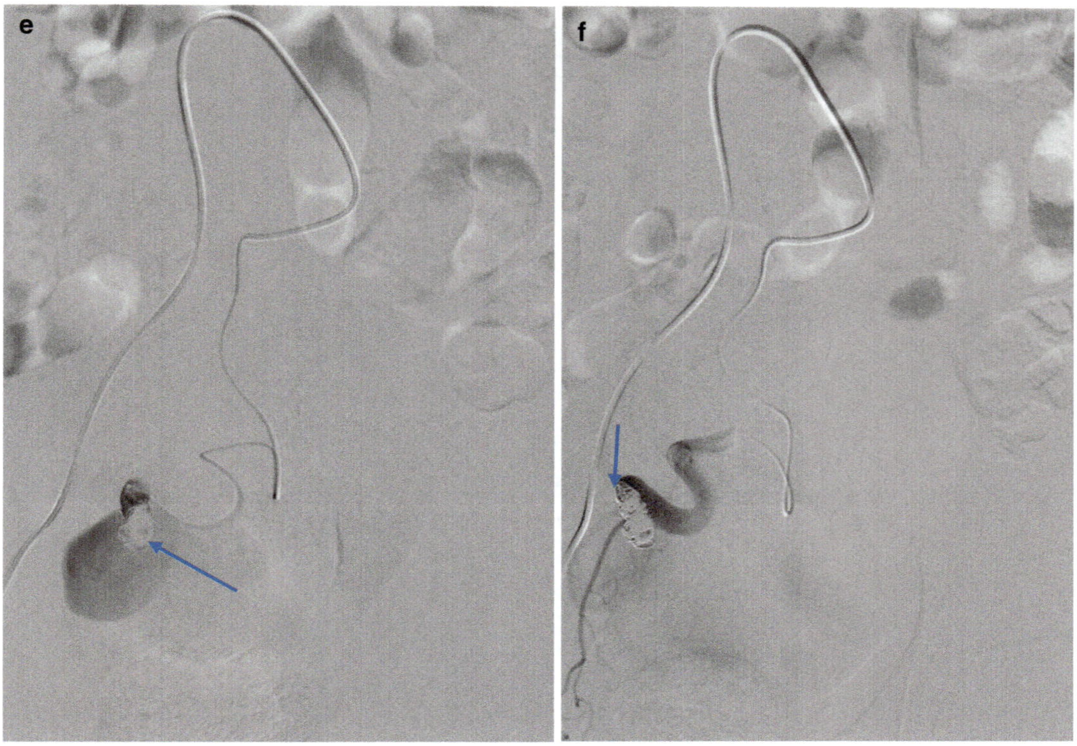

Fig. 4.50 (continued)

4.2.10 Renal Artery-I

> **Key Points**
> - Familiarization with balloon- or stent-assisted coil aneurysm embolization should be undertaken.
> - Detachable micro-coils should be used.
> - Stent grafts with diameters of 5 or 6 mm should be kept in stock.

4.2.10.1 Aetiology and Clinical Presentation

A 73-year-old patient with arterial hypertension and an incidentally discovered left renal artery aneurysm presented to our department. No other significant disease was reported. Baseline contrast-enhanced CT showed a left renal artery aneurysm 26 mm in diameter. The patient was asymptomatic. Control contrast-enhanced CT 6 months later showed enlargement of the aneurysm up to 29 mm (Fig. 4.53).

4.2.10.2 Pre-interventional Diagnosis

Control contrast-enhanced CT 6 months later showed enlargement of the aneurysm up to 29 mm (Fig. 4.52). Functional diagnostics confirmed that the left kidney contributed to 49% of the renal function; therefore, every effort was made to preserve renal function as much as possible (Fig. 4.53).

4.2.10.3 Endovascular Treatment

A 5 Fr renal-shaped catheter was inserted percutaneously through the right femoral artery for selective catheterization of the left renal artery. Angiography confirmed the diagnosis, and a microcatheter was coaxially advanced into the aneurysm. The microcatheter was placed deep

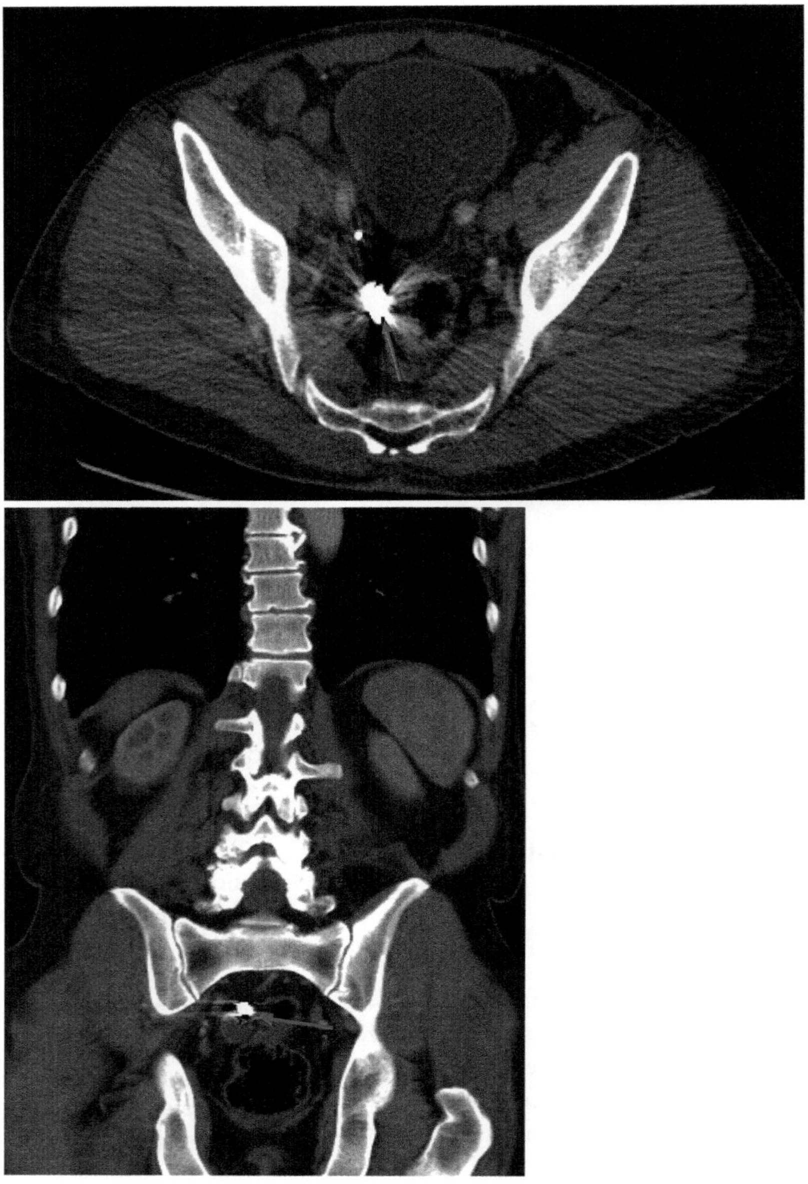

Fig. 4.51 Control contrast-enhanced CT scan 3 months after embolization showed a thrombosed aneurysm and a satisfactory result. Blue arrows indicate micro-coils

inside the aneurysm, and detachable micro-coils with diameters starting with 20 mm and followed by 18 mm, 16 mm and 14 mm and 10 mm were deployed. There were no complications during the intervention. The patient was discharged from the hospital the next day with unchanged renal creatinine and eGFR.

4.2.10.4 Outcome

Control contrast-enhanced CT 3 months after the embolization indicated a stable status and complete thrombosis of the renal aneurysm (Figs. 4.54 and 4.55). The renal parenchyma showed contrast opacifications. The patient remains in good health.

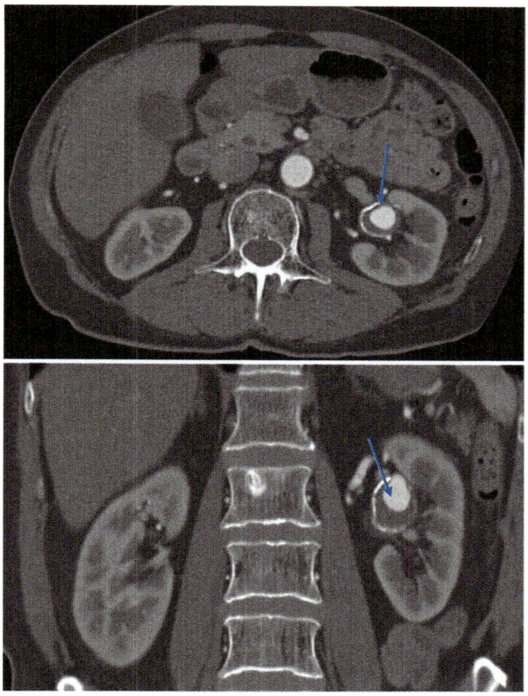

Fig. 4.52 An incidentally discovered 29 mm left renal artery aneurysm with calcification (arrows)

4.2.11 Renal Artery-II

> **Key Points**
> - Familiarization with balloon- or stent-assisted coil aneurysm embolization should be undertaken.
> - Detachable micro-coils should be used.
> - Stent grafts with diameters of 5 or 6 mm should be kept in stock.

4.2.11.1 Aetiology and Clinical Presentation

A 57-year-old patient presented with an incidentally discovered left polar renal artery aneurysm. The aneurysm measured 20 mm, and the polar artery had a diameter of 4.5 mm.

4.2.11.2 Pre-interventional Diagnosis

Contrast-enhanced CT showed a 20 mm saccular aneurysm of the left polar renal artery (Fig. 4.56). There was no rupture or ischaemia of the left kid-

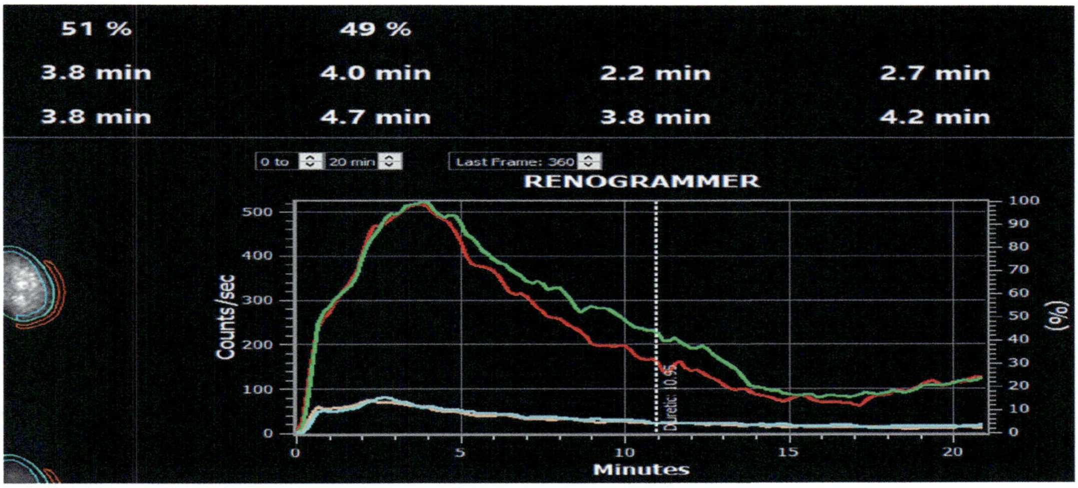

Fig. 4.53 Renography showed that the left renal artery contributed 49%

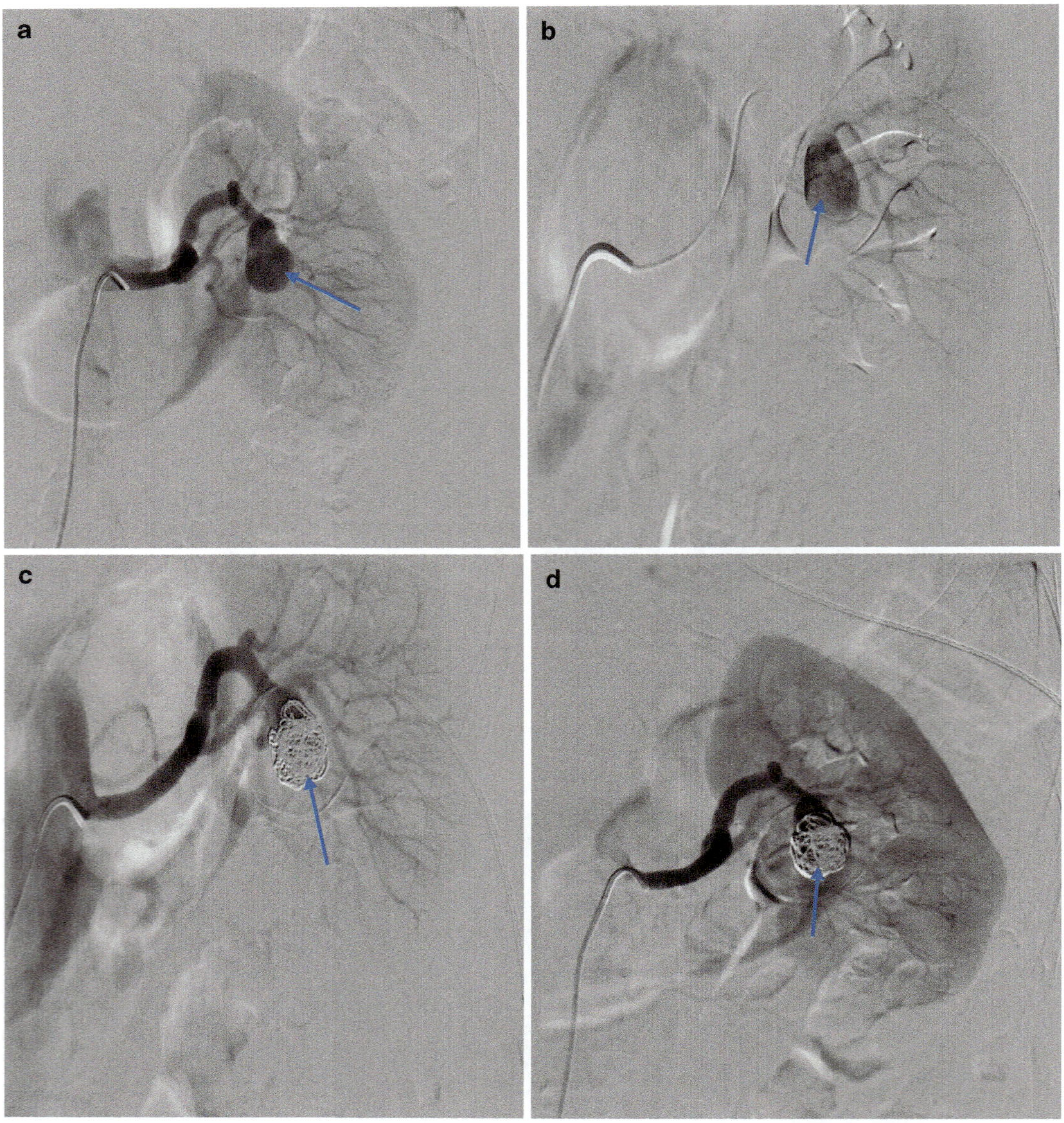

Fig. 4.54 Left renal artery angiography showing a renal aneurysm (blue arrows) (**a**). (**b**) advancement of a microcatheter into the aneurysm. (**c**, **d**) deployment of detachable micro-coils with a satisfactory outcome- (blue arrows)

ney. Renography showed that the left kidney was responsible for 61% of the renal function, and the right kidney was responsible for 39%. Therefore, the intention was to treat the aneurysm with a stent graft instead of occlusion (Fig. 4.57).

4.2.11.3 Endovascular Intervention

All insertions were made percutaneously through the right femoral artery. Diagnostic angiography confirmed the diagnosis. A 6 Fr sheath was advanced into the polar artery. A stent graft with a diameter of 5 mm and a length of 28 mm was advanced over a 0.035-in. guidewire and deployed without difficulty (Fig. 4.58). A bolus of 5000 IU heparin was administered. The percutaneous puncture was closed with StarClose closure devices.

4.2.11.4 Outcome

The patient was discharged from the hospital the next day. A control contrast-enhanced CT scan 3 months after the intervention showed satisfactory

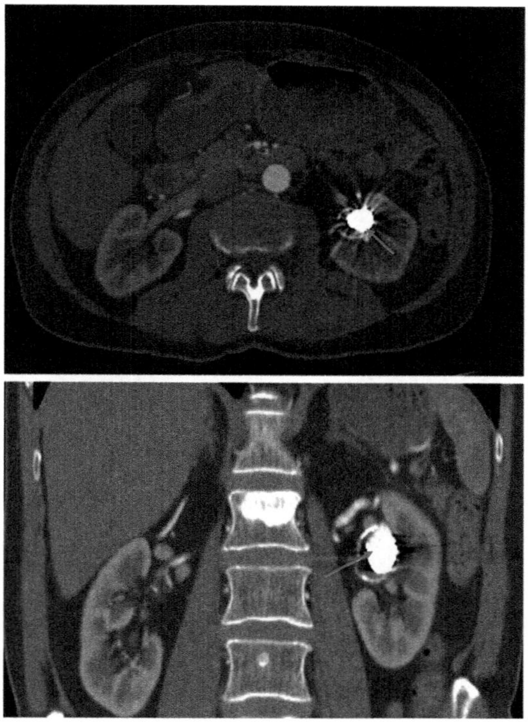

Fig. 4.55 Control contrast-enhanced CT 3 months after embolization with a satisfactory result and complete thrombosis of the thrombosis. Arrows indicate micro-coils

results (Fig. 4.59), and unchanged function of the left kidney was observed on control renography (Fig. 4.60).

4.3 Visceral Artery Occlusive Diseases

4.3.1 Superior Mesenteric Artery-I

Key Points

- Attempts should be made to revascularize the SMA if possible and if clinical status allows it, and bowel viability should be assessed after revascularization.
- Liberal use of brachial access is encouraged.
- For ostial stenosis, balloon-expandible bare metal or stent grafts should be used.

4.3.1.1 Aetiology and Clinical Presentation

A 71-year-old patient complained of crampy pain in the abdomen and diarrhoea that began a few days ago. The patient was admitted to the emergency department with signs of peritonitis. The white blood cell count was highly elevated (23 /L × 10^9 /L), and CRP was 212 mg/L. Acute explorative laparotomy was performed, and an ischaemic jejunum was removed. The rest of the small and large bowel was ischaemic, and the liver and spleen also had impaired circulation. The patient was planned for a second look.

4.3.1.2 Pre-interventional Diagnosis

Contrast-enhanced CT was performed the next day, before the second look, and showed an occluded superior mesenteric artery and severe stenosis and calcification around the coeliac trunk. There was a 35 mm abdominal aortic aneurysm (Fig. 4.61). The inferior mesenteric artery was open. It was decided to perform recanalization of the superior mesenteric artery before the second look.

4.3.1.3 Endovascular Treatment

A 5 Fr multipurpose catheter was inserted percutaneously through the left brachial artery for selective catheterization of the superior mesenteric artery (SMA). A 0.035 in. guidewire was used for recanalization of the SMA, and after recanalization and pre-dilatation with a 4 mm balloon, the stenosis of the SMA could be appreciated (Fig. 4.62). A balloon-expandible stent with a diameter of 7 mm and length of 39 mm was deployed across the stenosis with a satisfactory result. There were no embolic or ischaemic complications during or after the intervention. The patient underwent a second look the next day, and there was no need for additional surgical bowel resection. The status improved gradually without complications.

4.3.1.4 Outcome

The patient was discharged from the hospital with double antiplatelet medication to be taken in

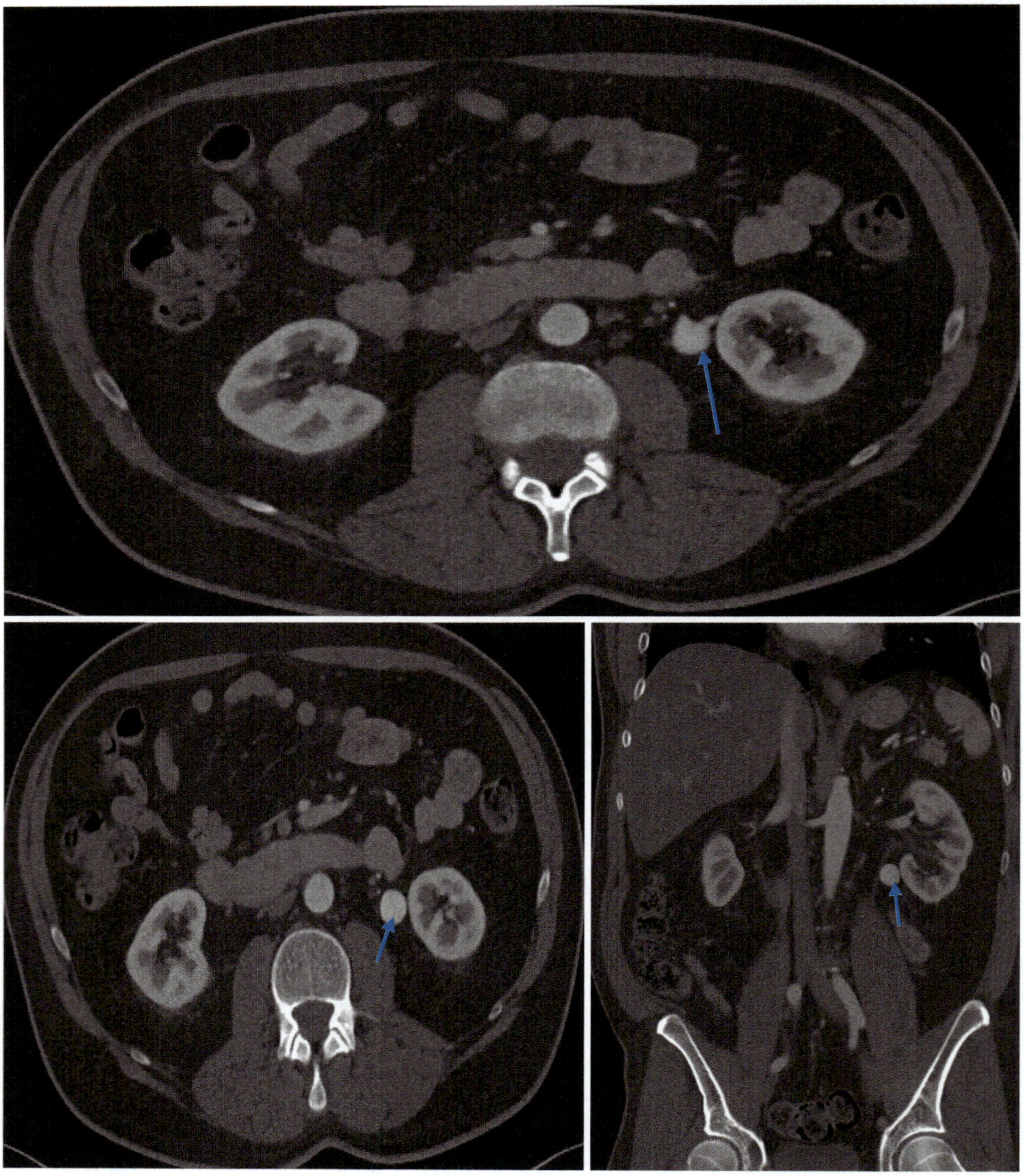

Fig. 4.56 Contrast-enhanced CT with incidentally discovered left renal artery aneurysm (arrows)

the first 3 months. After 3 months, only monotherapy with antiplatelet medication was to be taken. Three months later, control non–contrast-enhanced CT (Fig. 4.63) showed a good result and an open SMA stent. No new ischaemic complications occurred during the follow-up.

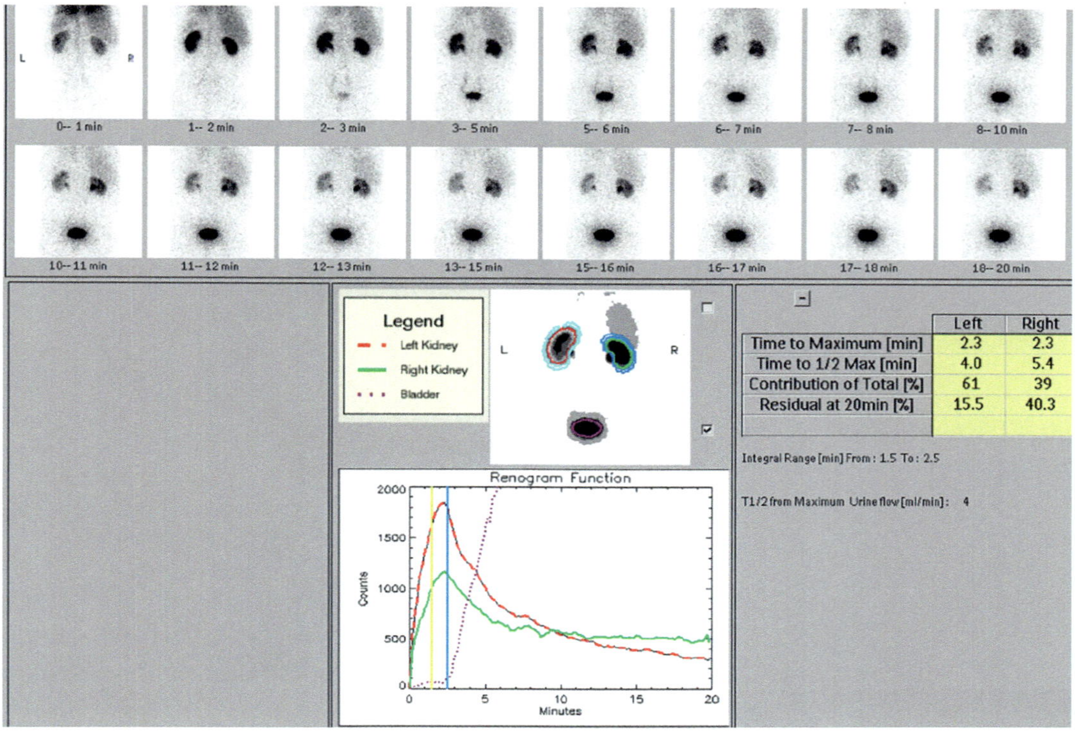

Fig. 4.57 Renography showed that the left kidney contributed 61% of the renal function

4.3.2 Superior Mesenteric Artery-II

Key Points

- Attempts should be made to revascularize the SMA if possible and if clinical status allows it, and bowel viability should be assessed after revascularization.
- Liberal use of brachial access is encouraged.
- For ostial stenosis, balloon-expandible bare metal or stent grafts should be used.

4.3.2.1 Aetiology and Clinical Presentation

A 69-year-old patient with resting pain on both legs and an ankle-brachial index of 36% bilaterally was scheduled for aortic bifemoral bypass surgery due to severe occlusive diseases in the aorta and the pelvic and femoral arteries. The preoperative contrast-enhanced CT scan revealed severe stenosis of the superior mesenteric artery (SMA), but the patient did not have symptoms of bowel ischaemia.

4.3.2.2 Pre-interventional Diagnosis

Contrast-enhanced CT showed severe calcifications in the aorta, occluded left pelvic arteries and severe stenosis and calcifications in the femoral arteries. The celiac trunk and SMA had stenosis and calcifications (Fig. 4.64). The inferior mesenteric artery was occluded. The patient did not have symptoms of visceral ischaemia. Aortic vascular reconstruction was performed. The patient underwent open aorta surgery, but afterward, the patient experienced severe abdominal pain, increased CPR and white blood cell count, and, according to pre-operative CT, a worsening of the SMA occlusion.

4.3.2.3 Endovascular Treatment

A 5 Fr Berenstein catheter was inserted percutaneously through the left brachial artery for selective catheterization of the superior mesenteric artery (SMA), revealing complete occlusion of

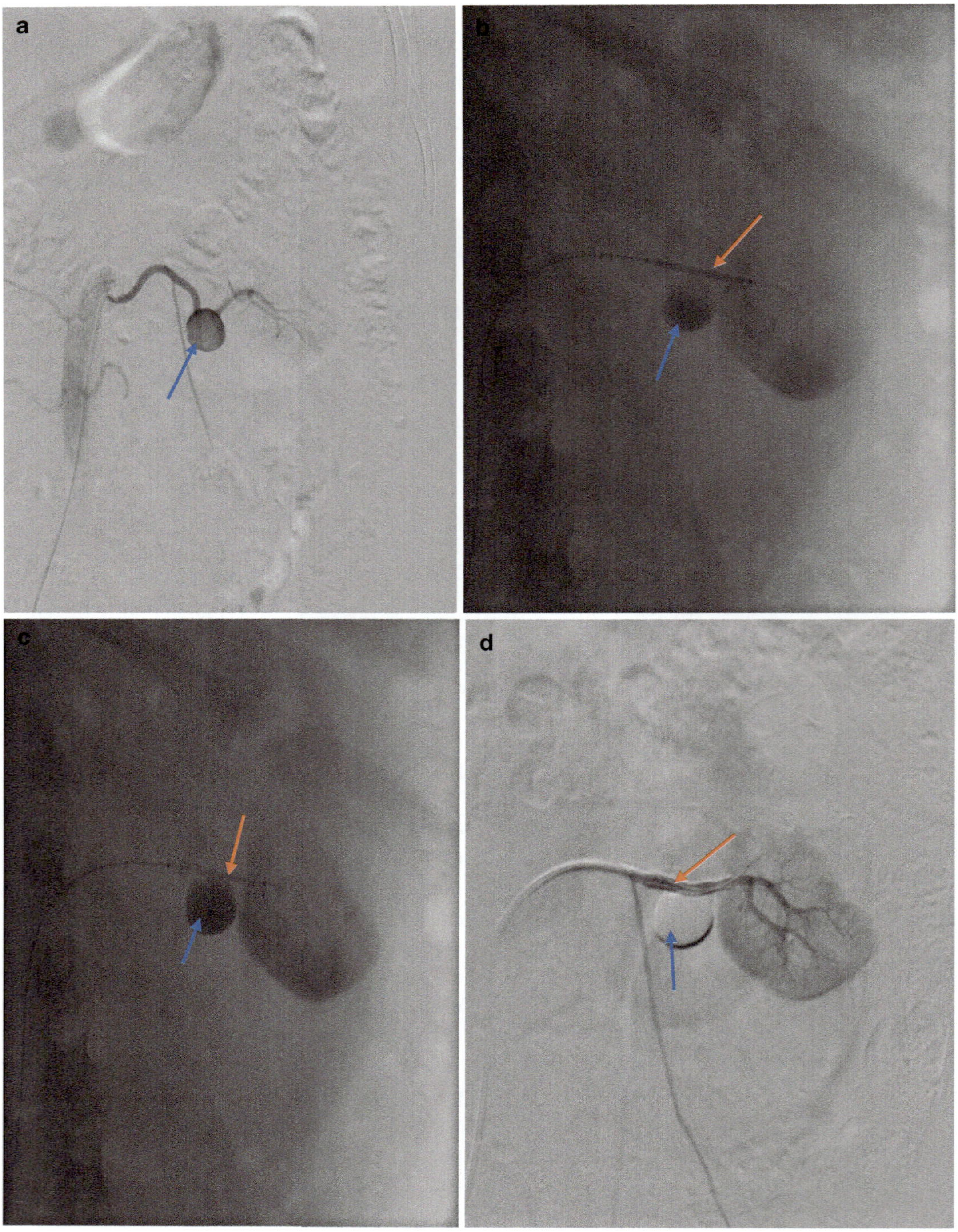

Fig. 4.58 Selective angiography of the left accessory renal artery showing an aneurysm- (blue arrow) (**a**). (**b–d**) advancement and deployment of the 5 mm-diameter stent graft (orange arrows) produced a satisfactory result

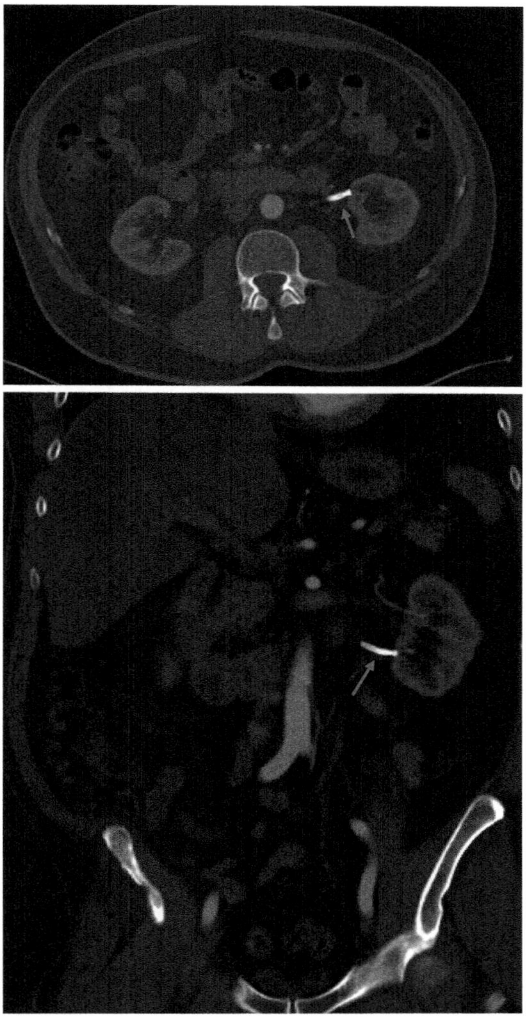

Fig. 4.59 Control contrast-enhanced CT scan 3 months after the intervention showed a satisfactory result. Blue arrows indicate the stent graft

the artery. A 0.035 in. guidewire was used for recanalization of the SMA, and after recanalization and pre-dilatation with a 6 mm balloon, the stenosis in the SMA was performed proximally (Fig. 4.65). A balloon-expandible stent with a diameter of 8 mm and a length of 39 mm was deployed across the stenosis with a satisfactory result. There were no embolic or ischaemic complications during or after the intervention.

4.3.2.4 Outcome

The patient was discharged from the hospital after a prolonged postoperative stay but without significant complications. The patient is to take double antiplatelet medication for the first 3 months, and then only monotherapy with antiplatelet medication. Three months later, control non–contrast-enhanced CT (Fig. 4.66) showed a good result and an open SMA stent. No new ischaemic complications occurred during the follow-up. The ankle-brachial index increased to 68%, and the patient was without pain.

4.3.3 Inferior Mesenteric Artery

Key Points

- If the patient experienced severe pain during the PTA, further dilatation should be stopped.
- It is always possible to bring the patient back to an OR the next day.
- Smaller diameter stents or balloons should be considered.

4.3.3.1 Aetiology and Clinical Presentation

An 81-year-old patient underwent aorto-inferior mesenteric bypass a decade ago due to occlusive diseases of the celiac trunk and superior mesenteric artery. The only open visceral vessel was the inferior mesenteric artery, which showed severe stenosis and calcifications. The vascularization of the entire bowel depends on the inferior mesenteric artery and a well-developed collateral network. The surgery went well, and the patient was asymptomatic until recently. The patient complained of abdominal pain and classic abdominal angina with worsening of the pain after a meal.

4.3.3.2 Pre-interventional Diagnosis

Abdominal aortography showed significant stenosis of the aorto-inferior mesenteric artery bypass and retrograde feeling of the superior mesenteric artery and celiac trunk via an inferior mesenteric artery (Fig. 4.67). Balloon angioplasty and stent deployment procedures were scheduled.

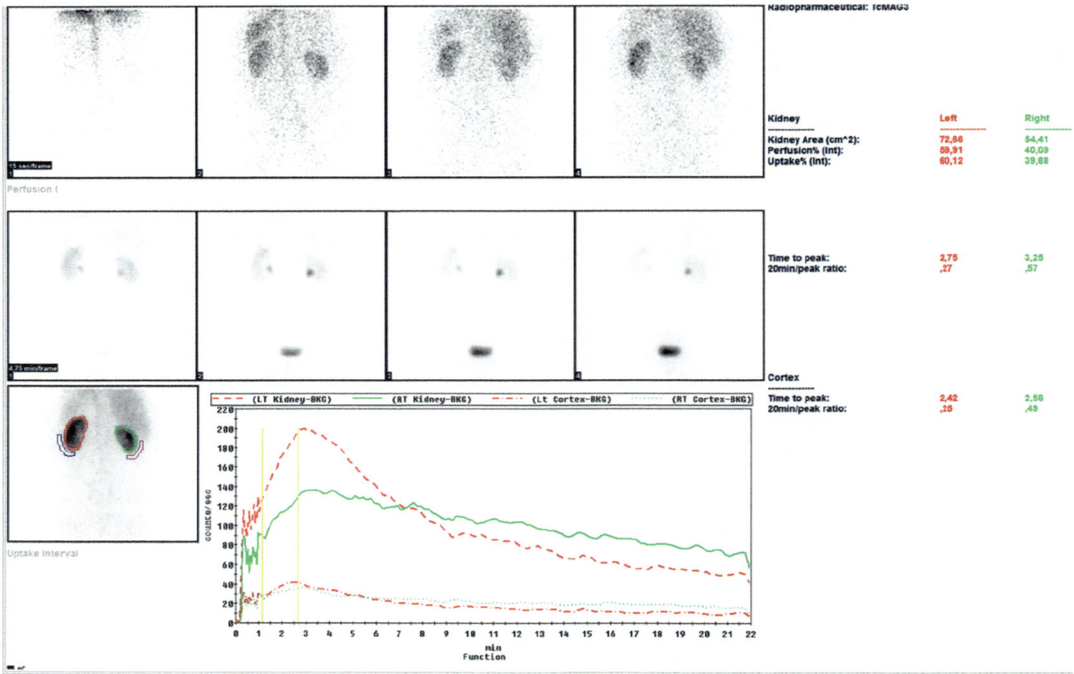

Fig. 4.60 Control renography showing unchanged function of the left kidney

4.3.3.3 Endovascular Treatment

Under local anaesthesia, a 5 Fr sidewinder catheter was advanced percutaneously through the right femoral artery into the inferior mesenteric artery. A 0.035 in. guidewire quickly navigated the stenosis, and direct stent deployment with a balloon-expandible stent 10 mm in diameter and 29 mm in length was performed. (Fig. 4.68). The patient experienced severe abdominal pain during stent deployment but remained haemodynamically stable. Repeat angioplasty of the residual stenosis was not performed due to patient pain. The intervention was abrupt, and the patient did not experience any further complaints. A second attempt was made a few days later, a new stent 9 mm in diameter was deployed without difficulties, and only minimal residual stenosis was appreciated on the final angiography (Fig. 4.69). The patient did not experience pain during the second intervention.

4.3.3.4 Outcome

The patient did not experience any complications during the follow-up and indicated no abdominal pain or any other complaints. The patient is currently receiving antiplatelet monotherapy.

4.3.4 Renal Artery

> **Key Points**
> - Captopril renography is advisable before the decision to treat renal artery stenosis.
> - Patients with recurrent flushing lung oedema and renal stenosis should be treated with angioplasty if possible.
> - Familiarization with the monorail system is important.

4.3.4.1 Aetiology and Clinical Presentation

A patient known to have long-standing arterial hypertension treated with three medications recently experienced worsening control of

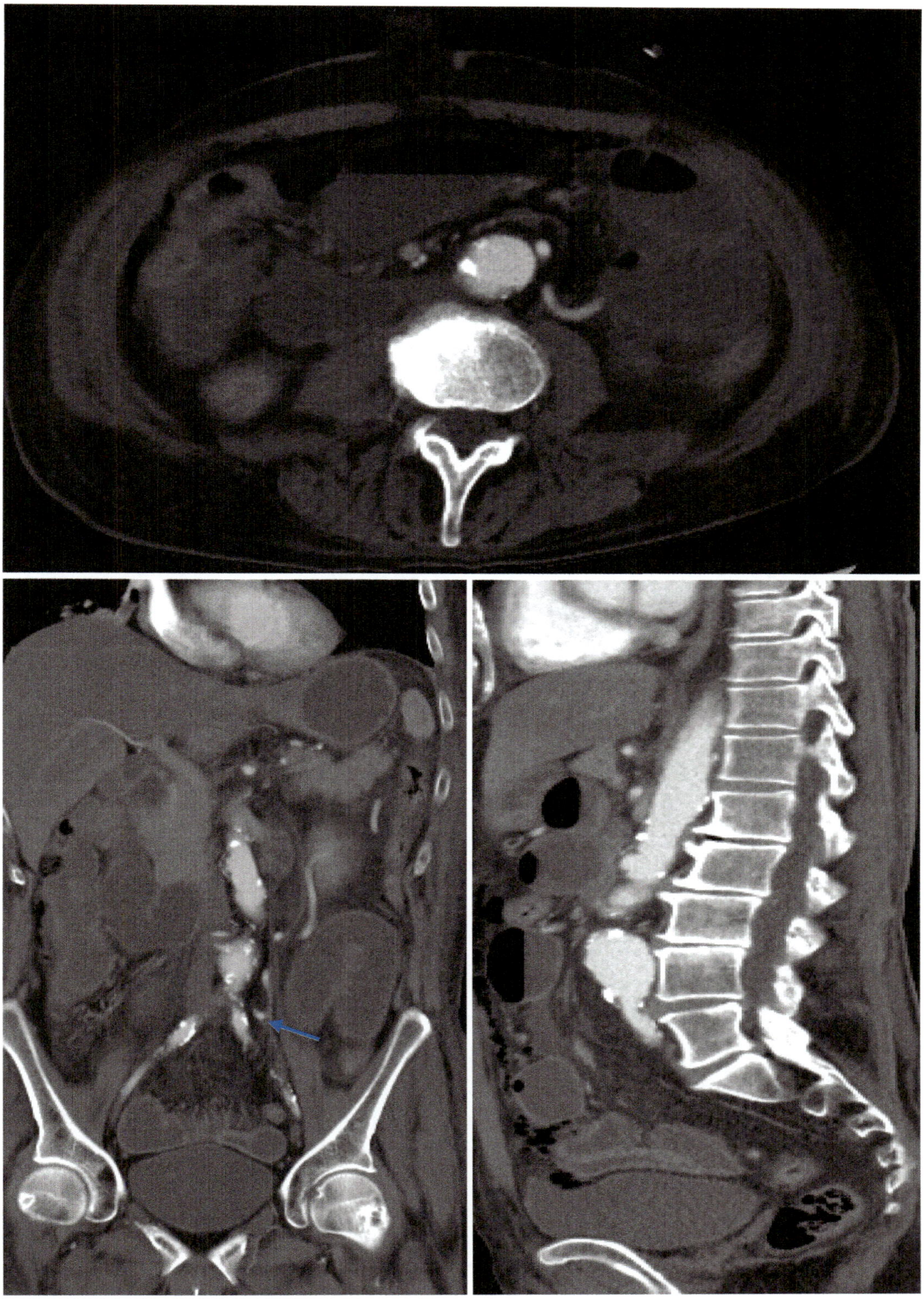

Fig. 4.61 Contrast-enhanced CT showing an occluded superior mesenteric artery and sub-occlusion of the celiac trunk. The inferior mesenteric artery was open (blue arrow). The free air in the abdomen is the result of a recent laparotomy

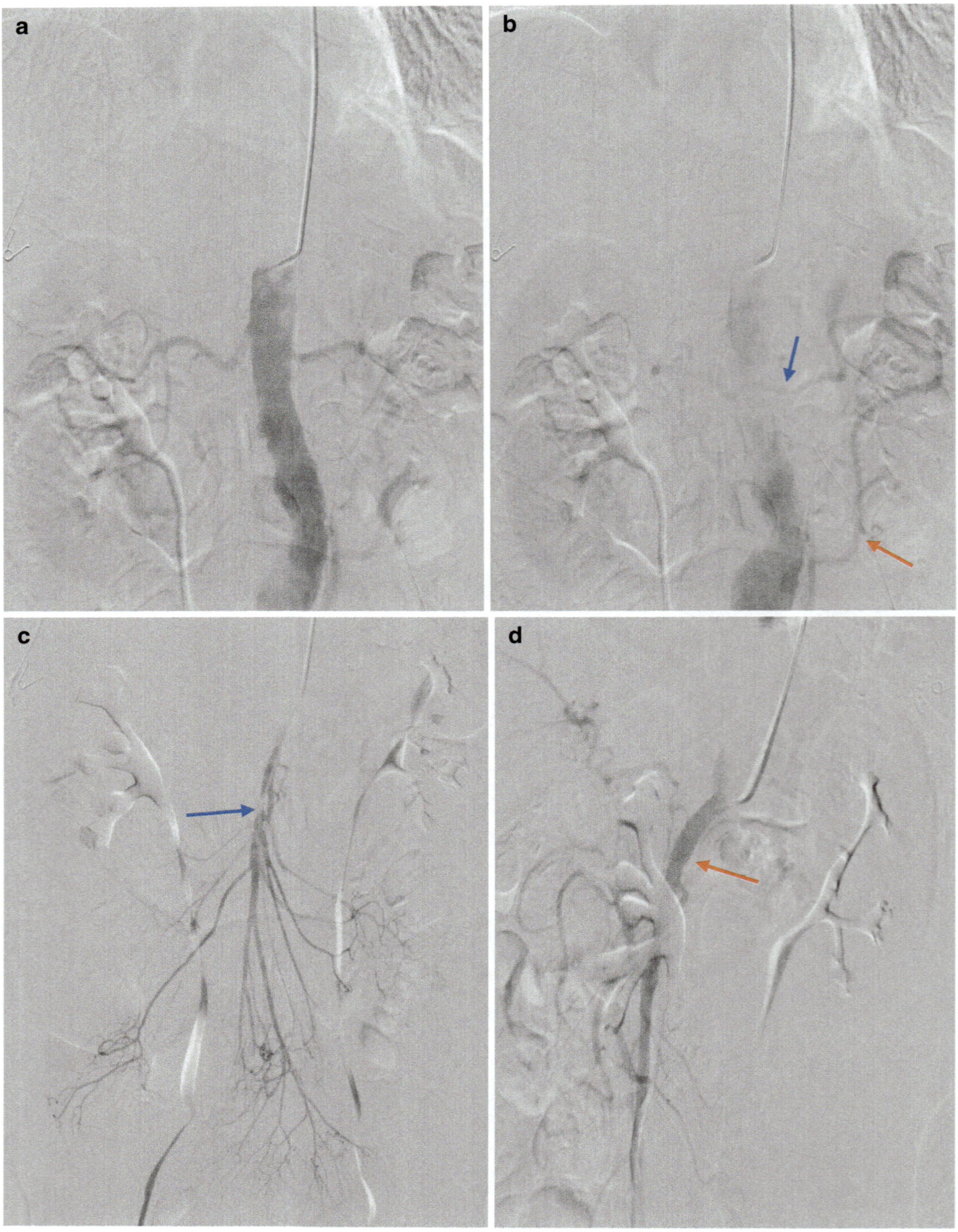

Fig. 4.62 Left brachial artery access. Angiography confirmed occlusion of the superior mesenteric artery (SMA). The celiac trunk (blue arrow) and inferior mesenteric artery (orange arrow) are open (**b**). (**c**) after recanalization of the SMA, the stenosis was observed (blue arrow). (**d**) control angiography after stent deployment shows an excellent result (orange arrow)

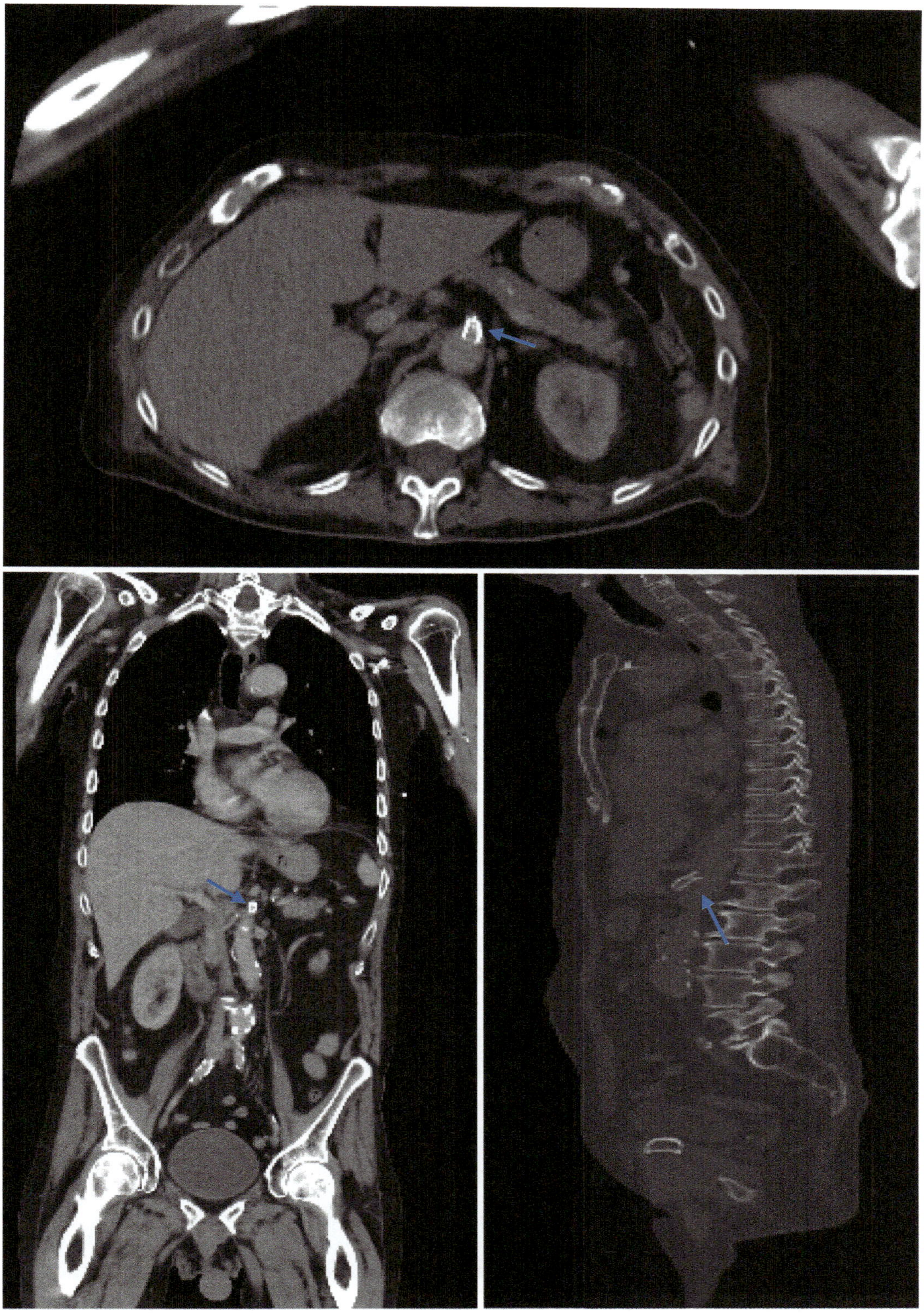

Fig. 4.63 Control contrast-enhanced CT 3 months after recanalization showing an open stent and no new ischaemic events. Blue arrows indicate the stent

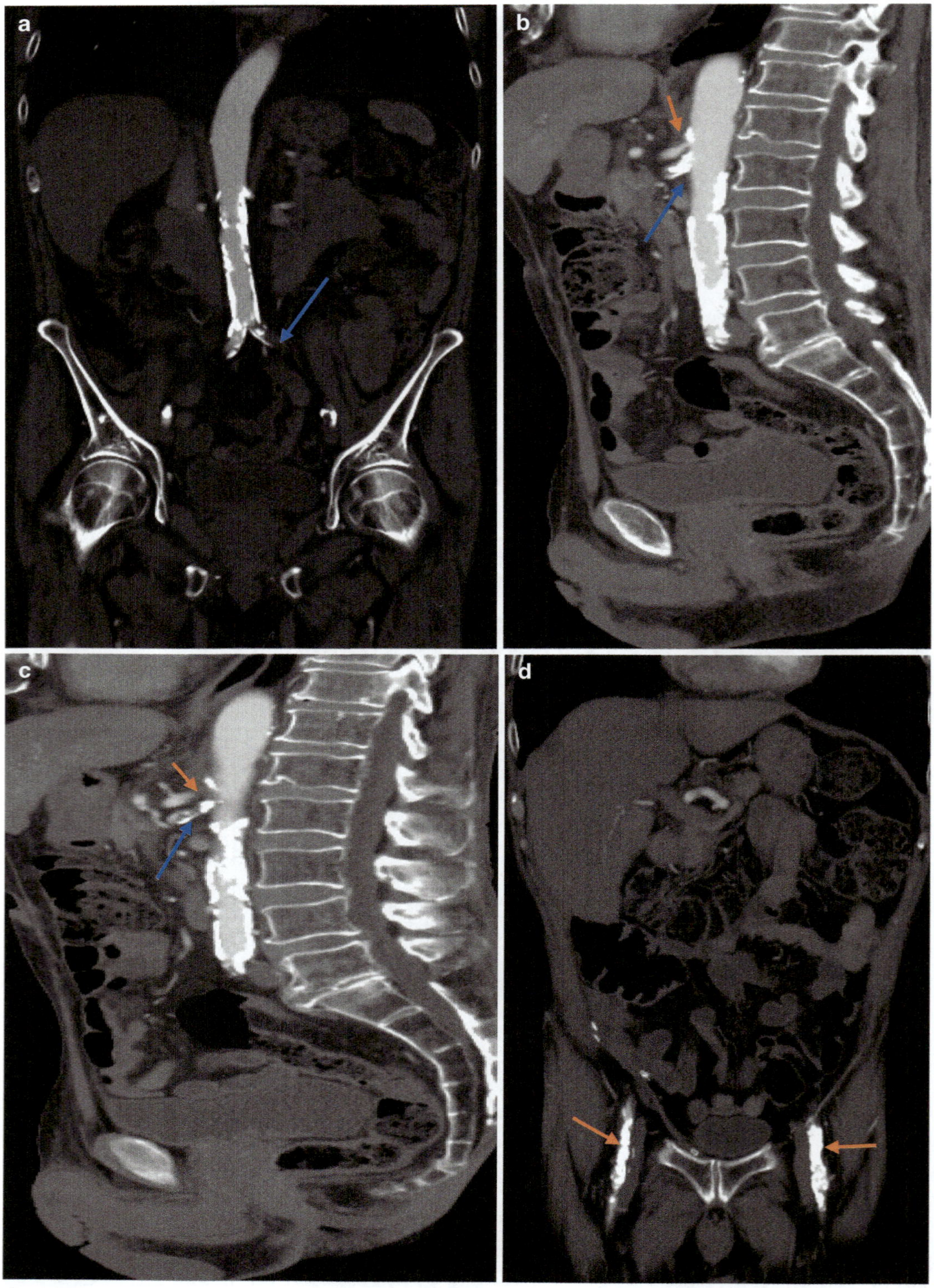

Fig. 4.64 (**a**) severe calcification in the aorta and peripheral arteries with occlusion of the left iliac artery (blue arrow). (**b, c**) occlusion of the SMA-(blue arrows). Orange arrows indicate stenosis of the celiac trunk. (**d**) severe stenosis and calcification in both femoral arteries- (orange arrows)

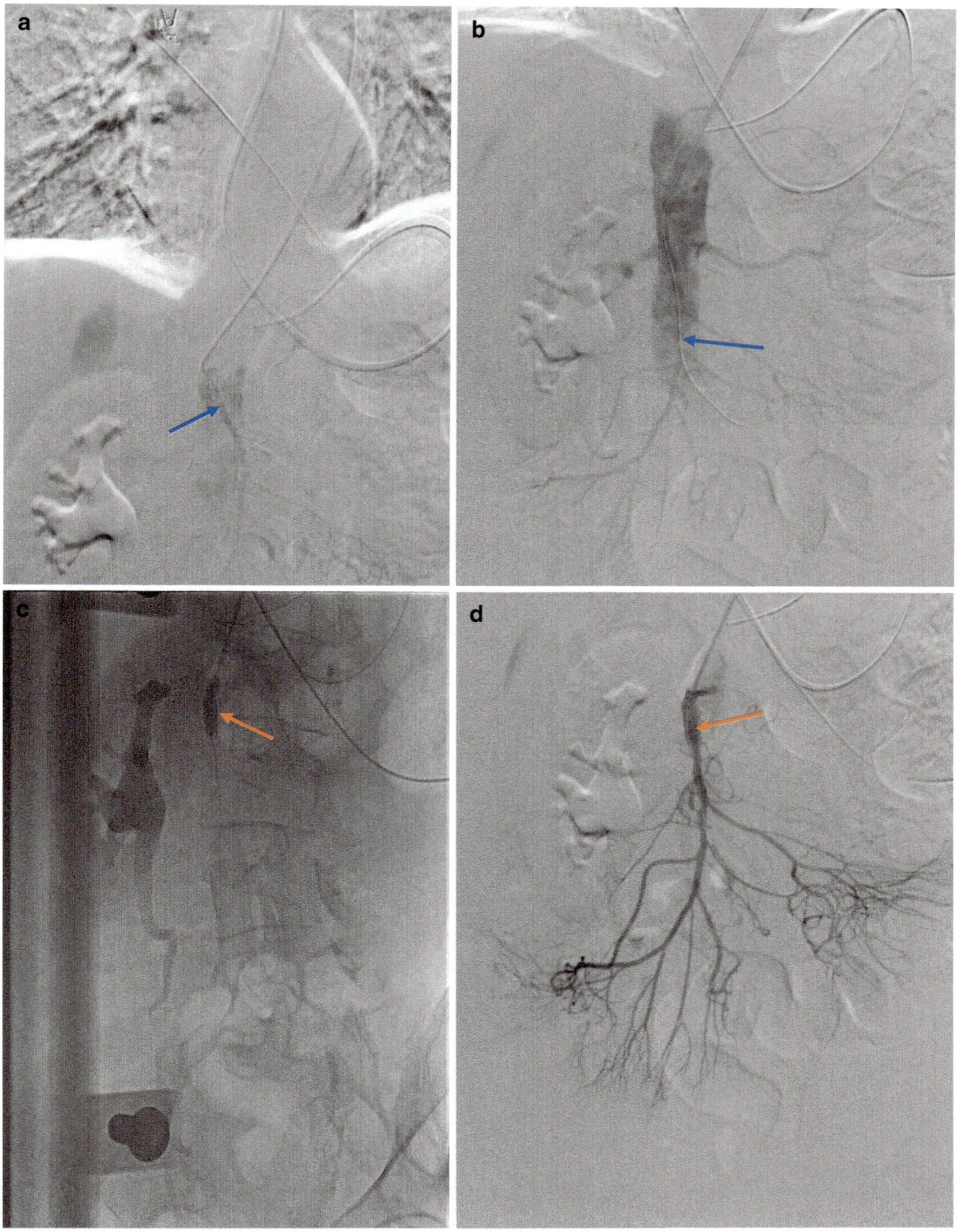

Fig. 4.65 Selective catheterization of the occluded SMA (arrow) (**a**). (**b**) advancement of the 0.035 in. guidewire distally (arrow). (**c**) pre-dilatation with a 6 mm balloon (arrow). (**d**) control image after stent deployment shows a good outcome (arrow)

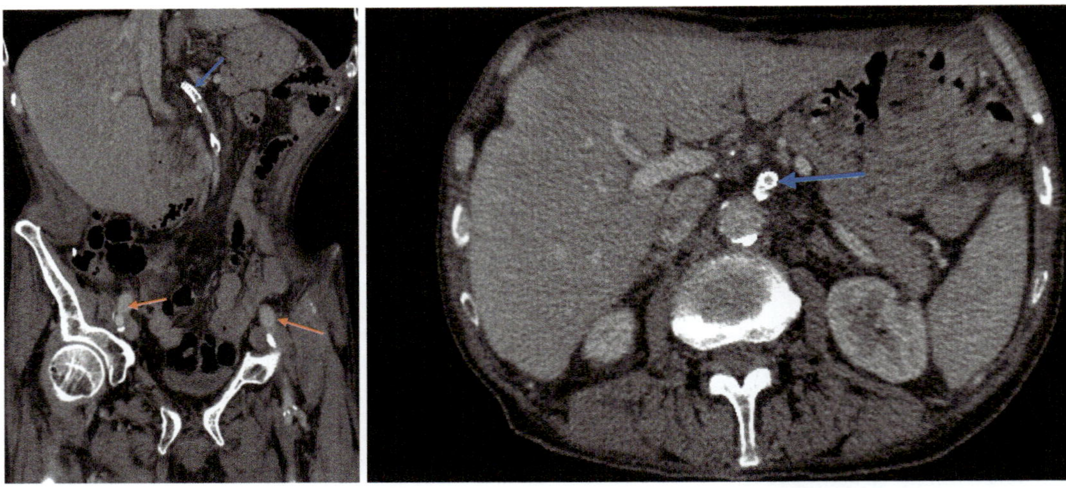

Fig. 4.66 Control CT scan 3 months after recanalization shows a satisfactory result and an open SMA stent (arrows). Orange arrows indicate aorto-bifemoral bypass

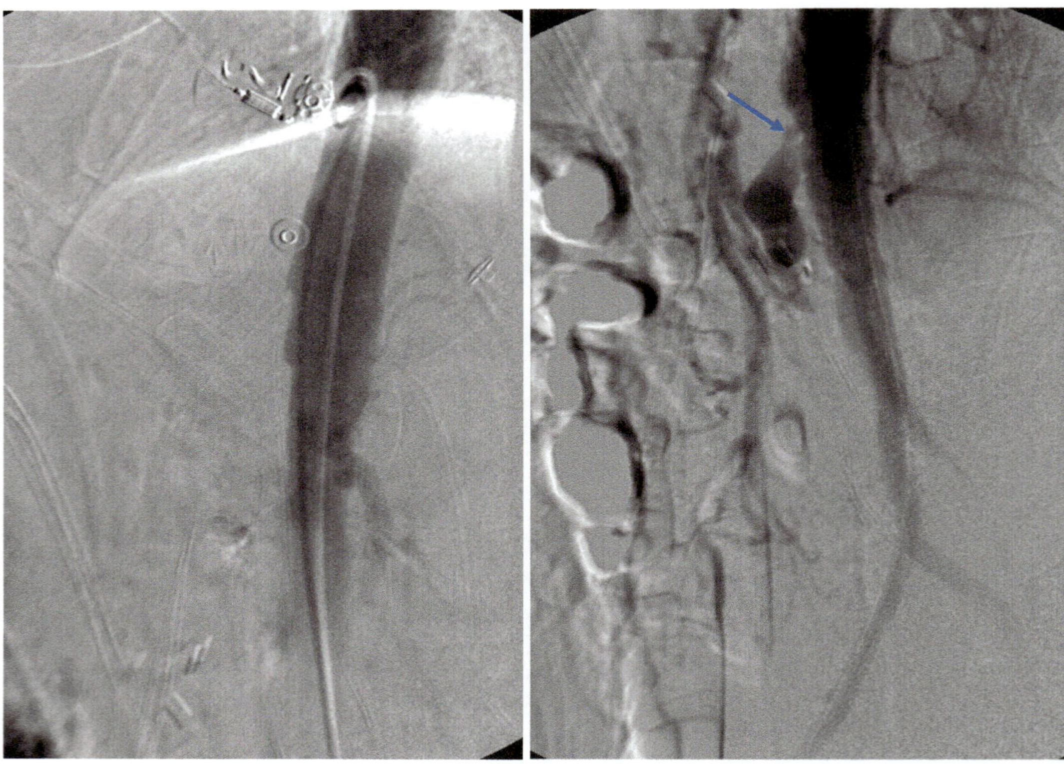

Fig. 4.67 Angiography shows significant stenosis of the inferior mesenteric artery bypass (arrow)

blood pressure. The blood pressure was 200/110 mmHg on admission. Intravenous nicardipine infusion was initiated and helped lower the blood pressure to 150/100 mmHg. Functional angiotensin II receptor blocker renography showed increased transit time on the right side (Fig. 4.70). The left kidney contributed 60% of the renal function.

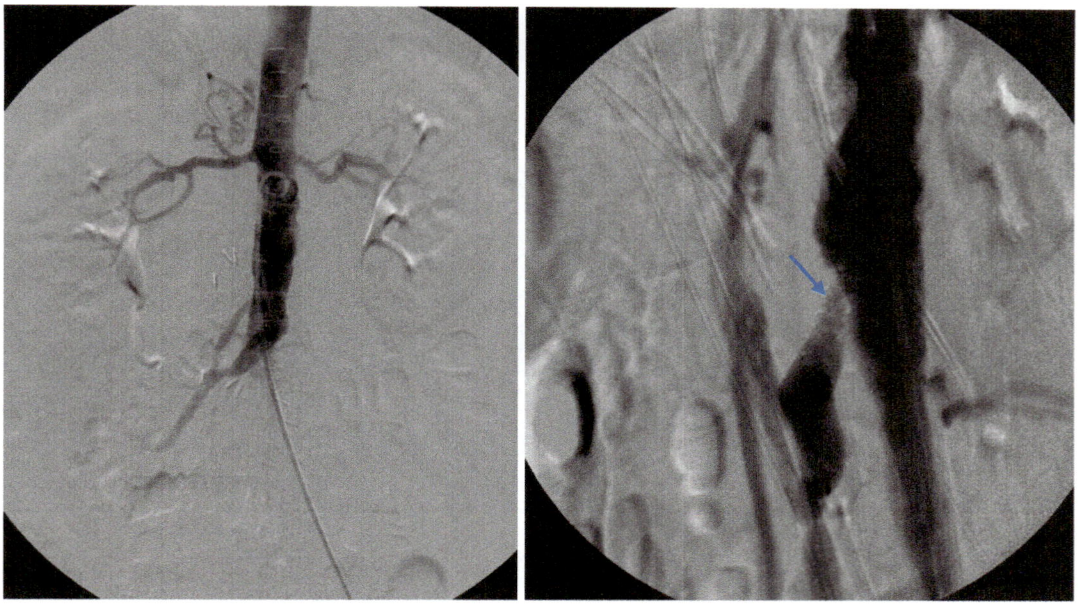

Fig. 4.68 Details from the first angioplasty and stent deployment. Arrow indicates the deployed stent and residual stenosis. The patient experienced severe pain during angioplasty; therefore, the residual stenosis was not treated during this angioplasty

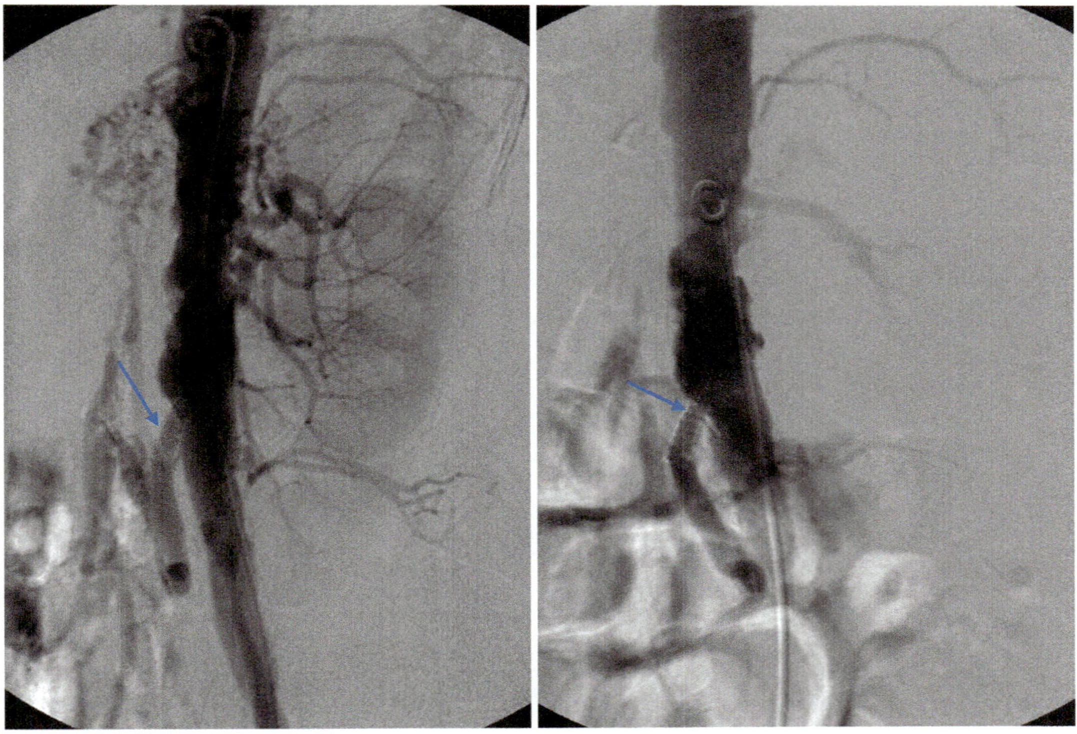

Fig. 4.69 The second angioplasty and additional stent deployment resulted in a much better outcome and minimal residual stenosis (arrow)

4.3.4.2 Pre-interventional Diagnosis

Contrast-enhanced CT showed significant stenosis of both renal arteries with ostial calcifications. There are two renal arteries on the left side, and only the first artery had stenosis (Fig. 4.71). Bilateral renal angioplasty was planned.

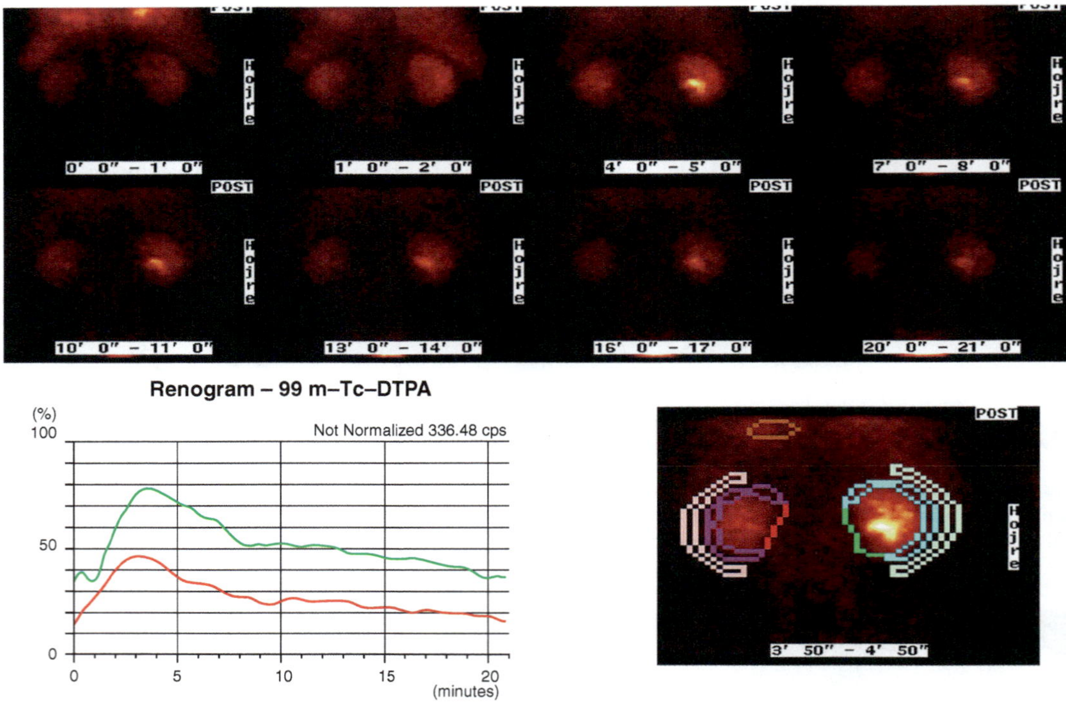

Fig. 4.70 Functional renography shows a prolonged transit time, especially on the right side. The left kidney contributed 60% of the renal function

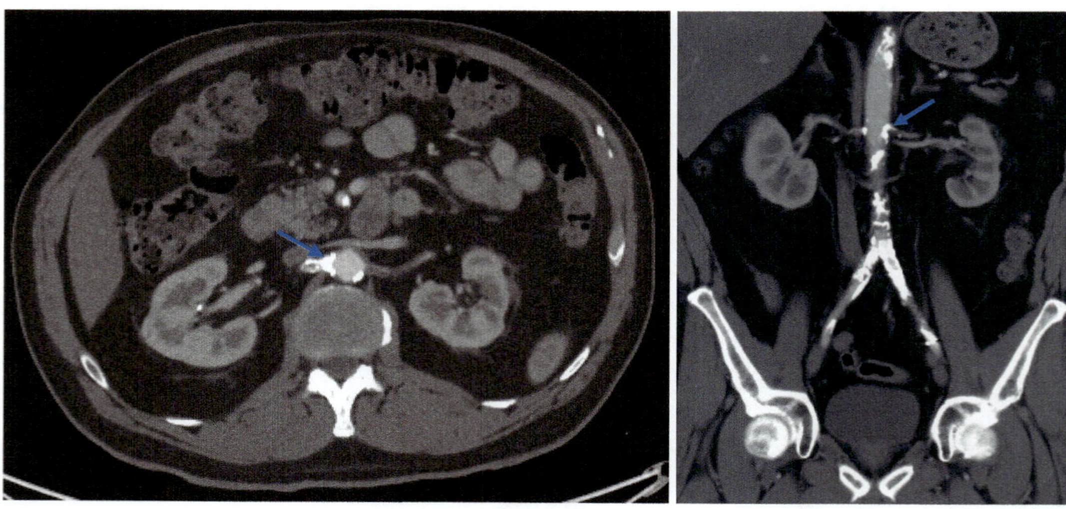

Fig. 4.71 Contrast-enhanced CT shows substantial bilateral renal artery stenosis (arrows). On the left side, there are two renal arteries, and the proximal artery shows significant stenosis

4.3.4.3 Endovascular Treatment

Under local anaesthesia, abdominal aortography performed percutaneously via right femoral artery access confirmed stenosis of both renal arteries (Fig. 4.72). A 5 Fr renal catheter was inserted into the left renal artery. A 0.035 in. guidewire quickly navigated to the stenosis, and a 6 Fr renal guiding catheter was advanced into the first left renal artery. A 0.018 in. guidewire was advanced across the stenosis, and a monorail system with a renal sent diameter of 5.5 mm and length of 15 mm was deployed. After that, with

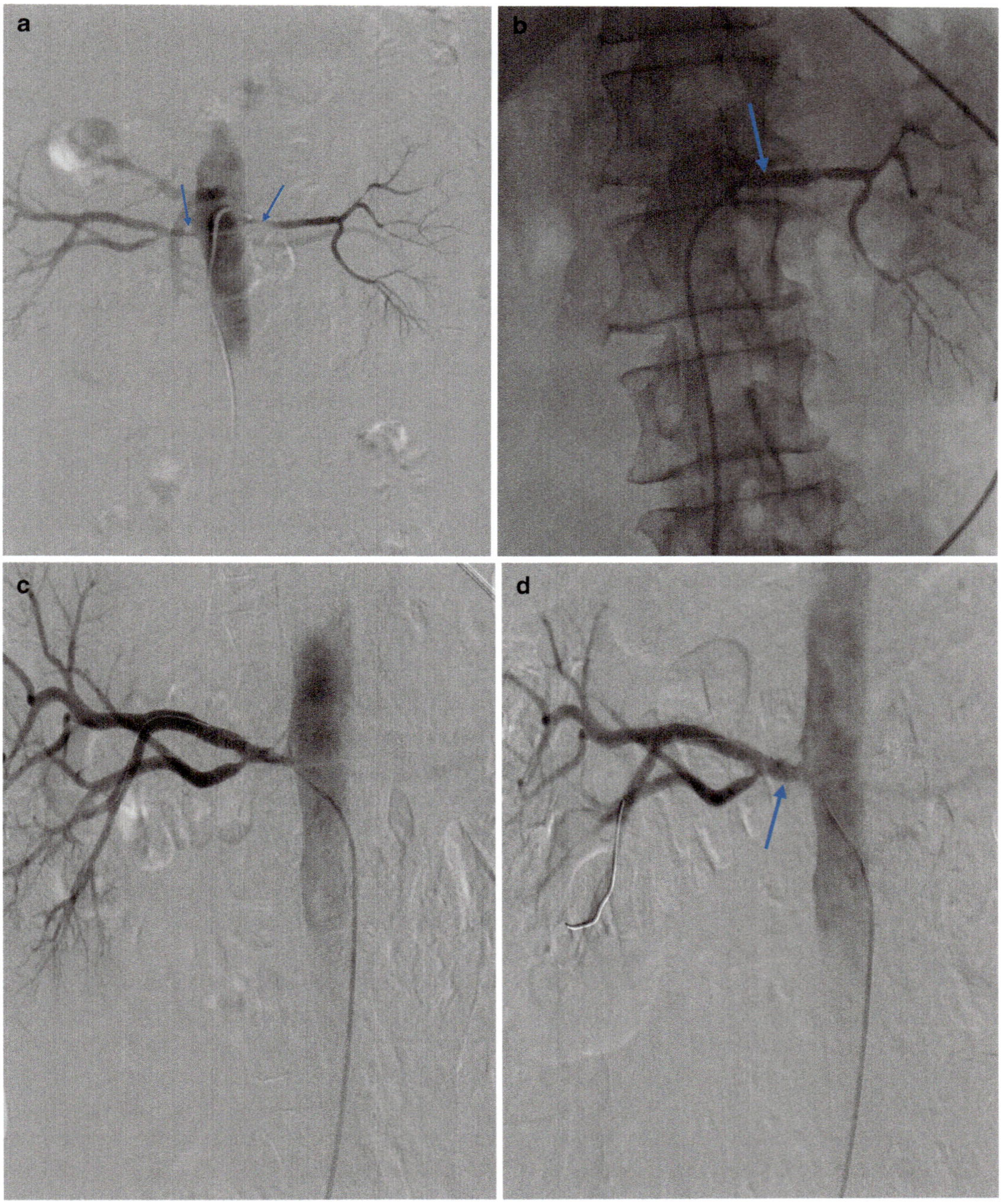

Fig. 4.72 (**a**) angiography reveals substantial bilateral renal stenosis (arrows). (**b**) deployment of a stent in the left renal artery. (**c, d**) deployment of a stent in the right renal artery, producing an excellent result

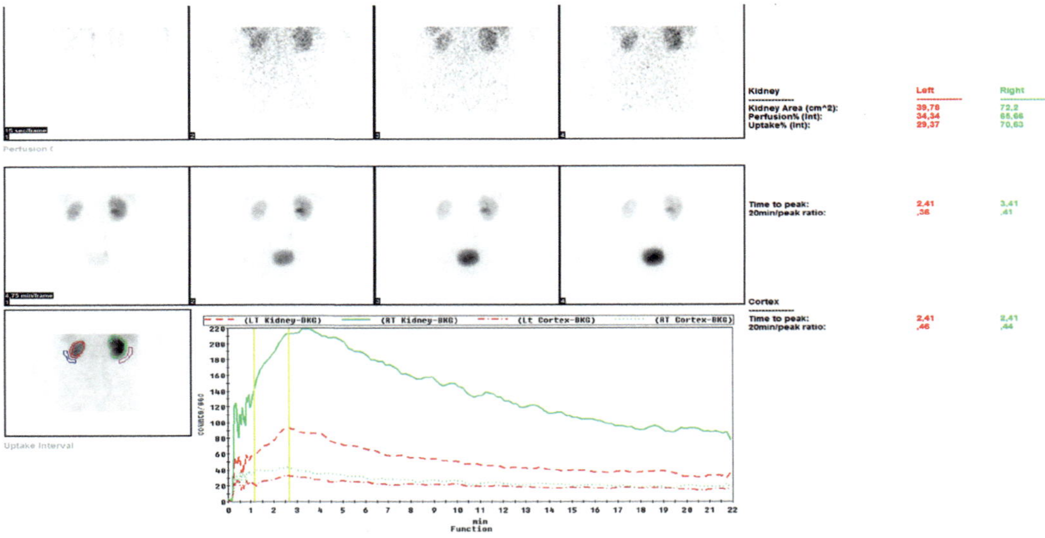

Fig. 4.73 Control renography showing functional improvement of right kidney and worsening of left kidney function

the same technique, the right renal artery was treated with a renal stent 6 mm in diameter and 12 mm in length with a good outcome.

4.3.4.4 Outcome

The patient did not experience any complications during the follow-up and had well-controlled blood pressure. Control renography showed improved right renal function but worsening of the left kidney function. The patient remained asymptomatic with stable creatinine and eGFR (Fig. 4.73).

4.4 Abdominal Arterial Bleeding

4.4.1 Coeliac Trunk-Left Gastric Artery

> **Key Points**
> - Endoscopic clips can help guide the embolization intervention.
> - Familiarization with different embolic material is important.
> - The micro-plug is a relatively new product that can be delivered through the microcatheter.

4.4.1.1 Aetiology and Clinical Presentation

A 68-year patient with known peptic ventricle ulcers had been previously treated endoscopically due to excessive bleeding. During the latest admission, an increase in the upper gastrointestinal bleeding made it impossible to treat endoscopically, and the patient became haemodynamically unstable with a drop in blood pressure to 90 mmHg.

4.4.1.2 Pre-interventional Diagnosis

Endoscopy examination a few months before the current bleeding (Fig. 4.74a) demonstrated non-bleeding peptic ulcers. Urgent endoscopy revealed ongoing bleeding and endoscopic treatment (Fig. 4.79b) after the patient was admitted. Endoscopic control was suboptimal due to persistent bleeding, and embolization was planned.

4.4.1.3 Endovascular Treatment

Under local anaesthesia, a 5 Fr sidewinder catheter was inserted percutaneously through the right femoral artery into the celiac trunk, and selective angiography of the left gastric artery was performed and confirmed the then-current bleeding from the artery (Fig. 4.75). A microcatheter was coaxially advanced into the bleeding branch, a micro plug with a diameter of 5 mm

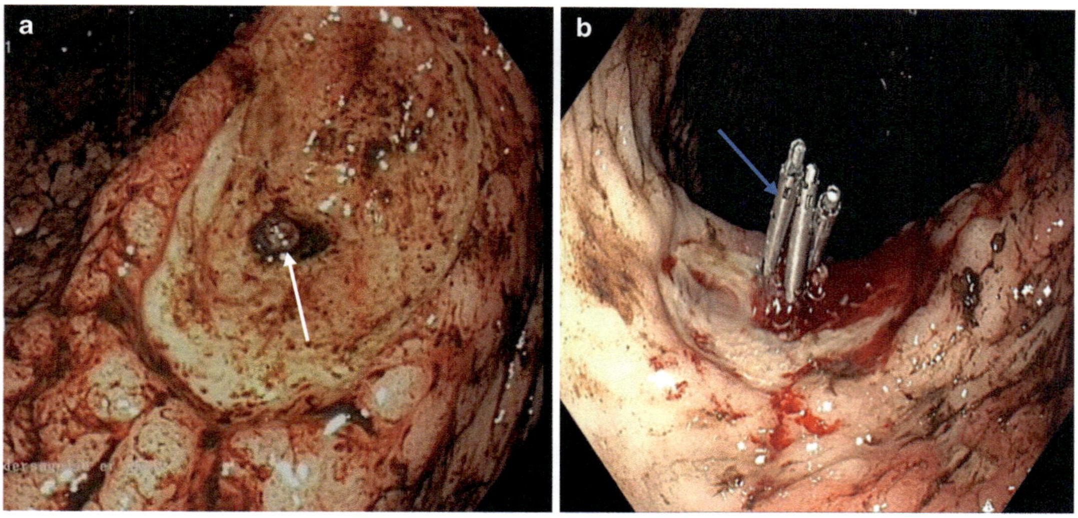

Fig. 4.74 (**a**) arrow indicates a peptic ulcer without ongoing bleeding. (**b**) latest image showing bleeding and endoscopic clips (arrows)

was deployed, and haemostasis was achieved immediately. The main left gastric artery and other branches remained open.

4.4.1.4 Outcome

The patient recovered very well, and no new bleeding events occurred. The patient was discharged from the hospital after 4 days.

4.4.2 Superior Mesenteric Artery-I

Key Points

- Aneurysms arising from the pancreaticoduodenal artery should be treated irrespective of the aneurysm size.
- All ruptured visceral aneurysms need to be treated, but endovascular treatment is usually not possible.
- A microcatheter should always be used in such cases.

4.4.2.1 Aetiology and Clinical Presentation

A 59-year healthy patient experienced sharp abdominal pain, and abdominal ultrasound showed free fluid in the abdomen. The patient was haemodynamically stable with a blood pressure of 110/80 mmHg. There were no other complaints.

4.4.2.2 Pre-interventional Diagnosis

A contrast-enhanced CT scan was performed and showed intraperitoneal bleeding and a small aneurysm arising from the pancreaticoduodenal artery. The likely small aneurysm ruptured, causing intraperitoneal haematoma. An embolization was planned (Fig. 4.76).

4.4.2.3 Endovascular Treatment

Under local anaesthesia, a 5 Fr sidewinder catheter was inserted percutaneously through the right femoral artery for selective angiography of the superior mesenteric artery, confirming a small aneurysm arising from the pancreaticoduodenal artery. A microcatheter was then advanced beyond the aneurysm, and embolization of the "back door" of the aneurysm was performed first with micro-coils 2 mm in diameter (Fig. 4.77). After that, the aneurysm and "front door" were occluded with micro-coils 3 mm in diameter.

4.4.2.4 Outcome

The patient did not experience any complications during the follow-up. Three months later, control non–contrast-enhanced CT (Fig. 4.78) showed

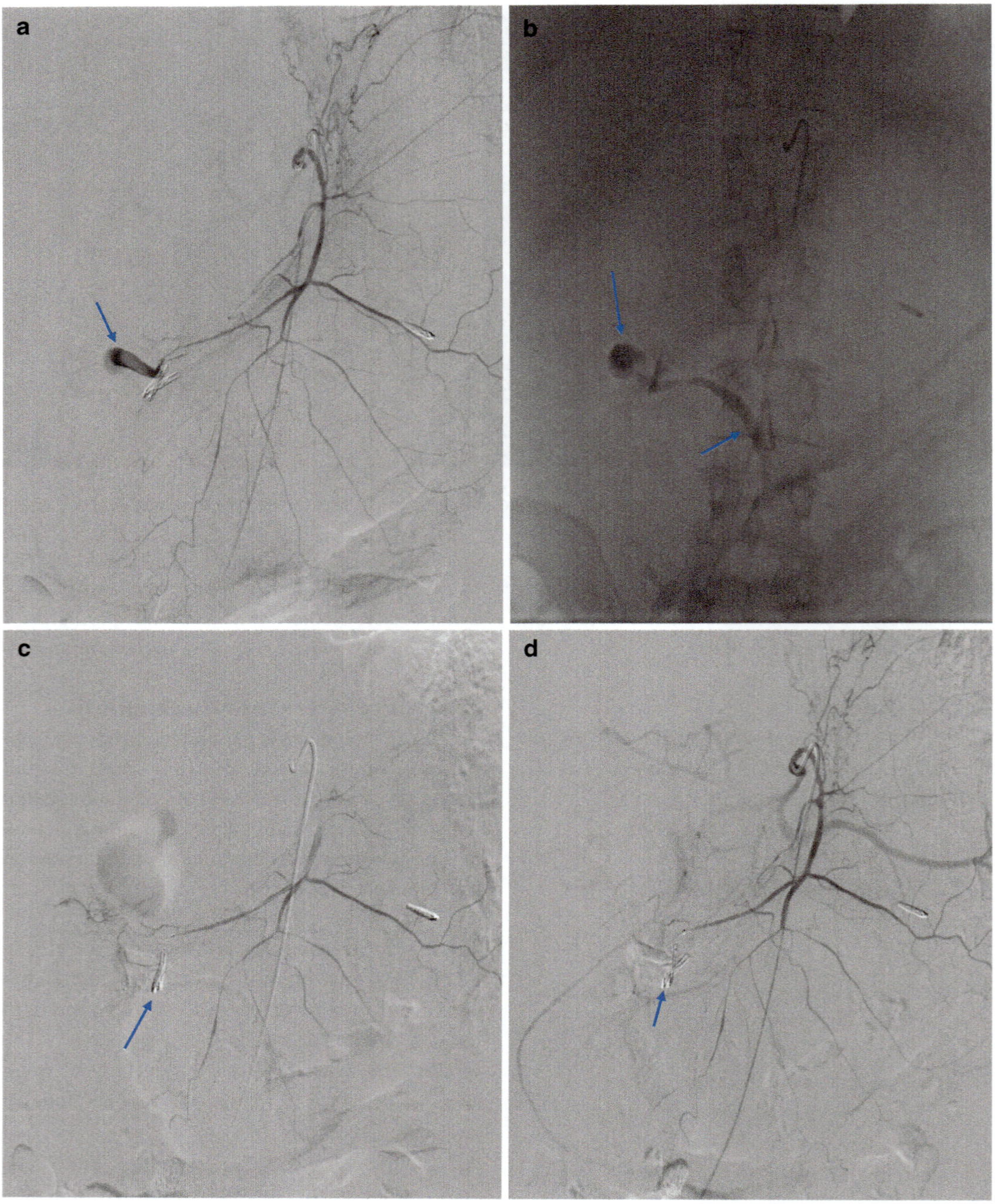

Fig. 4.75 (**a**) selective angiography of the left gastric artery showing active bleeding from one branch (arrow). (**b**) late phase image showing contrast extravasation (arrows). (**c**, **d**) deployment of a micro plug (arrows) and control image after embolization showing a good result

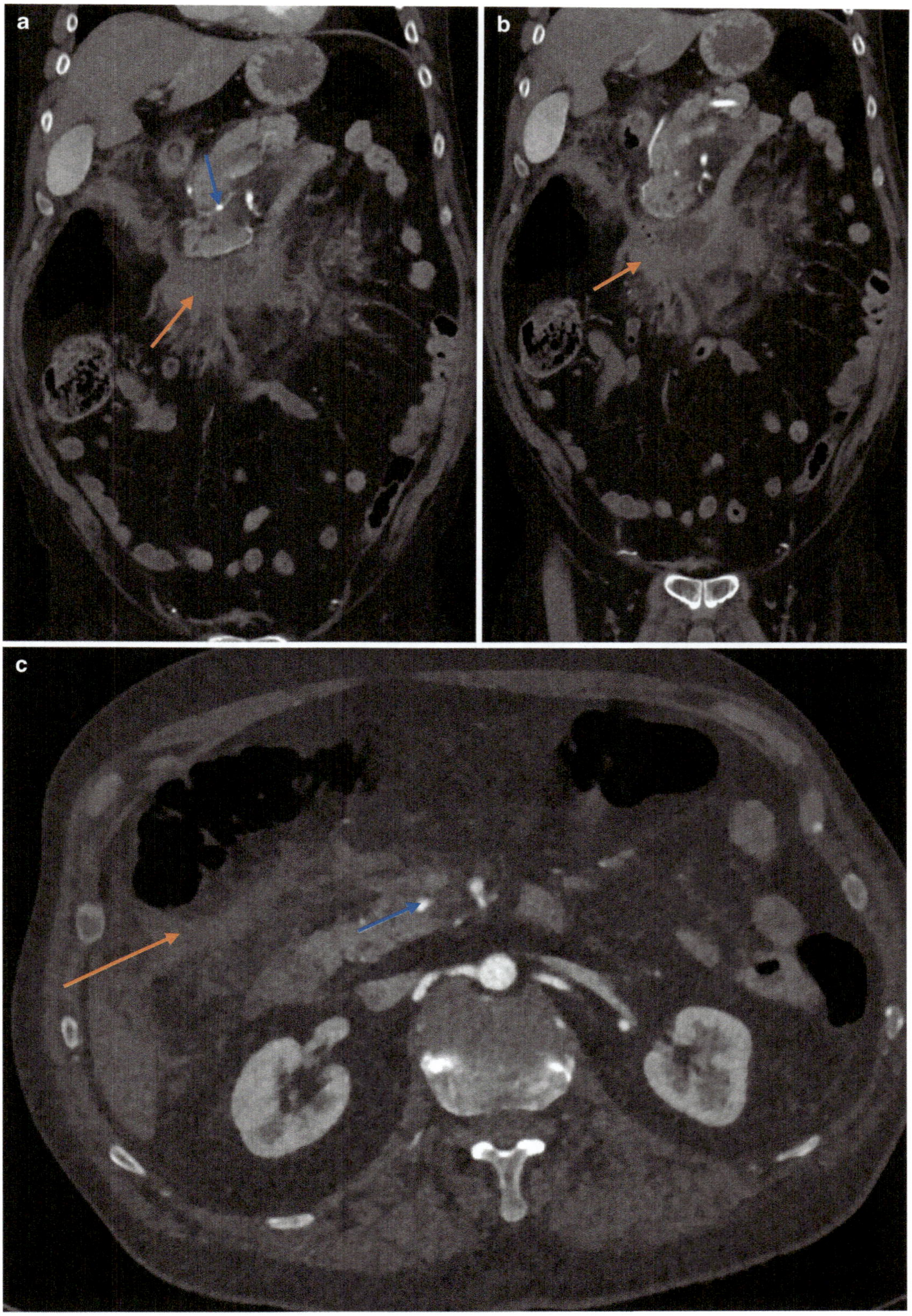

Fig. 4.76 Contrast-enhanced CT showing intraperitoneal bleeding (orange arrows). Blue arrows indicate a small aneurysm arising from the pancreaticoduodenal artery

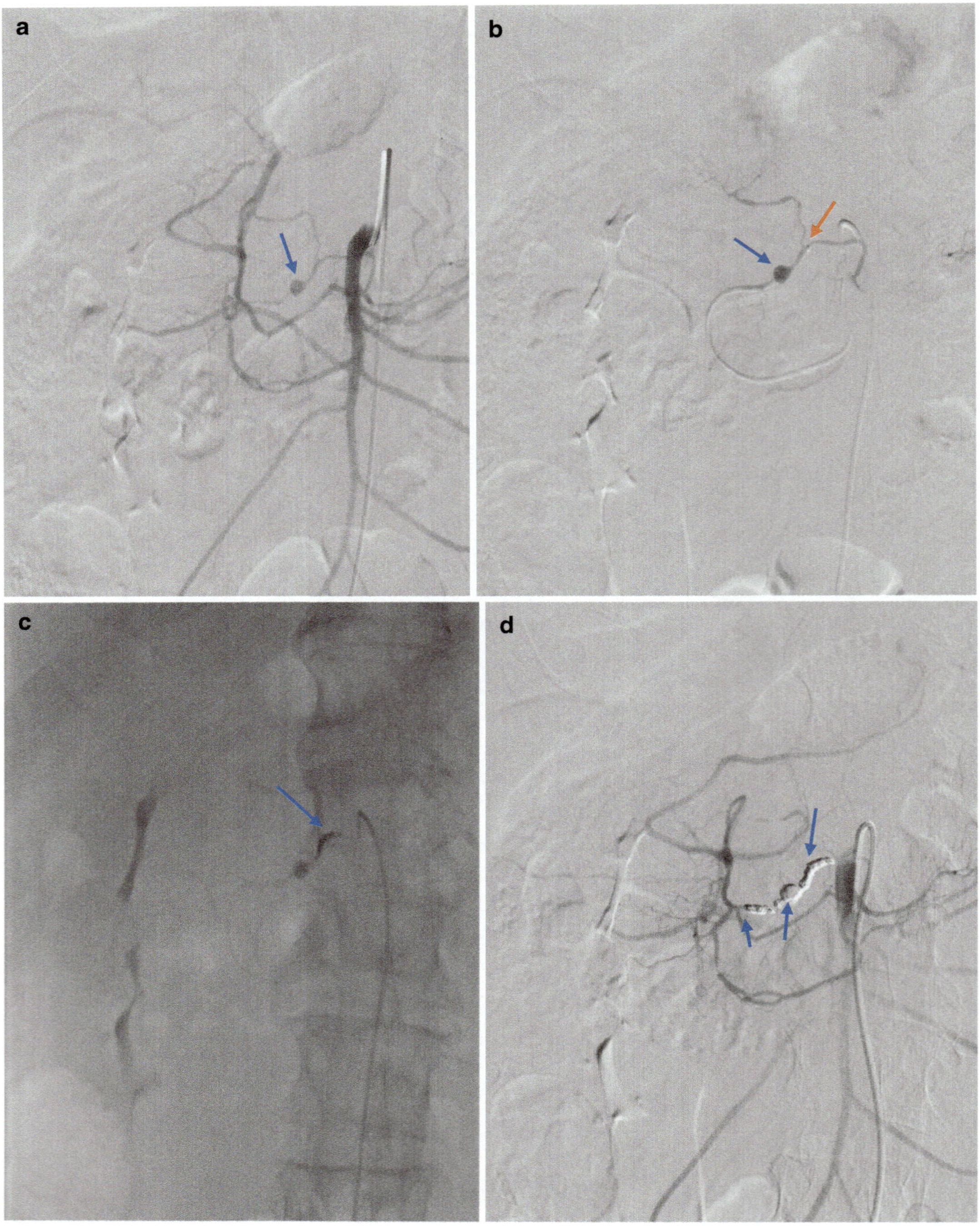

Fig. 4.77 (**a**) selective angiography of the SMA shows a small aneurysm arising from the pancreaticoduodenal artery (arrow). (**b**) advancement of a microcatheter beyond the origin of the aneurysm; orange arrow indicates the tip of the microcatheter. Blue arrow indicates the aneurysm. (**c**) embolization of the "back door" (arrows). (**d**) control image after embolization of the "back and front doors" (arrows)

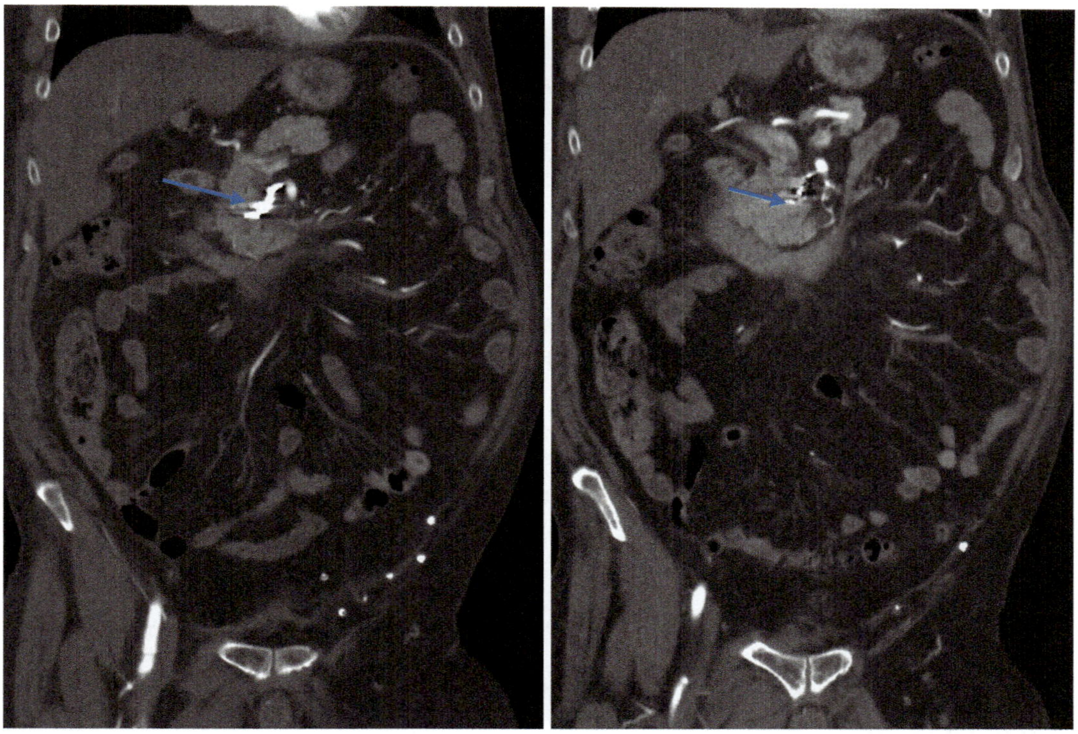

Fig. 4.78 Control CT scan 3 months after embolization. Almost complete resorption of the haematoma and a satisfactory result were obtained. Arrows indicate micro-coils

almost complete resorption of the haematoma. The small aneurysm is now complete occluded. No other aneurysms were visible.

4.4.3 Superior Mesenteric Artery-II

Key Points

- There is a rich collateral network between the visceral mesenteric vessels.
- The small branches, especially in cases of bleeding, are prone to spasm.
- A microcatheter should always be used in such cases.

4.4.3.1 Aetiology and Clinical Presentation

An 82-year-old patient complained of sharp acute pain in the right lower abdominal quadrant. Shortly after the pain subsided, the patient became unresponsive and hypotensive. Emergency services were administered, and the patient responded to resuscitation and was admitted to the emergency department. The patient had a previous ischaemic cerebral attack with complete remission and was on clopidogrel treatment.

4.4.3.2 Pre-interventional Diagnosis

Acute contrast-enhanced CT showed rupture of a branch arising from the SMA and intraperitoneal haematoma (Fig. 4.79). On sagittal projection, it was not possible to see the superior mesenteric artery. Emergency embolization was planned.

4.4.3.3 Endovascular Treatment

Under local anaesthesia, a sidewinder catheter was inserted percutaneously into the right femoral artery for selective angiography of the superior mesenteric artery (SMA). Angiography showed the right hepatic artery arising from the SMA, which lacked flow in the distal portion and demonstrated a possible small thrombus within (Fig. 4.80). After that, selective angiography of the inferior mesenteric artery showed an open

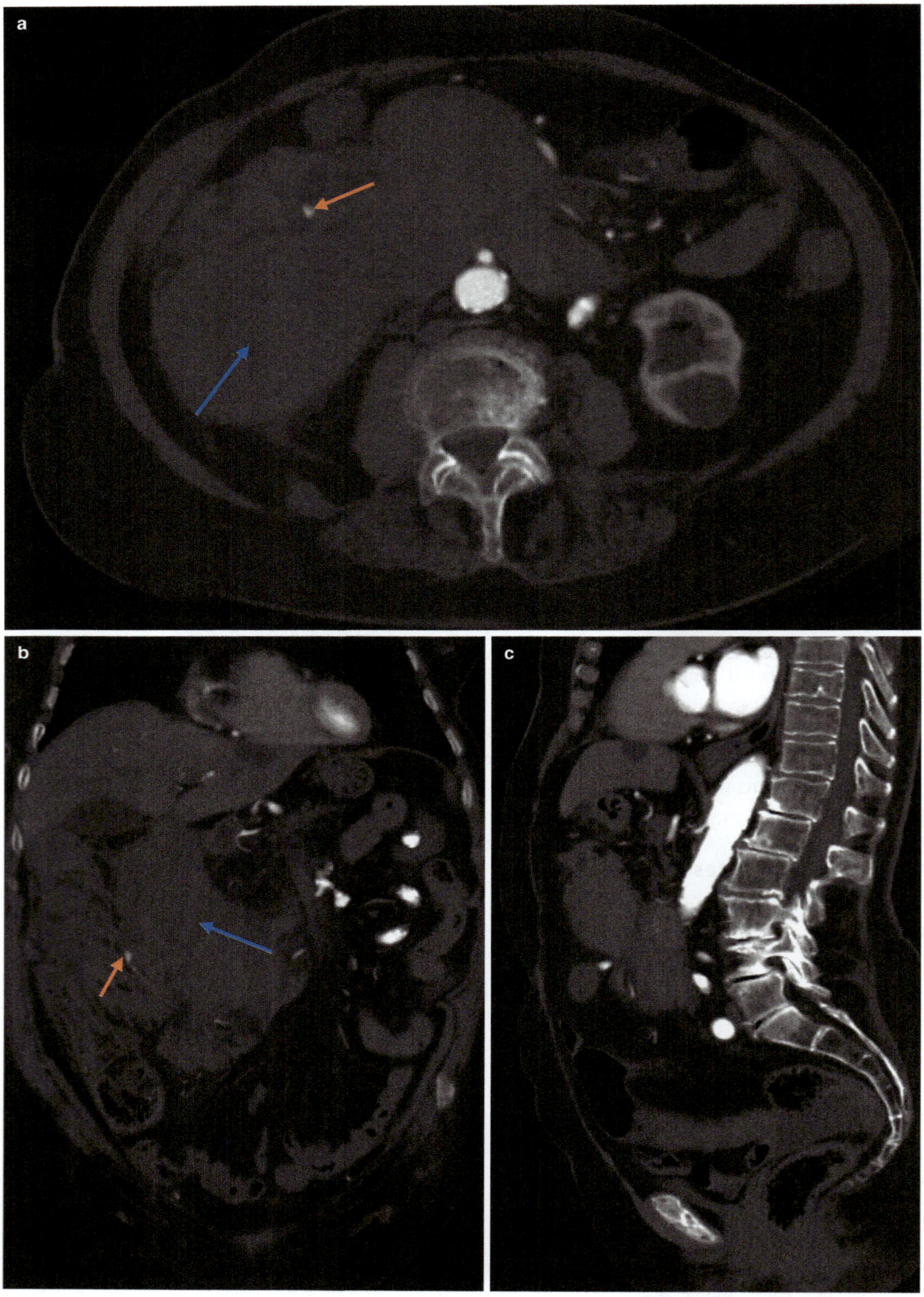

Fig. 4.79 Contrast-enhanced CT showing a bleeding branch arising from the mesenteric artery (orange arrows) in panels (**a**, **b**). Blue arrows indicate an intraperitoneal haematoma. (**c**) the superior mesenteric artery is not visible

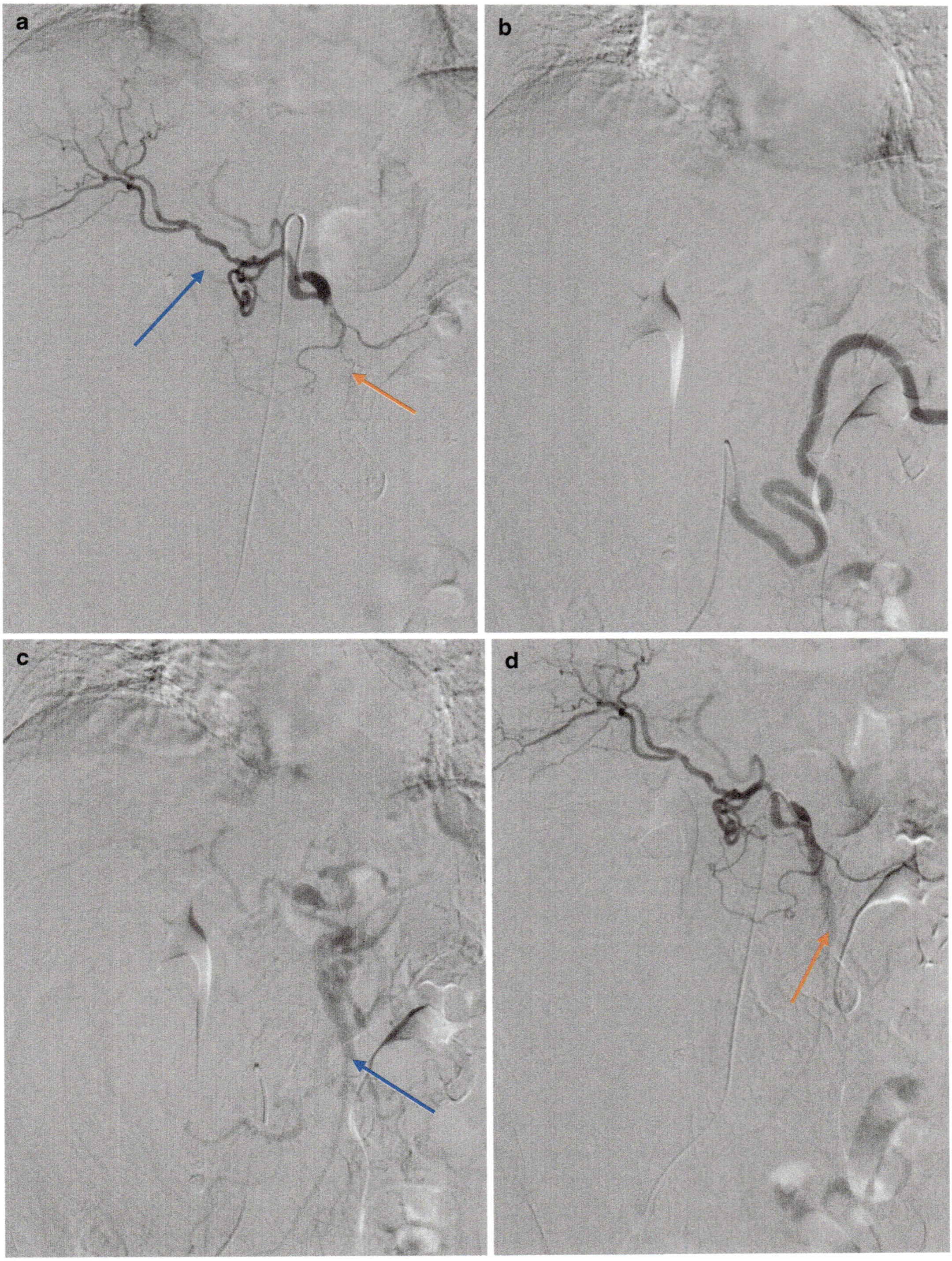

Fig. 4.80 (**a**) blue arrow indicates that the right hepatic artery arises from the SMA. Orange arrow indicates slow flow in the SMA and possible thrombosis. (**b**) selective angiography of the inferior mesenteric artery. (**c**) open SMA angiography via the inferior mesenteric artery; blue arrow indicates the SMA. (**d**, **e**) advancement of the catheter into the SMA and depiction of the bleeding site from a small branch arising from the ileocolic artery (blue arrow). (**f**) control image after the bleeding was arrested with a micro-plug; orange arrow indicates the micro-plug

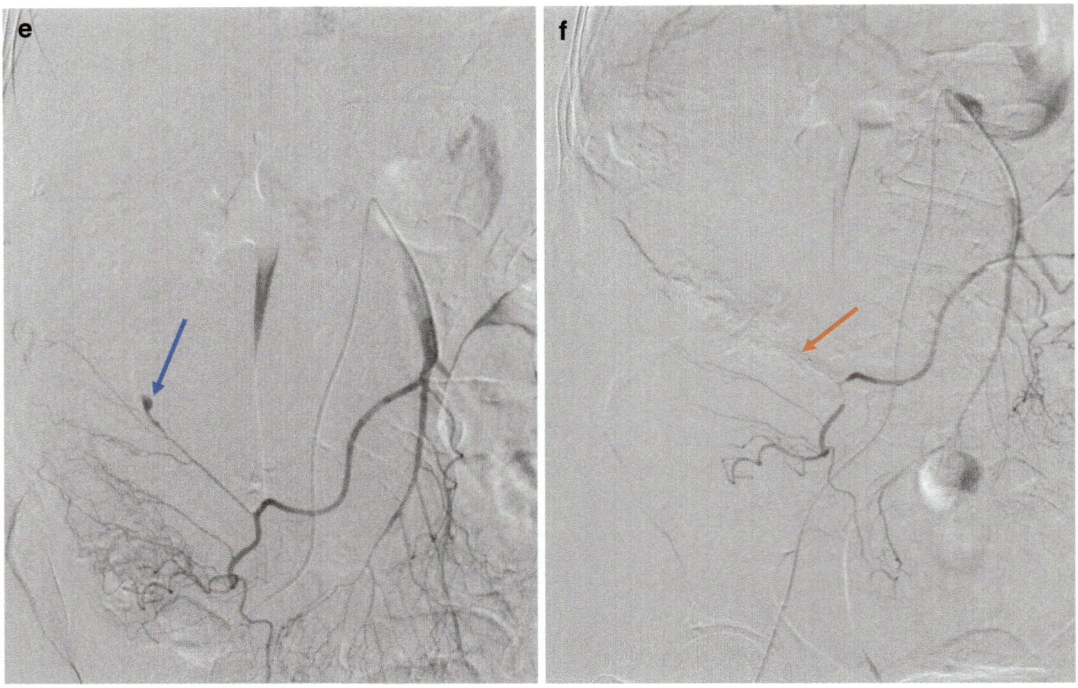

Fig. 4.80 (continued)

SMA, and again, a catheter was advanced into the SMA. After further advancement of the catheter, angiography confirmed an open SMA and bleeding from one branch on the right side. Then, a microcatheter was advanced into the bleeding branch, and a 3 mm micro-plug was used for embolization with excellent results. There was no significant stenosis or thrombus of the SMA, and the artery was open. The intervention went well, and the patient did not experience worsening of the haemodynamic status or develop compartment syndrome. The patient was discharged 6 days after embolization.

4.4.3.4 Outcome

The patient recovered well and has not experienced new bleeding events. There were no ischaemic complications, and the patient was symptom free. Control contrast-enhanced CT before discharge (Fig. 4.81) showed that the size of the haematoma had not changed and that the artery was well embolized.

4.4.4 Inferior Mesenteric Artery

Key Points

- Bleeding from the lower gastrointestinal tract requiring endovascular treatment can and should be diagnosed with CT.
- A microcatheter should always be used.
- Usually, small micro-coils 2 and 3 mm in diameter are required for super-selective, safe embolization.

4.4.4.1 Aetiology and Clinical Presentation

A 74-year-old patient was admitted to the hospital due to increased bleeding into the stool. The patient had previously experienced discrete lower gastrointestinal bleeding, but this time, heavy bleeding was observed, and the patient's blood pressure was 90/60 mmHg. Haemoglobin was

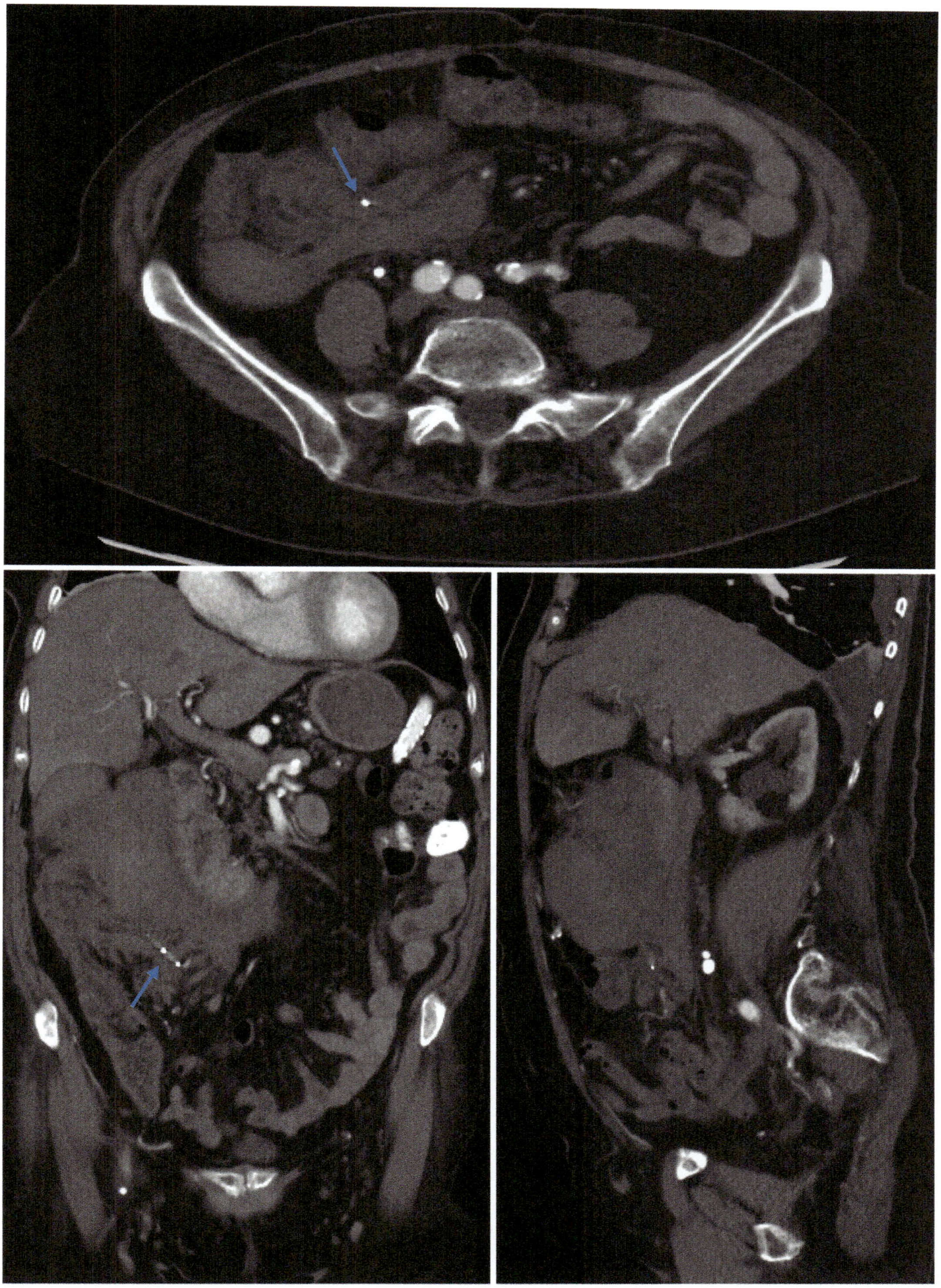

Fig. 4.81 Control contrast-enhanced CT before discharged showing a satisfactory result. Arrows indicate the micro-plug

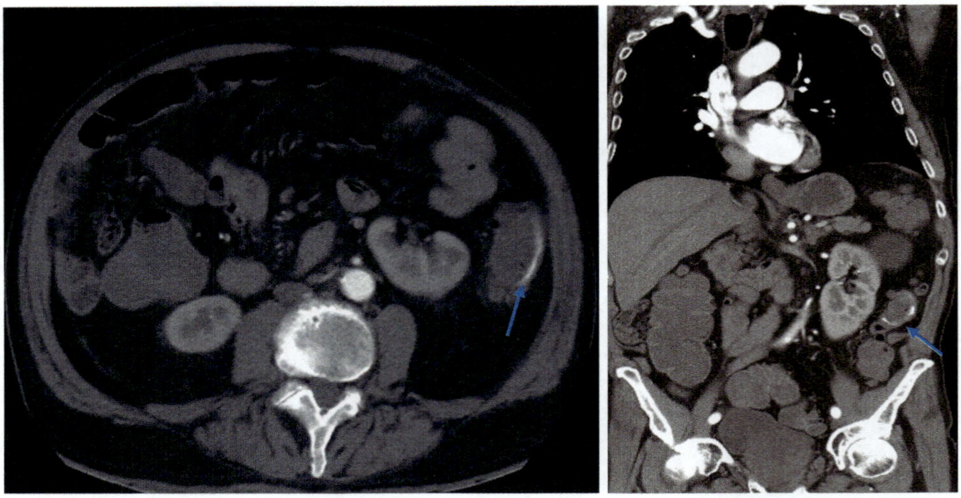

Fig. 4.82 Contrast-enhanced CT showing bleeding into the descending colon (arrows)

low (4.5 mmol/L). The patient was known to have colonic diverticulosis, and bleeding from the diverticulum was suspected.

4.4.4.2 Pre-interventional Diagnosis

Contrast-enhanced CT confirmed bleeding from the sigmoid diverticulum and the left branch of the colic artery (Fig. 4.82).

4.4.4.3 Endovascular Treatment

Under local anaesthesia, a 5 Fr sidewinder catheter was inserted percutaneously through the right femoral artery for selective angiography of the inferior mesenteric artery. Angiography confirmed that the bleeding site was in the left peripheral branch of the colic artery (Fig. 4.83). A microcatheter was then advanced very quickly, and the target branches were occluded with small micro-coils 2 mm in diameter.

4.4.4.4 Outcome

The patient did not experience any complications, especially ischaemic complications. Control contrast-enhanced CT 3 months after embolization (Fig. 4.84) showed a satisfactory outcome and no new bleeding.

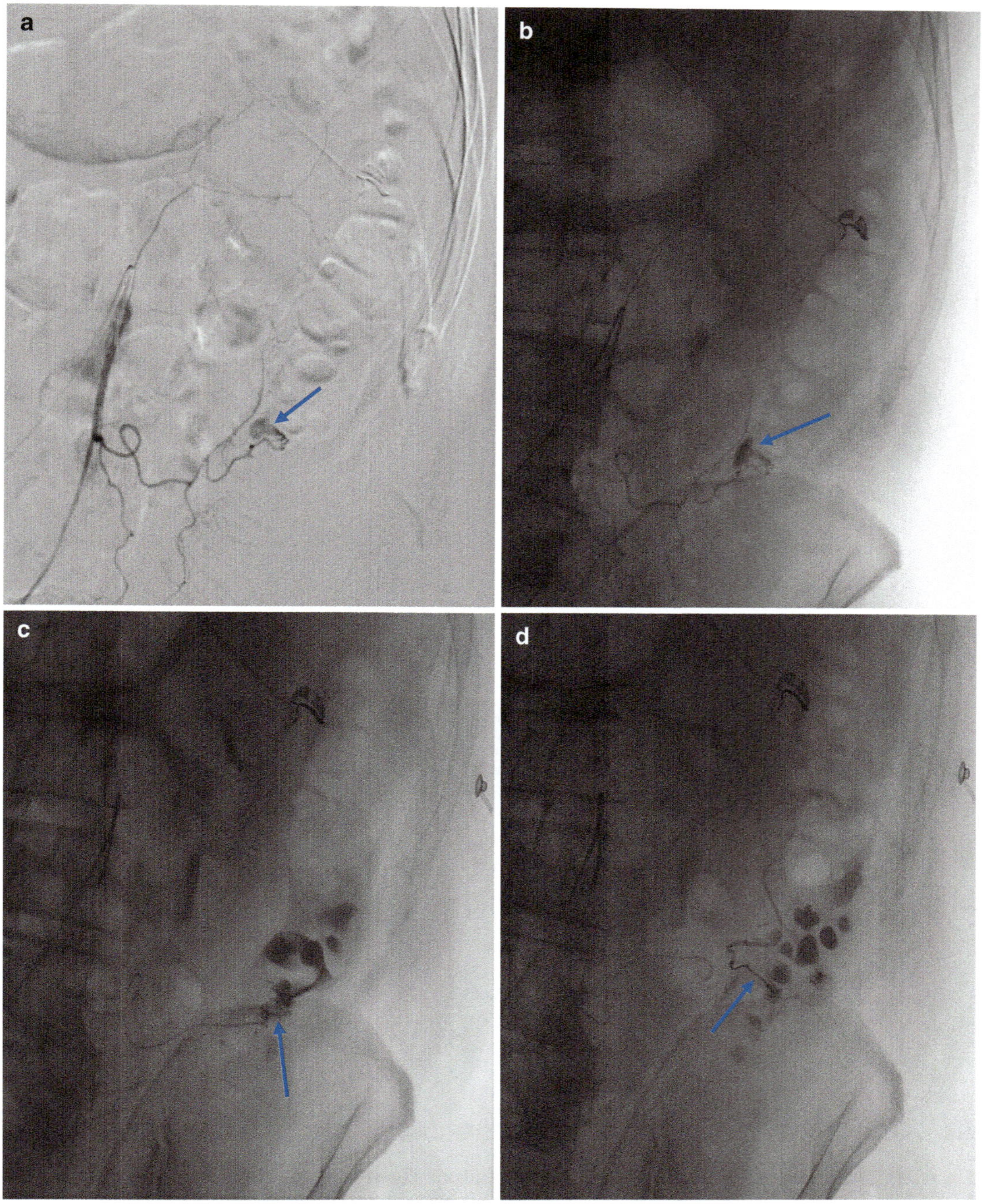

Fig. 4.83 (**a**, **b**) arrows indicate active bleeding from the mural branches of the left colic artery. (**c**) advancement of a microcatheter as close as possible to the bleeding point; arrow indicates the tip of the microcatheter. (**d**, **e**) control angiography showing arrested bleeding and occlusion only of the bleeding artery

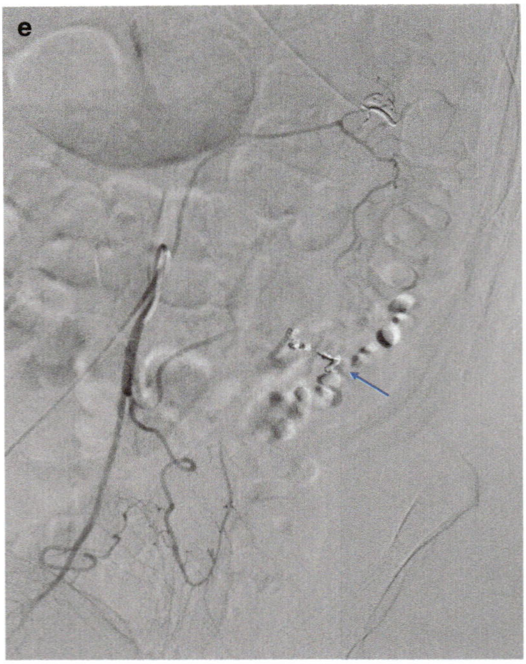

Fig. 4.83 (continued)

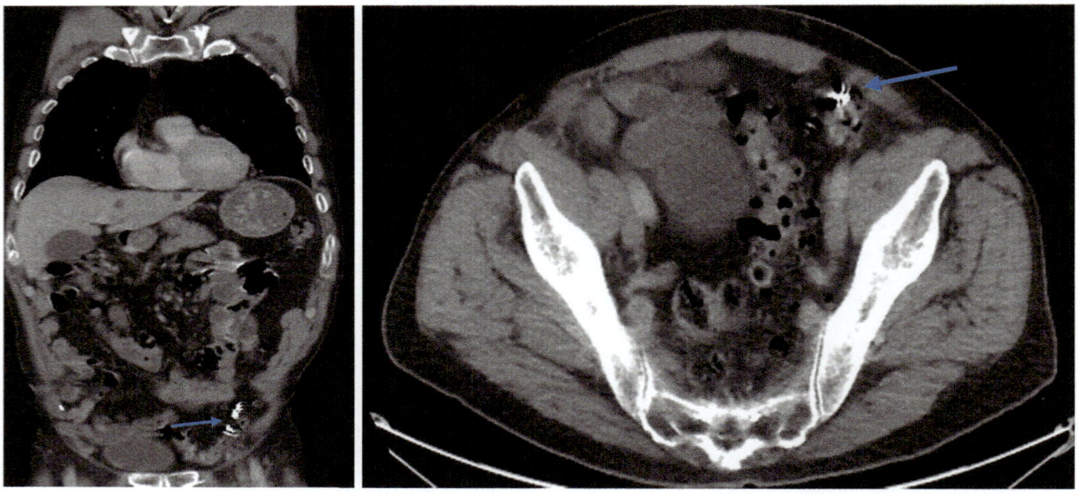

Fig. 4.84 Control contrast-enhanced CT 3 months after embolization showing a satisfactory result; arrows indicate micro-coils

Pelvic Vascular Emergencies

5

Contents

S. Duvnjak, *Endovascular Treatment of Arterial Emergencies*,
https://doi.org/10.1007/978-3-030-68832-5_5

5.1 External Iliac Artery Bleeding

Key Points

- The access vessels should be carefully assessed; usually, the problem is with the external iliac artery.
- If rupture occurs, the guidewire should be kept in place while the stent graft is deployed.
- Excessive post-dilatation of the stent graft should be avoided while maintaining the balloon inside it.

5.1.1 Aetiology and Clinical Presentation

A 72-year-old patient with chronic pulmonary obstructive disease and hypertension with an incidentally discovered 5.7 cm abdominal aortic aneurysm (AAA) was scheduled for elective repair. The patient had a normal renal function.

5.1.2 Pre-interventional Diagnosis

Contrast-enhanced CT showed a 57 mm AAA suitable for endovascular repair (EVAR). The iliac arteries had calcifications and stenosis. The common iliac artery on the right side had a diameter of 14 mm, and that on the left side had a diameter of 17 mm (Fig. 5.1). The lumen of the external iliac arteries was approximately 6–7 mm.

5.1.3 Endovascular Intervention

Under general anaesthesia, a bifurcated stent graft was advanced through the surgically exposed right femoral artery and deployed without difficulty (Fig. 5.2). A contralateral iliac limb stent graft with a diameter of 20 mm distally was used on the left side. Post-dilatation on the right side was performed with balloon angioplasty with a balloon 14 mm in diameter. A 16 mm-diameter limb was used for the right leg. The patient dropped in blood pressure, and angiography showed a ruptured right external iliac artery (Fig. 5.2). An iliac limb extension with a diameter of 16 proximally and 13 distally and a length of 82 mm was quickly deployed without occluding the right internal iliac artery. The patient responded quickly with pressure normalization. There were no other complications.

5.1.4 Outcome

The patient had an uneventful recovery in the intensive care unit and at the department. There

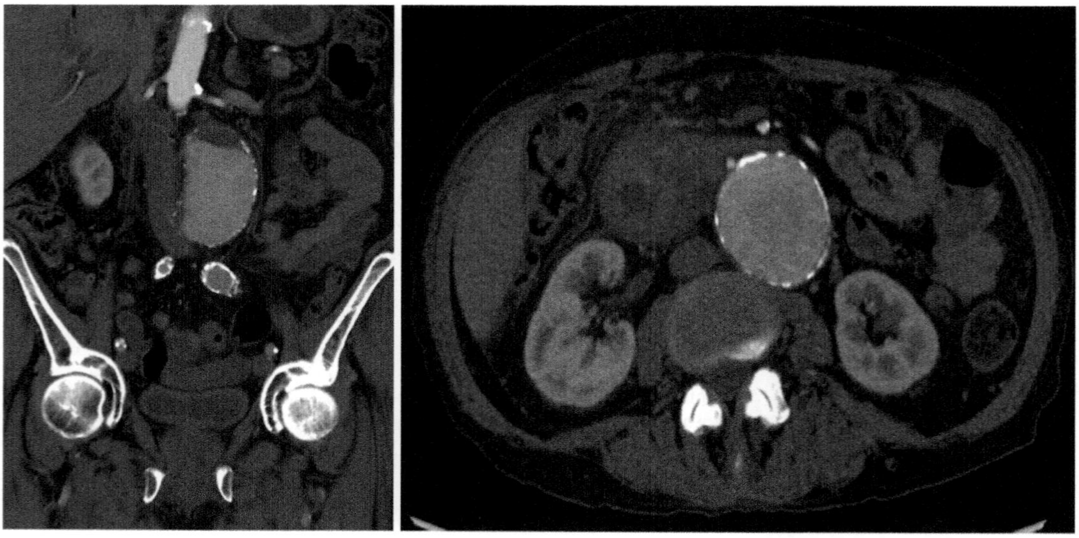

Fig. 5.1 Contrast-enhanced CT showing an incidentally discovered 57 mm AAA, suitable for EVAR

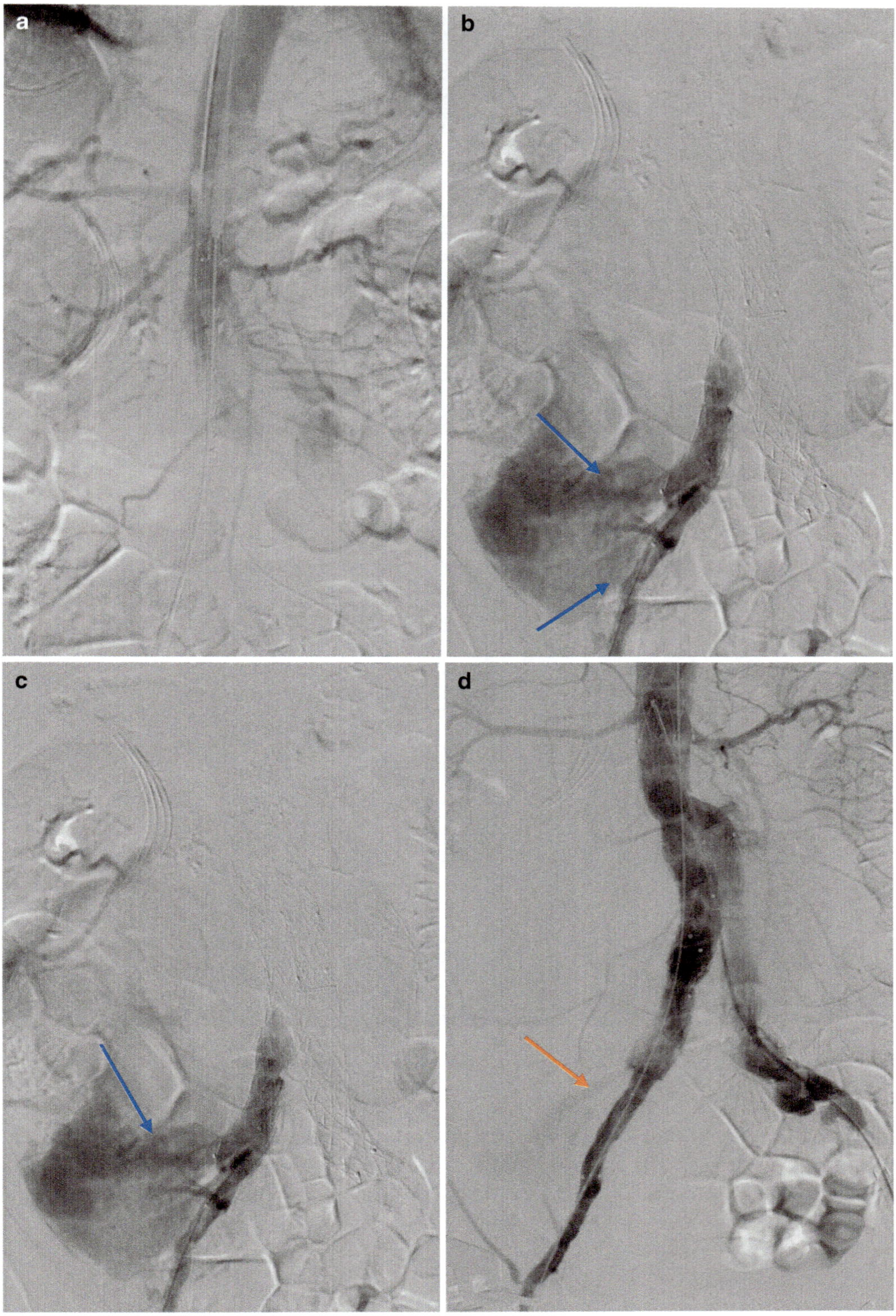

Fig. 5.2 Details from EVAR intervention. (**a**) advancement of a bifurcated stent graft. (**b** and **c**) rupture of the right external iliac artery after post-dilatation with a 14 mm balloon (arrows). (**d**) control imaging after deployment of an additional iliac limb extension with a 16 mm proximal and 13 distal diameter (orange arrow)

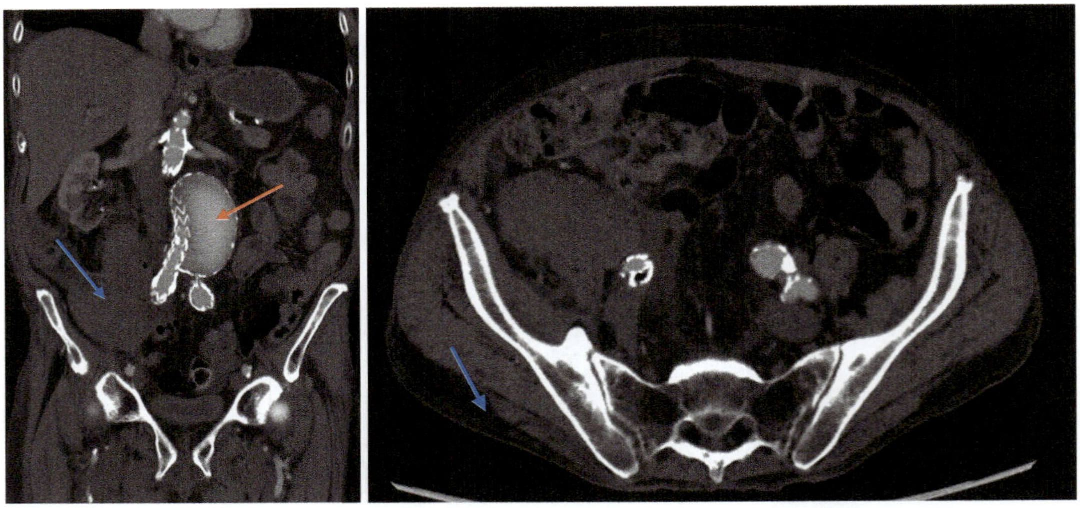

Fig. 5.3 Control scanning the next day after the EVAR. There was no bleeding. Haematoma can be seen in the right retroperitoneum (blue arrows). Contrast is observed inside the AAA due to the recent intervention (orange arrow)

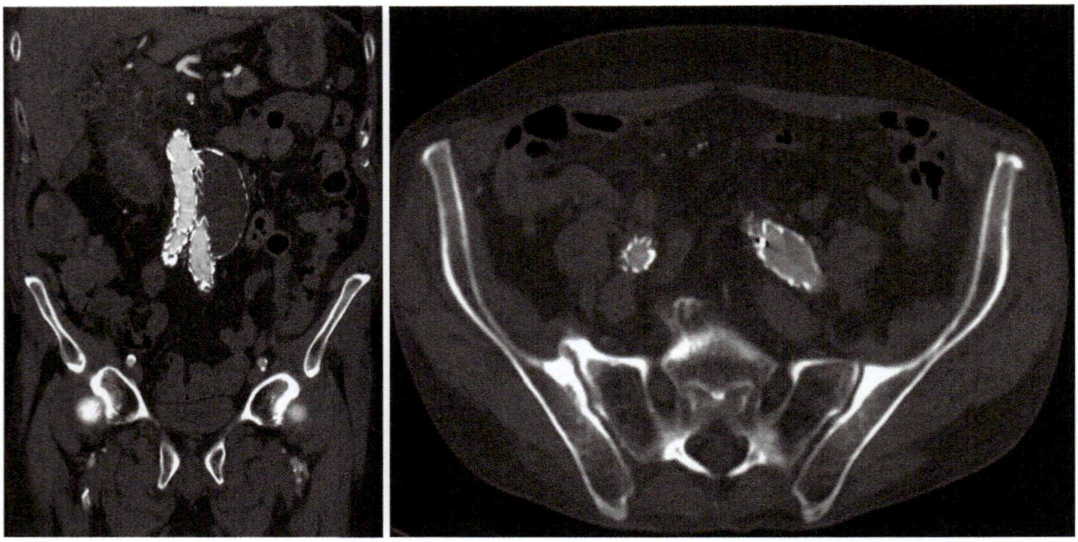

Fig. 5.4 Three months later, control CT showed a satisfactory result and haematoma resorption

was no significant drop in haemoglobin and no compartment syndrome. The control CT performed the next day showed a satisfactory result, and no endoleak was observed through the non-occluded right internal iliac artery (Fig. 5.3). Control imaging 3 months later showed complete haematoma resorption and no complications (Fig. 5.4).

5.2 Internal Iliac Artery Bleeding

Key Points

- A complicated surgery and infection can cause arterio-enteric fistula formation.
- Embolization is preferred if possible in severe cases to control bleeding.
- Antibiotic treatment is usually required in the long-term, and further complications can occur.

5.2.1 Aetiology and Clinical Presentation

A 69-year-old patient underwent complex uterine surgery due to cancer. After that, sigmoideum resection and stoma creation were performed. Two weeks after the complicated surgery, the patient was highly febrile, and abscesses were observed at the top of the vagina, which were treated with antibiotics and surgical revision. The patient suddenly presented with massive bleeding through the vagina after the last abscess revision.

5.2.2 Pre-interventional Diagnosis

Contrast-enhanced CT showed bleeding on the left side and active contrast extravasation from the left internal iliac branch (Fig. 5.5). That was abscess and collection around the vaginal top.

5.2.3 Endovascular Intervention

The right femoral artery was punctured. The left internal iliac artery was selectively catheterized, and angiography confirmed bleeding from the anterior division (Fig. 5.6). A microcatheter was then advanced, and micro-coils 3 mm in diameter were used to embolize the bleeding site, resulting in complete bleeding control and occlusion of the anterior division.

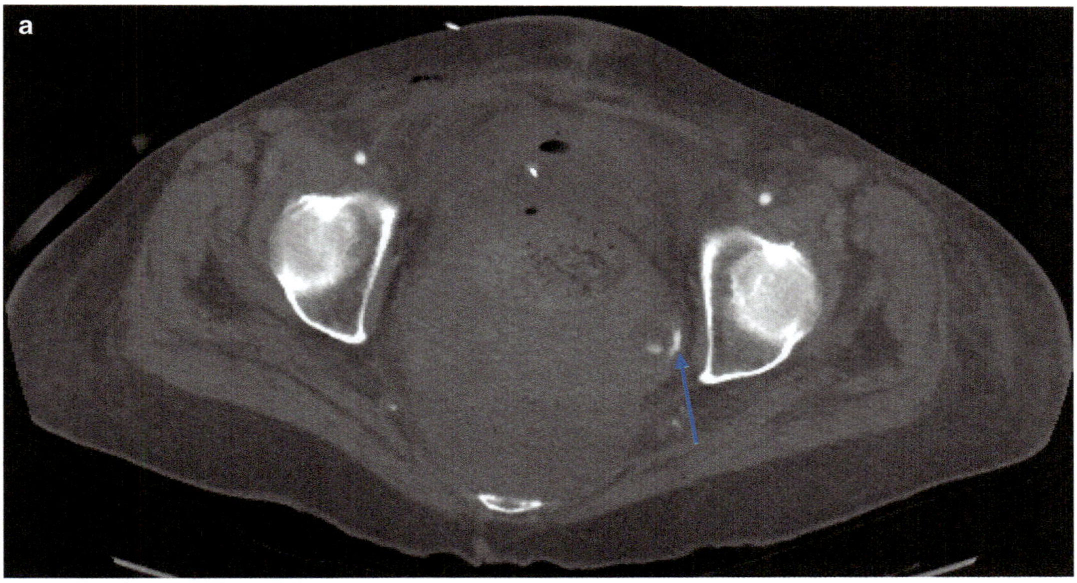

Fig. 5.5 Contrast-enhanced CT showing active bleeding from the left internal iliac artery branches (**a**–**c**) (blue arrows). Orange arrows indicate abscess collection at the top of the vagina (**b**)

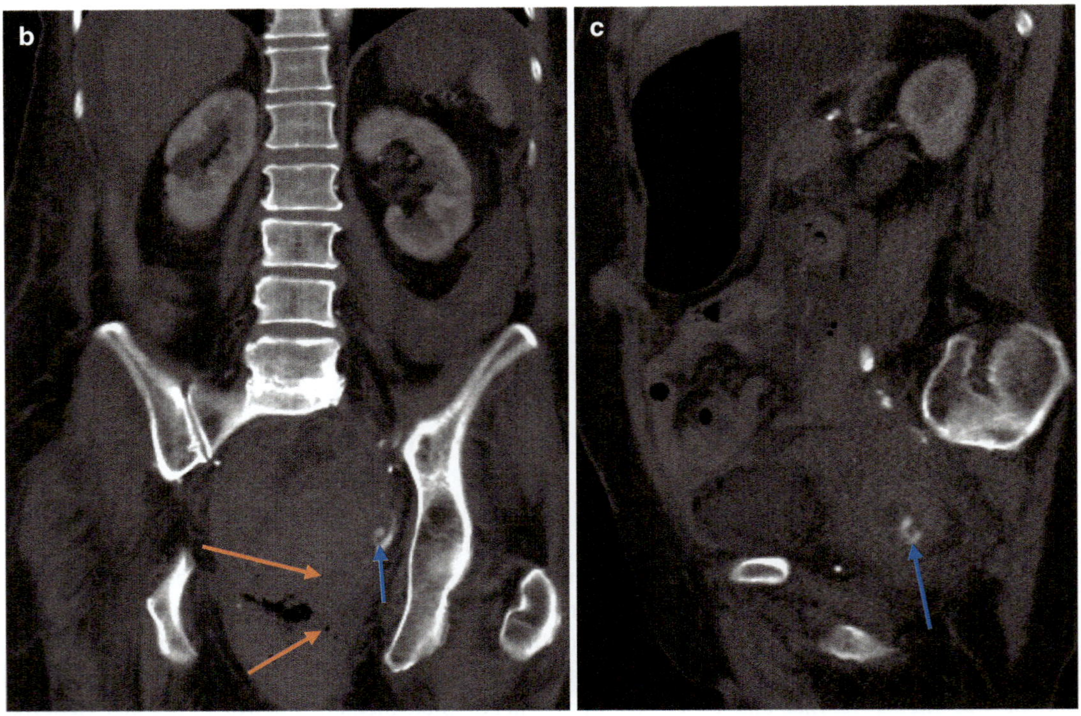

Fig. 5.5 (continued)

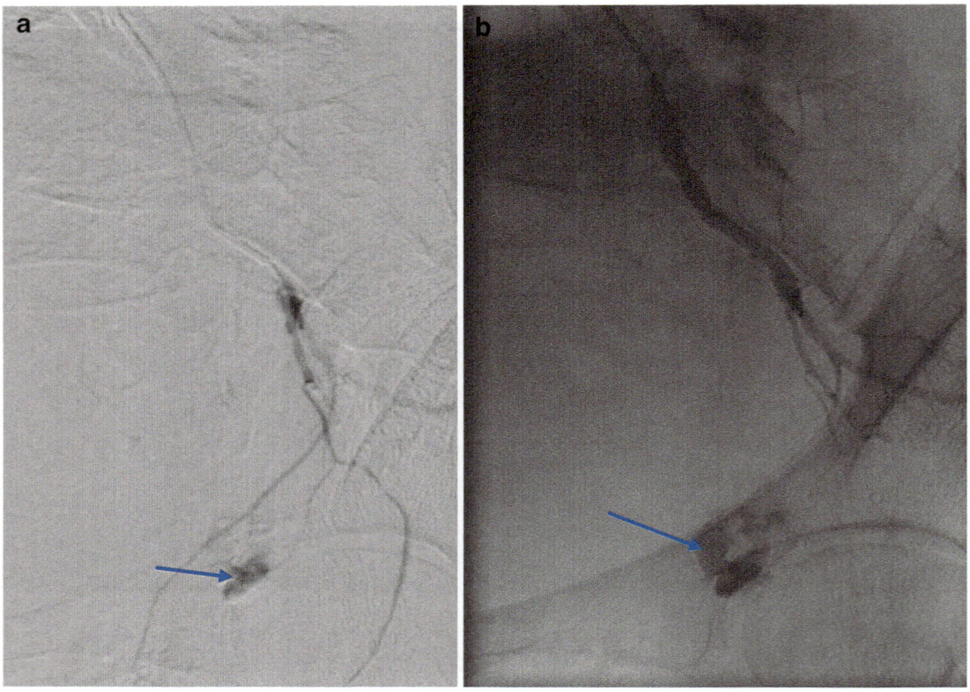

Fig. 5.6 Crossover technique. Angiography of the left internal iliac artery confirmed bleeding from the anterior division (blue arrows) (**a** and **b**). Orange arrow shows fistula to the bowel/vagina (**c**). Control after micro-coil embolization (black arrows), resulting in control of the bleeding (**d** and **e**). Final bilateral pelvic angiography was performed to evaluate other eventual bleeding points. There were no other sources of bleeding (**e**)

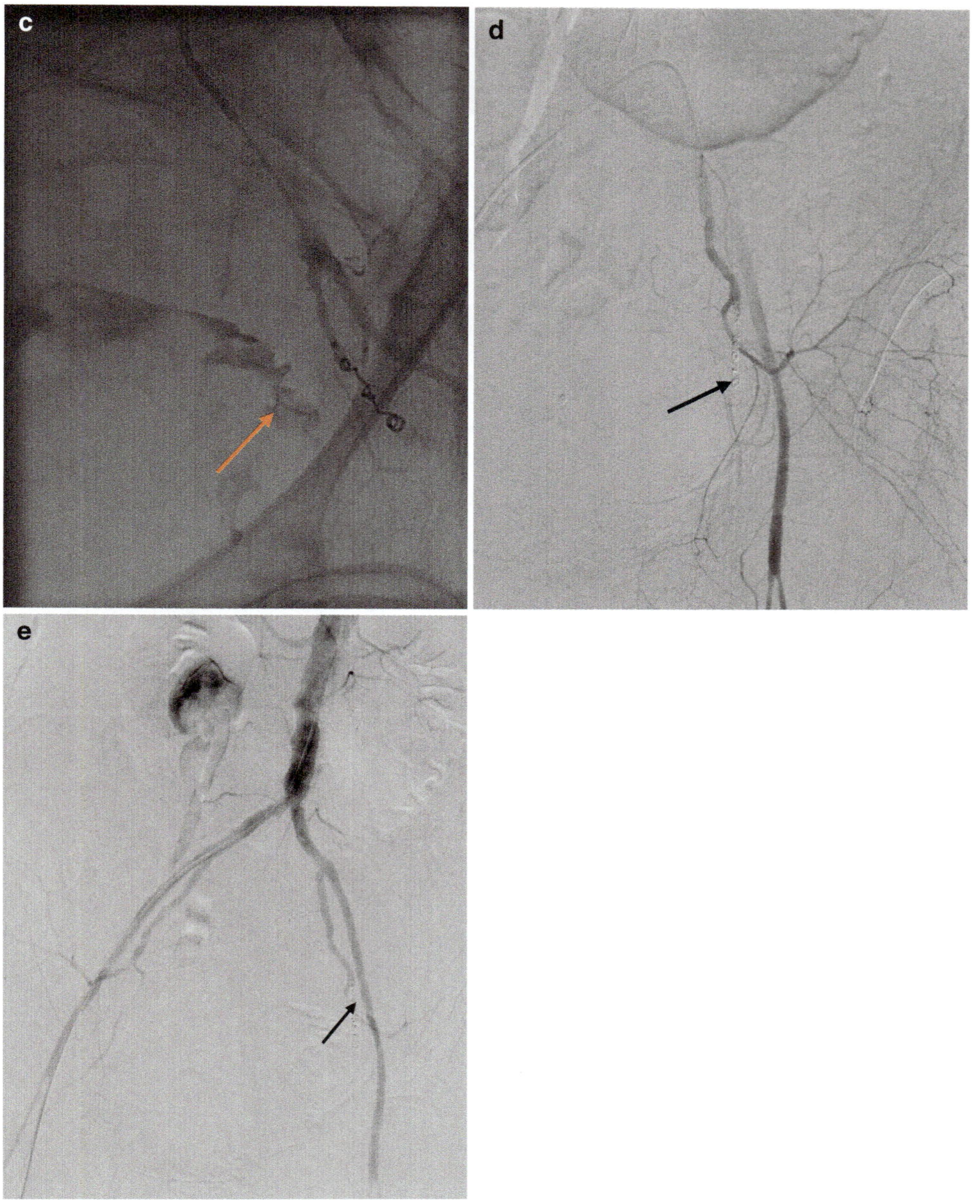

Fig. 5.6 (continued)

5.2.4 Outcome

The patient remains in the hospital, and recovery over the last few months has been gradual. No new bleeding has been observed from the pelvis or through the vagina. Control CT 3 months after the procedure showed significant improvement with some residual abscess collection on the left side in the pelvis (Fig. 5.7).

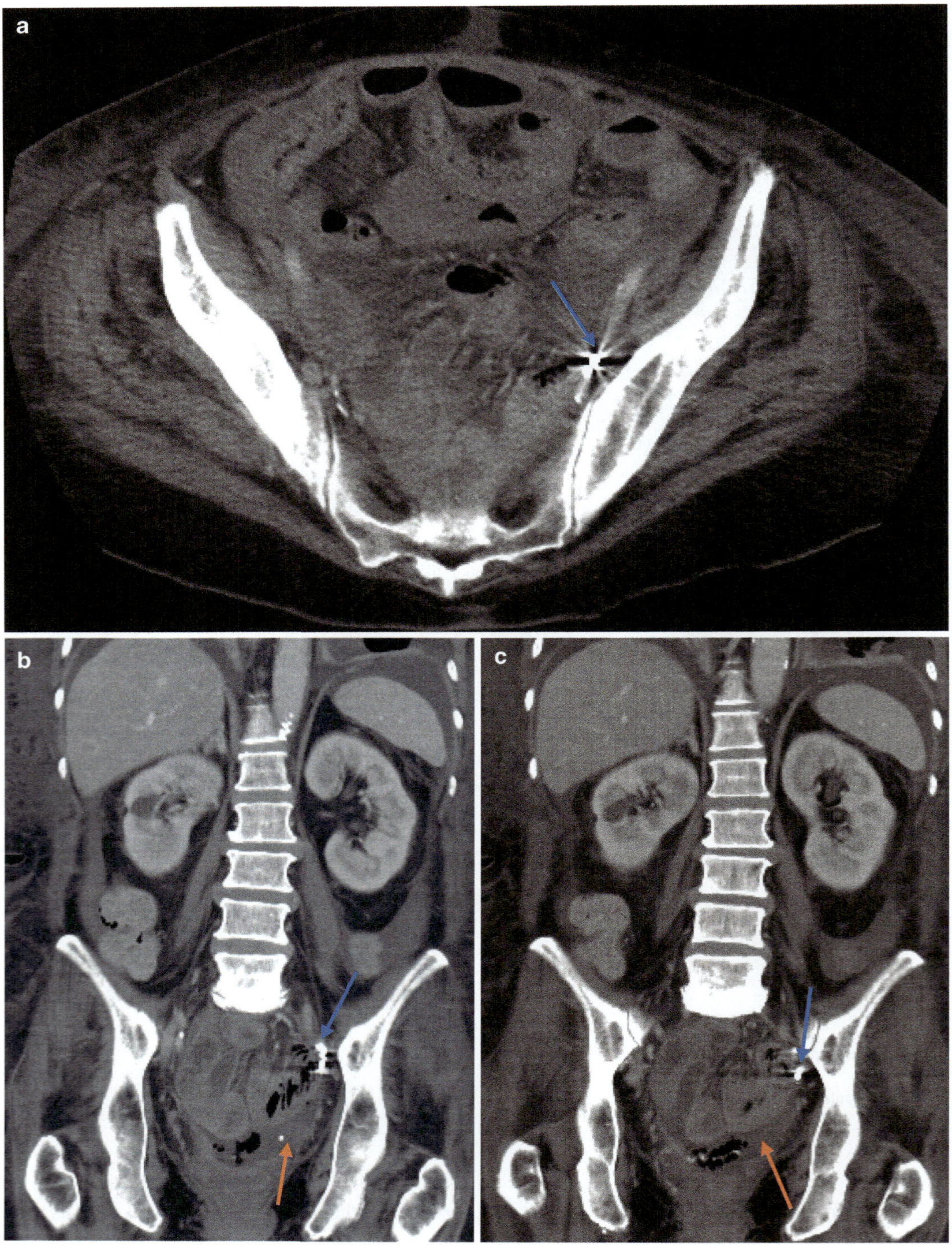

Fig. 5.7 Control contrast-enhanced CT 3 months after embolization. Blue arrows indicate micro-coils (**a**). Orange arrows indicate residual abscess collection on the left side (**b–c**)

5.3 Uterine Artery Bleeding-I

Key Points

- Uterine artery pseudoaneurysms are very easily treated with micro-coil embolization.
- In a majority of cases, both uterine arteries usually need to be occluded, but sometimes is possible to perform embolization on only one side.
- The intervention is well-tolerated.

5.3.1 Aetiology and Clinical Presentation

A 29-year-old patient underwent an abortion 3 months prior. The patient experienced recurrent uterine bleeding several times after the surgery. Clinically, the patient was haemodynamically stable, but the bleeding was a social problem and impacted the quality of life of the patient.

5.3.2 Pre-interventional Diagnosis

Contrast-enhanced CT showed a pseudoaneurysm in the right uterine artery and focal hyperdense changes in the left part of the uterus (Fig. 5.8). An enlarged uterus, a retroperitoneal haematoma and abdominal packing could be seen on CT.

5.3.3 Endovascular Intervention

Selective catheterization of the right internal iliac artery was performed percutaneously through the left femoral artery and confirmed a pseudoaneurysm arising from the right uterine artery (Fig. 5.9). Then, super-selective catheterization was performed with a microcatheter advanced into the right uterine artery, and micro-coils 3 mm in diameter were used for embolization. The left uterine artery was occluded with multiple 3 mm micro-coils afterwards to prevent filing of the pseudoaneurysm via the collateral network.

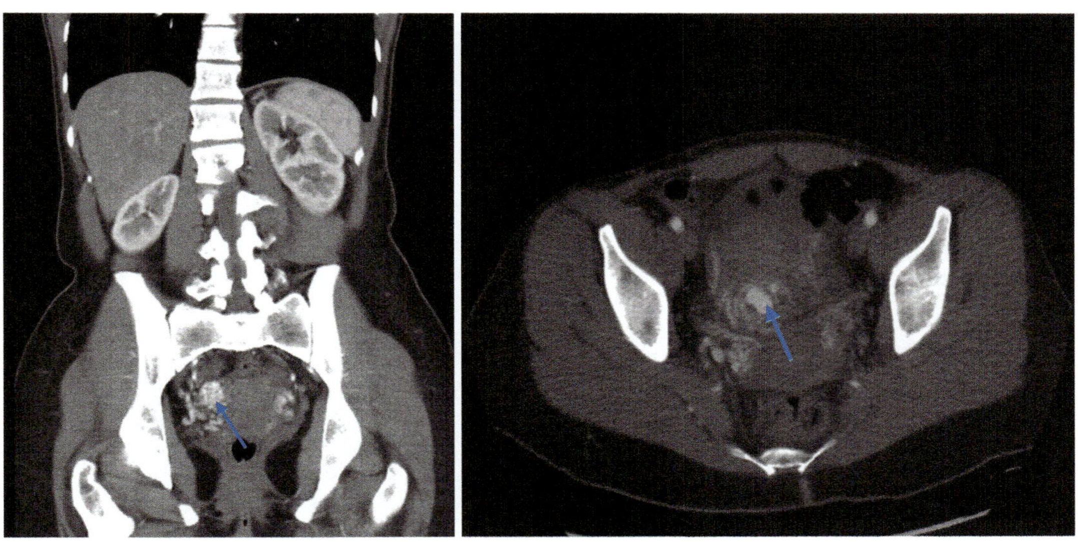

Fig. 5.8 Contrast-enhanced CT showing a pseudoaneurysm of the right uterine artery (arrows)

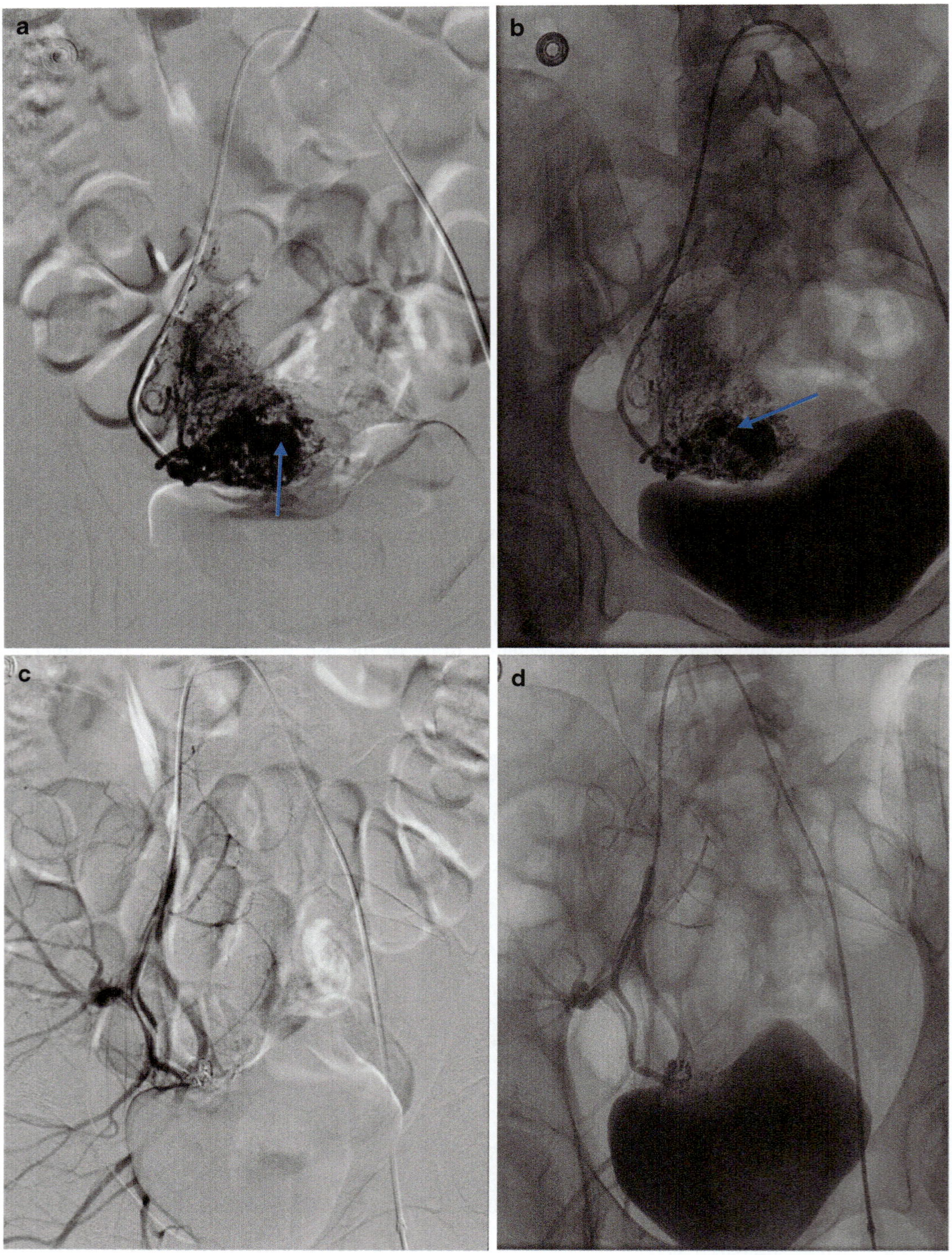

Fig. 5.9 Details from the embolization. (**a**–**d**) selective catheterization of the right uterine artery and embolization of the artery with micro-coils; arrows indicate the pseudoaneurysm. (**d**, **e**) embolization of the left uterine artery with micro-coils (**f**)

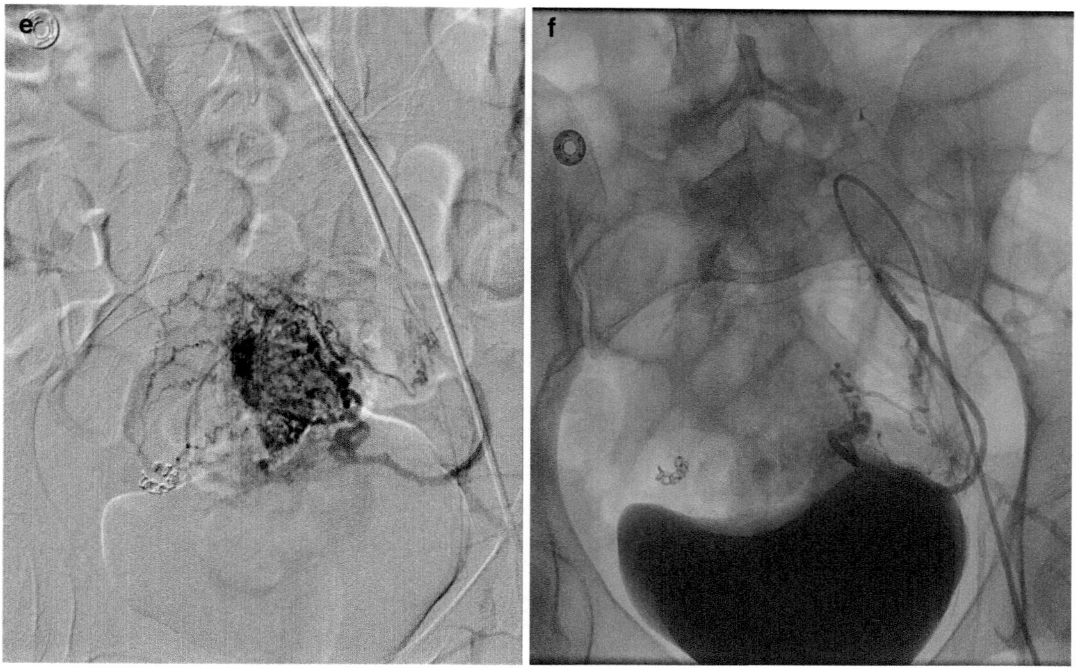

Fig. 5.9 (continued)

5.3.4 Outcome

The patient was discharged the next day without any complications. There were no new bleeding episodes or complaints in the follow-up period and control MR scanning showed restored uterus morphology (Fig. 5.10).

5.4 Uterine Artery Bleeding-II

Key Points

- Uterine artery pseudoaneurysms with arteriovenous fistulae are very easily treated with micro-coil embolization.
- In a majority of cases, both uterine arteries usually need to be occluded, but sometimes it is possible to perform embolization on only one side.
- The intervention is well-tolerated.
- Microspheres should never be used for such patients.

5.4.1 Aetiology and Clinical Presentation

A 34-year-old patient underwent a medical abortion 2 months prior. The patient was haemodynamically stable with recurrent metrorrhagia. There were no other complaints. Doppler ultrasound revealed a hypervascular uterine lesion.

5.4.2 Pre-interventional Diagnosis

Contrast-enhanced CT showed a hypervascular arterial lesion/pseudoaneurysm on the right side and a hypervascular region in the uterus suspected of early venous filling (Fig. 5.11).

5.4.3 Endovascular Intervention

Selective angiography of both uterine arteries revealed a pseudoaneurysm of the right uterine artery and early venous filling with a traumatic arteriovenous fistula (Fig. 5.12). Embolization was performed with micro-coils delivered

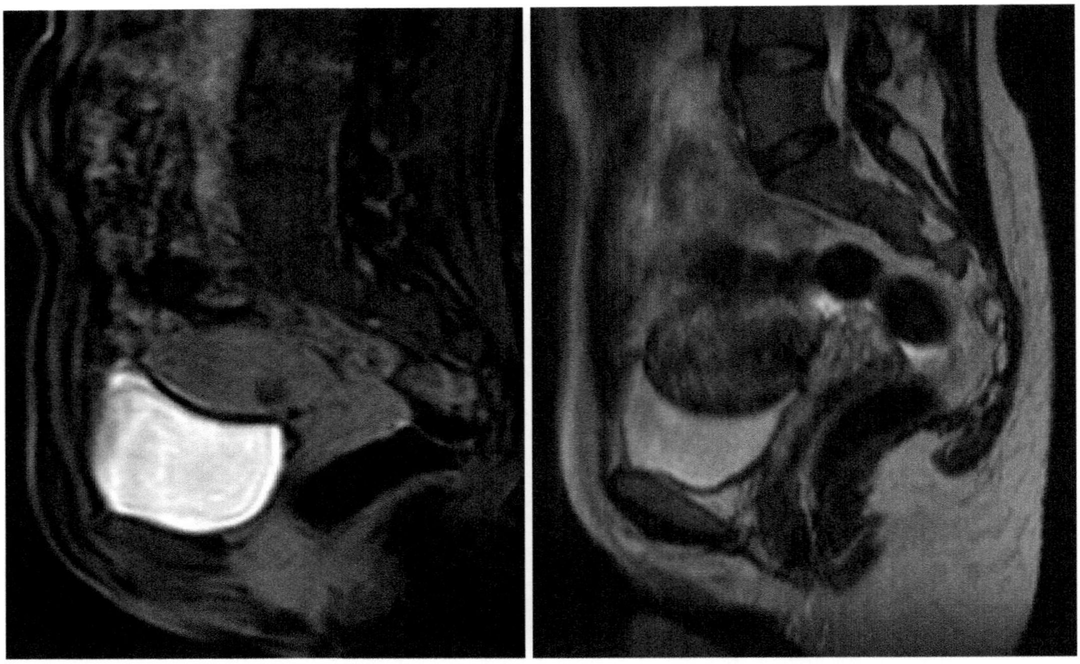

Fig. 5.10 Control T1- and T2-weighted MR sequences 3 months after the embolization showing a normal uterus morphology and no new signal changes

through a microcatheter with a good outcome. In such cases, microspheres are contraindicated due to the presence of the fistula to the venous system. Mechanical micro-coils are a very safe and relatively simple intervention (Fig. 5.13).

5.4.4 Outcome

The patient was discharged the next day without any complications. There were no new bleeding episodes or complaints in the follow-up period.

5.5 Uterine Artery Bleeding-III

Key Points

- Uterine artery pseudoaneurysms with arteriovenous fistulas are very easily treated with micro-coil embolization.
- In a majority of cases, both uterine arteries usually need to be occluded, but sometimes it is possible to perform embolization on only one side.
- The intervention is well-tolerated.
- Microspheres should never be used for such patients.

5.5.1 Aetiology and Clinical Presentation

A 26-year-old patient underwent acute sectioning complicated with bleeding and underwent re-operation 2 times thereafter. After the second operation, the bleeding persisted, and the patient received 18 portions of SAG-M blood. Abdominal packing was performed, and acute CT scanning was ordered.

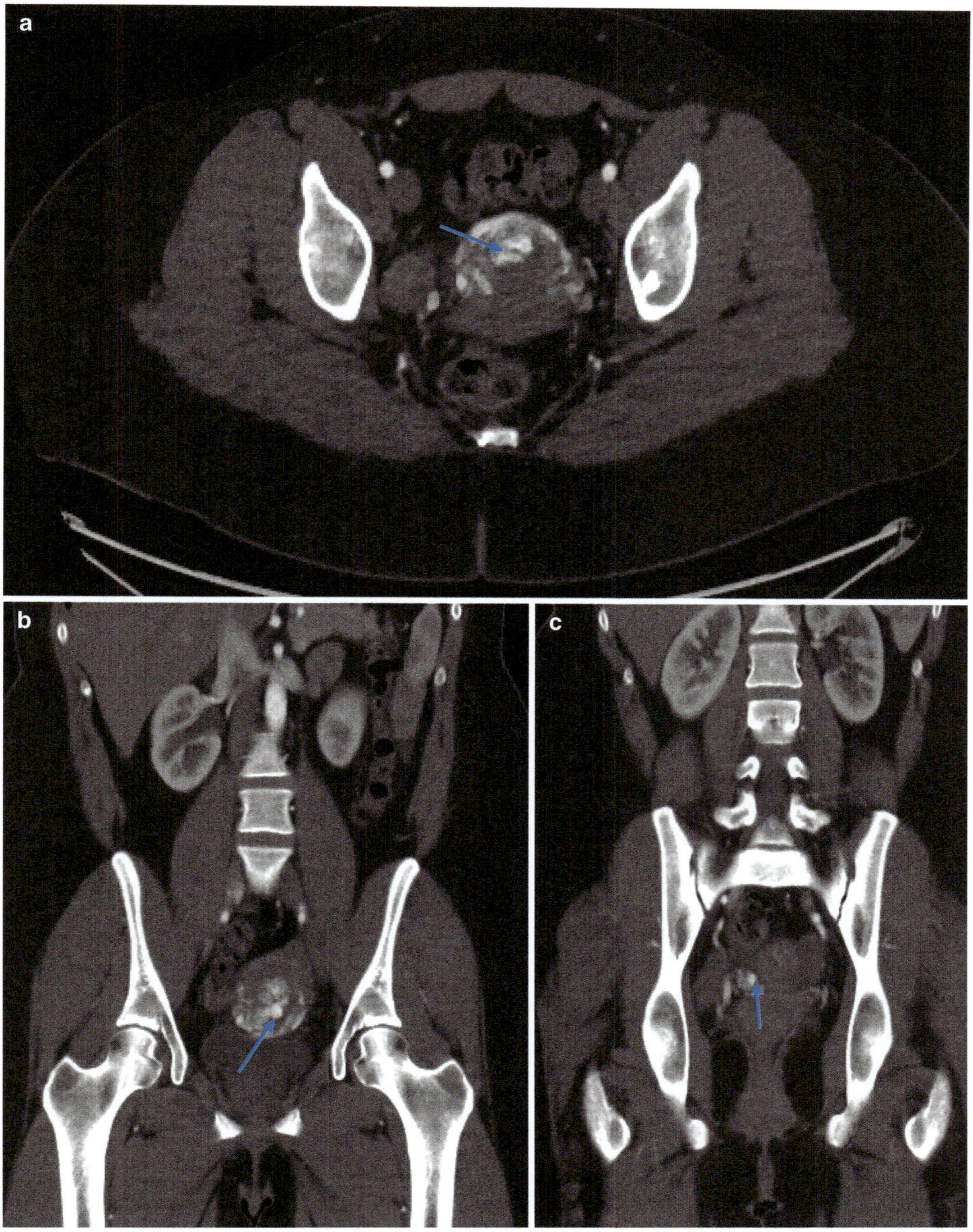

Fig. 5.11 Contrast-enhanced CT showing a right uterine artery pseudoaneurysm (blue arrows) and a hyperdense region suspected of being an arteriovenous fistula

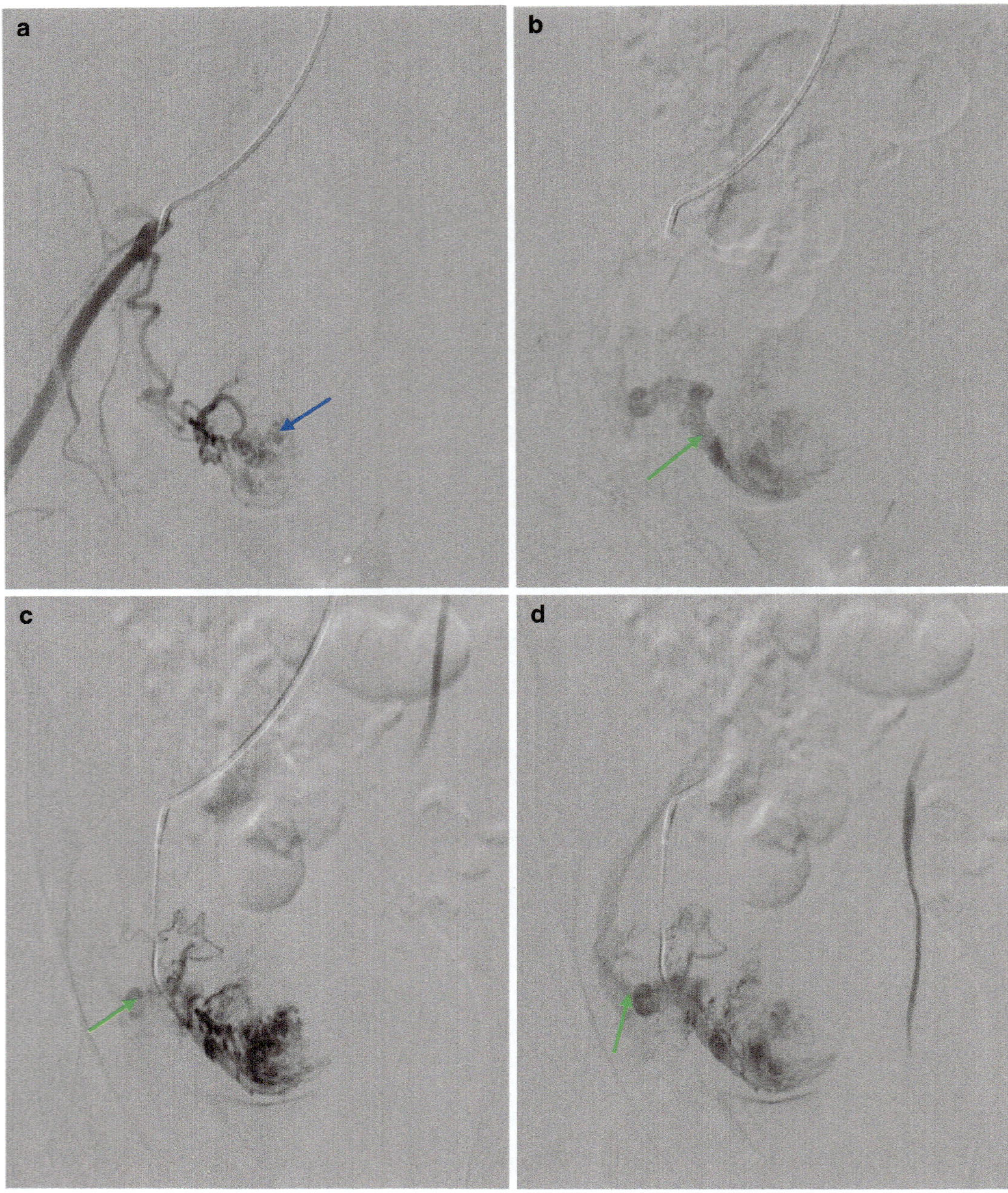

Fig. 5.12 Selective angiography of the right uterine artery showing a pseudoaneurysm (blue arrow) (**a**). Late phase image showing a fistula to the venous system (green arrows) (**b**–**d**). A microcatheter was advanced, and embolization with micro-coils (orange arrows) was performed (**e**–**h**). Selective angiography of the left uterine artery shows venous filling via the left uterine artery, and micro-coil embolization was performed (orange arrows) (**f**–**h**)

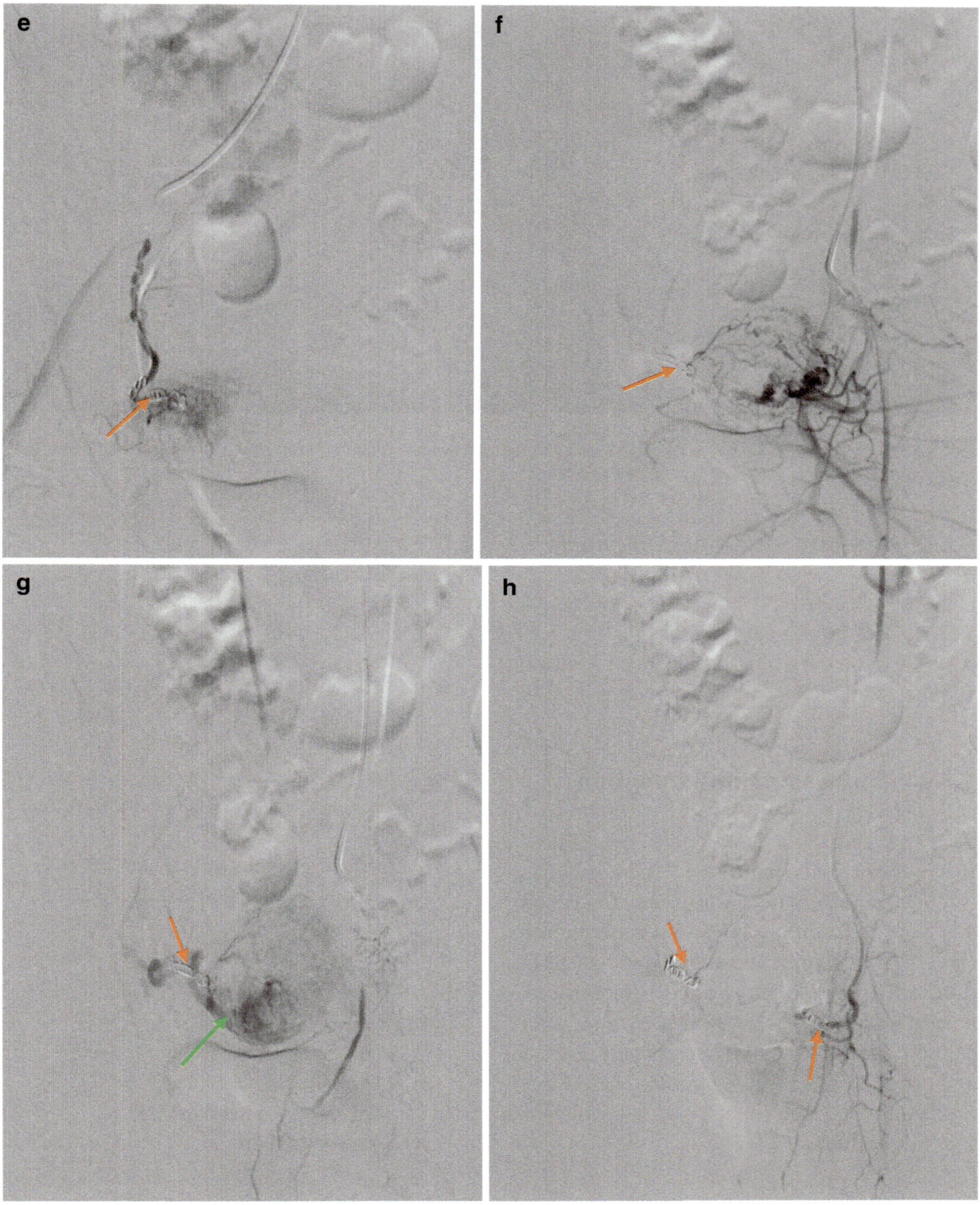

Fig. 5.12 (continued)

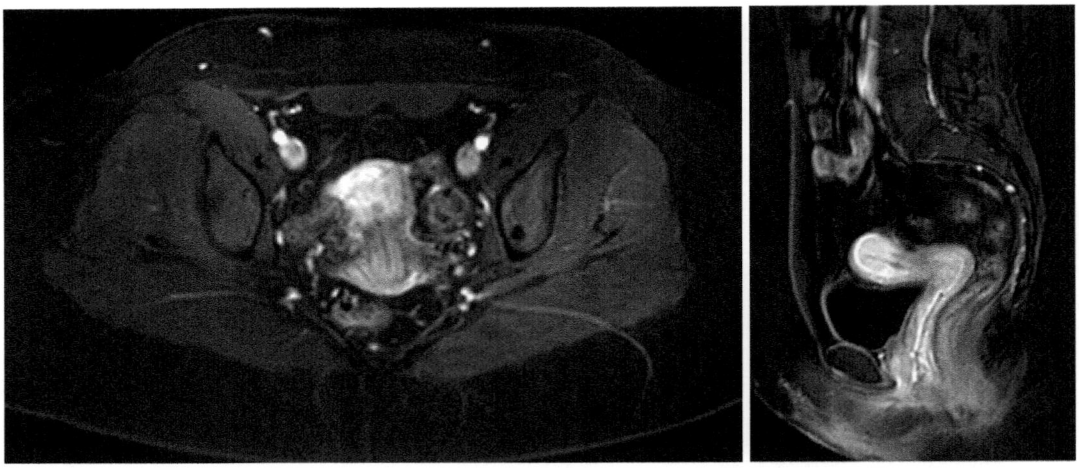

Fig. 5.13 Control T2-weighted axial and sagittal magnetic resonance imaging scans showing remodelling of the uterine cavity and no signal changes or vascular pathology

5.5.2 Pre-interventional Diagnosis

Contrast-enhanced CT showed bleeding from the internal iliac branch on the right side (Fig. 5.14). An enlarged uterus, a retroperitoneal haematoma and the abdominal packing can be seen on CT.

5.5.3 Endovascular Intervention

Selective catheterization of the right internal iliac artery was performed percutaneously through the left femoral artery, and the bleeding site from the right uterine artery was confirmed (Fig. 5.15). Then, super-selective catheterization was performed with a microcatheter advanced into the bleeding uterine artery. Micro-coils 3 mm in diameter were used for embolization and bleeding arrest. There was no problem with the left uterine artery, which was thus not occluded.

5.5.4 Outcome

The patient recovered gradually no new bleeding complications. Control CT 3 months after the embolization showed almost complete haematoma resorption (Fig. 5.16).

5.6 Arterio-Enteric Fistula Bleeding-I

Key Points

- Arterio-enteric fistulas are a severe complication with high mortality and morbidity.
- Usually, arterio-enteric fistulas occur a few years after the surgery but can occur earlier as well.
- In cases of gastrointestinal bleeding after surgery, arterio-enteric fistula should be considered.
- Stent graft deployment can serve as a temporary or definitive treatment in some cases.

5.6.1 Aetiology and Clinical Presentation

A 67-year-old patient underwent open surgery 4 years prior due to an abdominal aortic aneurysm. There were no other significant comorbidities. The patient was admitted with massive gastrointestinal bleeding and responded to initial resuscitation. The gastroscopy was inconclusive. An emergency CT scan was performed.

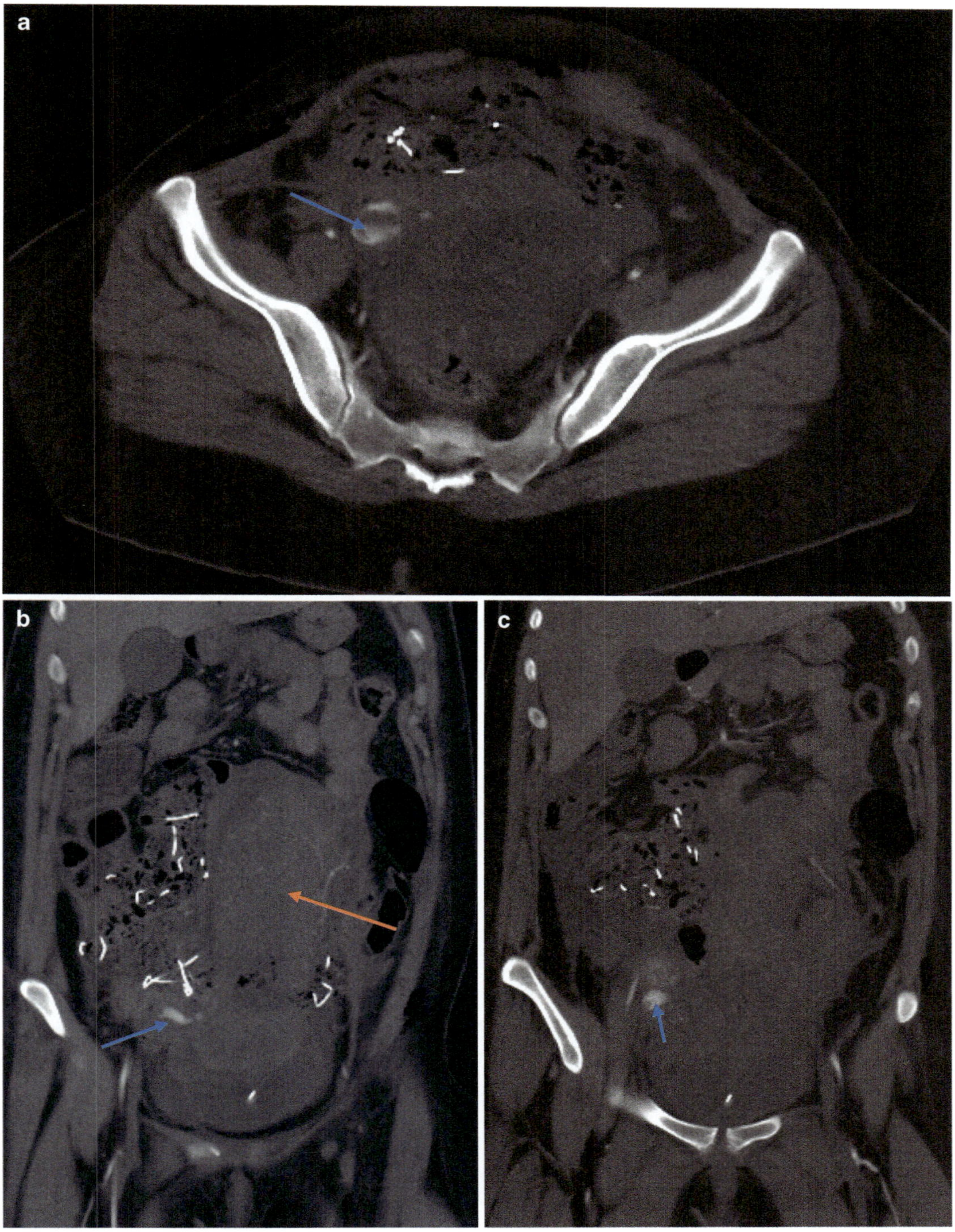

Fig. 5.14 Contrast-enhanced CT showing active bleeding from the right uterine artery (blue arrows). The uterus was enlarged (orange arrow)

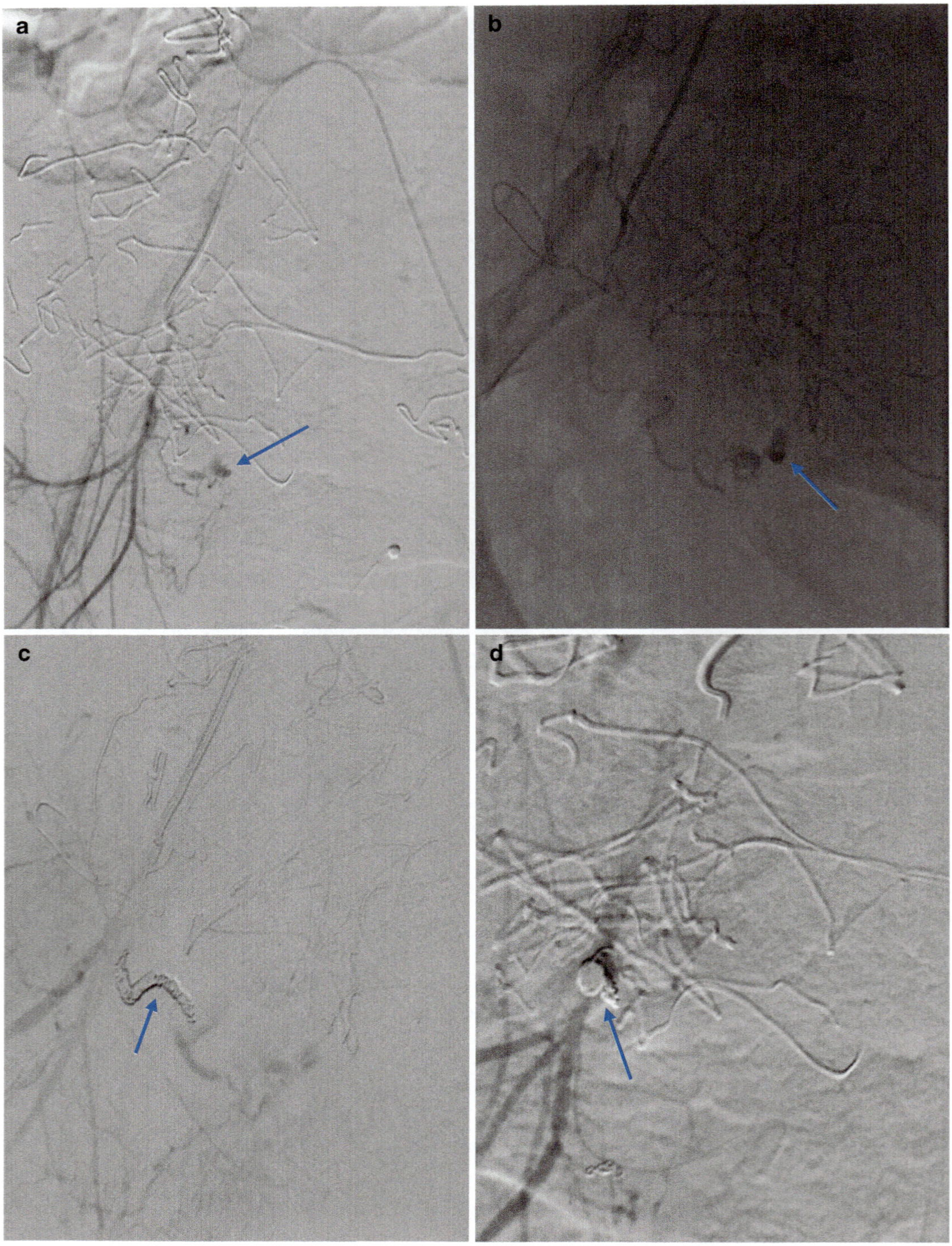

Fig. 5.15 Crossover technique. (**a** and **b**) selective angiography of the right internal iliac artery and right uterine artery show extravasation (blue arrows). (**c** and **d**) control images after micro-coil embolization with bleeding arrest

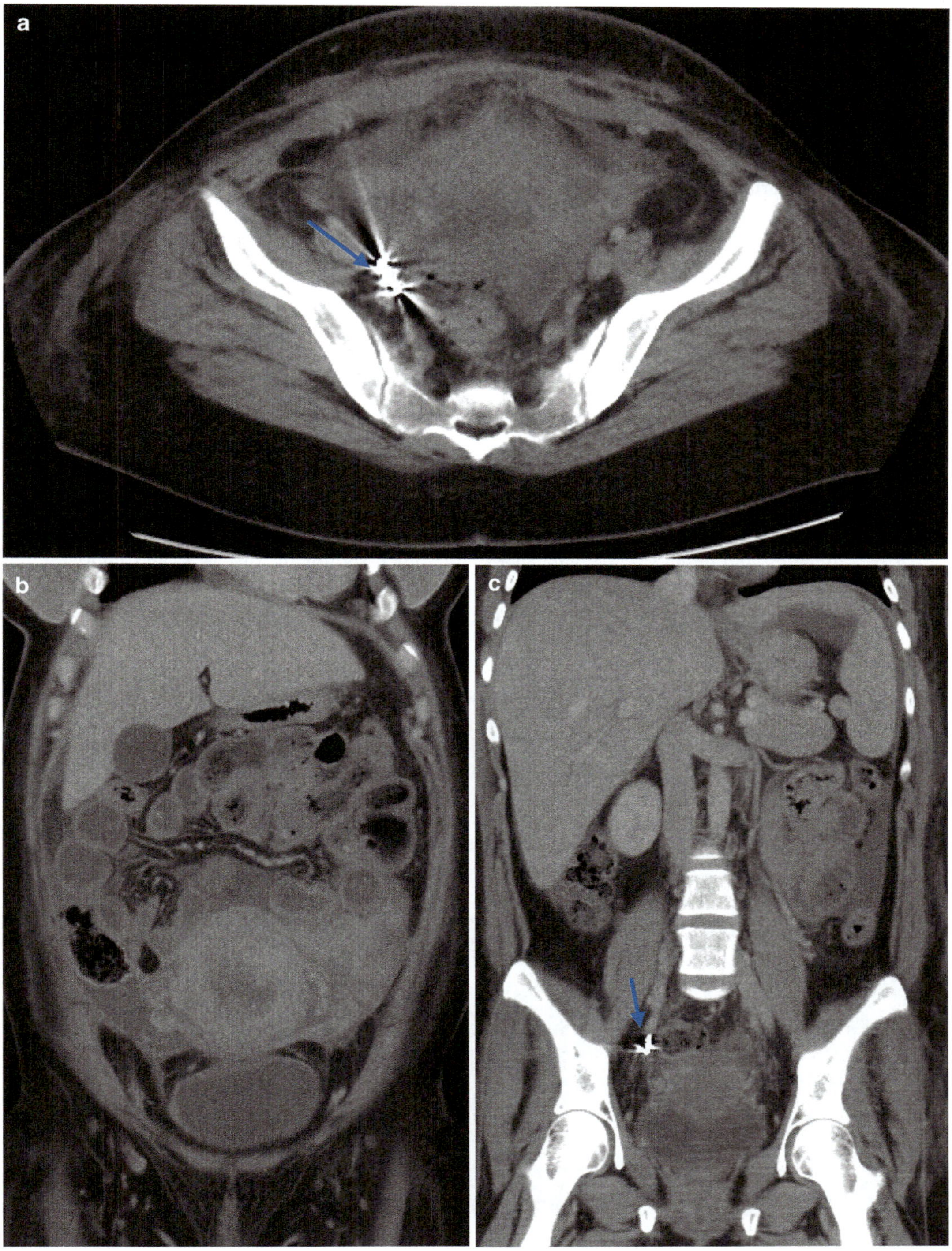

Fig. 5.16 Control CT 3 months after the procedure showed a satisfactory result. Arrows indicate the micro-coils

5.6.2 Pre-interventional Diagnosis

Contrast-enhanced CT showed an aorto-duodenal fistula between the proximal aortic anastomosis and duodenum (Fig. 5.17) and contrast extravasation into the duodenum. The length between the fistula and renal arteries was 22 mm, so acute endovascular treatment with an aortic stent graft tube was planned.

5.6.3 Endovascular Treatment

First, via the left femoral artery, a diagnostic catheter was percutaneously advanced into the suprarenal aorta, confirming the diagnosis of aorto-duodenal fistula (Fig. 5.18) and acting as the control angiography catheter during stent graft deployment. Then, via the right femoral artery, a 0.035-in. guidewire and diagnostic catheter were advanced percutaneously into the ascending aorta. The guidewire was exchanged for a super-stiff guidewire, and an aortic tube stent graft 25 mm in diameter and 70 mm in length was advanced and deployed infrarenally with excellent clinical and angiographic outcomes.

5.6.4 Outcome

The patient's haemodynamic status improved dramatically and without the need for subsequent blood transfusion. Broad-spectrum antibiotics were ordered and are currently being taken by the patient. The patient is waiting for definitive treatment with a new surgery and eventual aortic reconstruction with the deep vein as the graft material. The patient has not experienced a new bleeding episode. In some cases, endovascular treatment can serve as the definitive treatment. Nevertheless, in the present case, the patient had no other significant diseases, and endovascular treatment is usually used in emergency situations as the bridge to the final treatment.

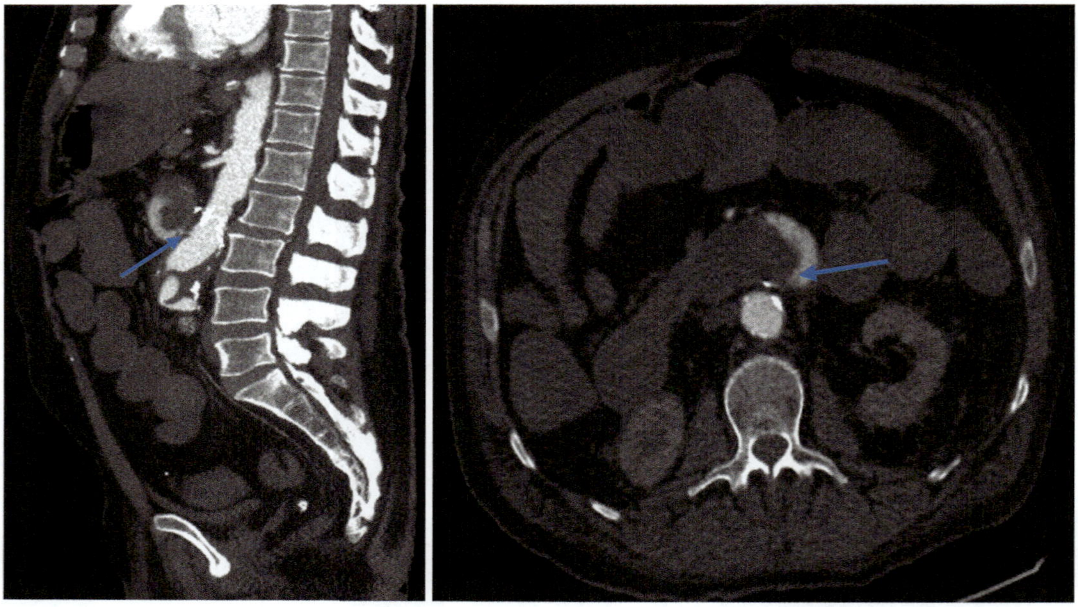

Fig. 5.17 Emergency contrast-enhanced CT showing an aorto-duodenal fistula after a previous aortic reconstruction surgery; arrows indicate the fistula and contrast extravasation into the duodenum

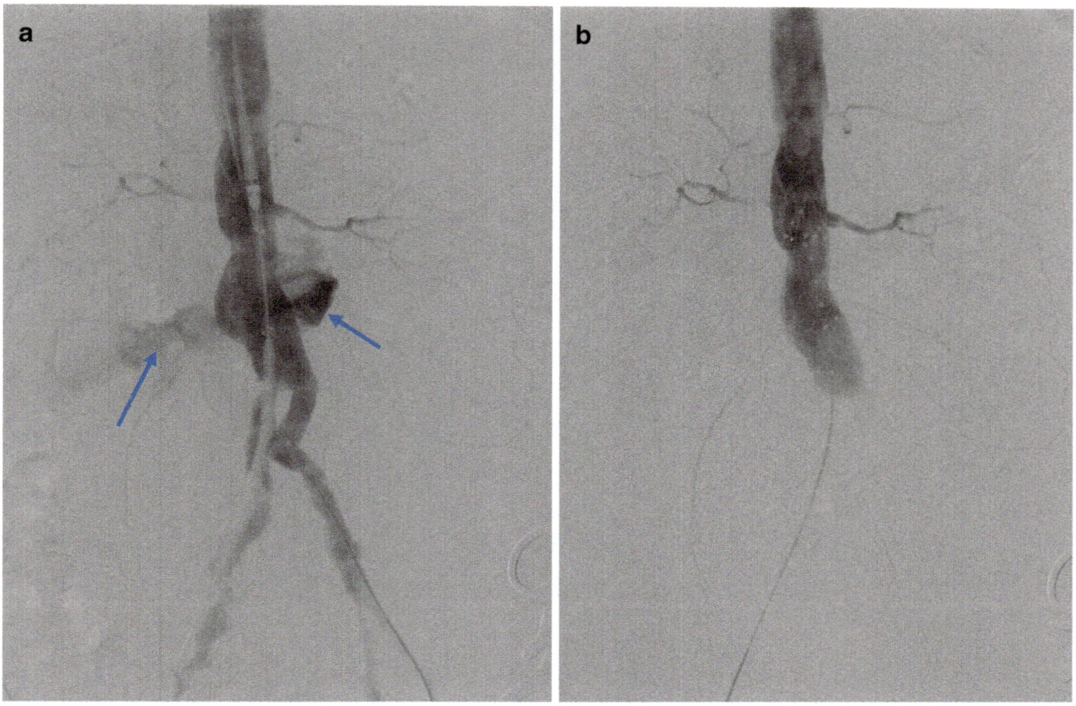

Fig. 5.18 (**a**) abdominal aortography during stent graft deployment with massive contrast extravasation (arrows). (**b**) control angiography after stent graft deployment showing arrested bleeding and open renal arteries

5.7 Arterio-Enteric Fistula Bleeding–II

Key Points

- Arterio-enteric fistulas are a severe complication with high mortality and morbidity.
- Usually, arterio-enteric fistulas occur a few years after the surgery but can occur earlier as well.
- In cases of gastrointestinal bleeding after the surgery, arterio-enteric fistulas should be considered.
- Stent graft deployment can serve as a temporary or definitive treatment in some cases.

5.7.1 Aetiology and Clinical Presentation

A 57-year-old patent underwent a complicated urostomy. During the surgery, the right external iliac artery was injured, a short vascular prosthesis was sewn in place, and the external iliac artery was repaired on the right side. A few weeks after the surgery, the patient complained about recurrent melena and pain in the abdomen. The patient was haemodynamically stable and showed no clinical signs of peritonitis. White blood count and CRP were high, 12,000 and 84, respectively.

5.7.2 Pre-interventional Diagnosis

A contrast-enhanced CT scan was performed and showed a right external iliac artery-bowel fistula (Fig. 5.19). Haematomas and infections were found around the fistula. Treatment with metronidazole and broad-spectrum antibiotics was initiated.

5.7.3 Endovascular Intervention

First, via the left femoral artery, a diagnostic catheter was advanced percutaneously over the aortic

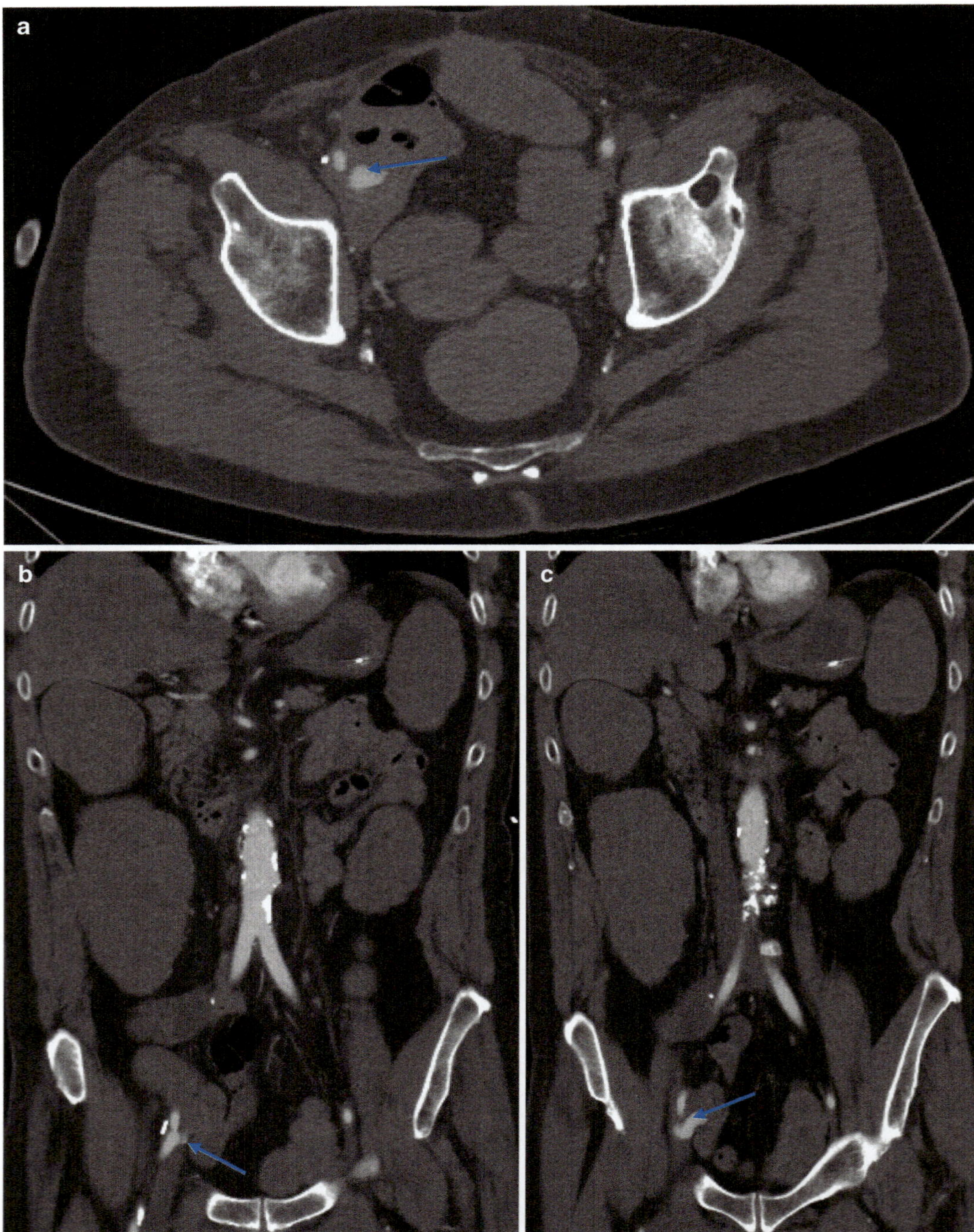

Fig. 5.19 Contrast-enhanced CT showing a right external iliac arterio-enteric fistula (blue arrows)

bifurcation into the right iliac artery, and the diagnosis was confirmed (Fig. 5.20). Then, via right femoral artery, a 0.035-in. guidewire was advanced percutaneously, some suspected temporary coagulum was removed, and the patient experienced a sudden drop in blood pressure. Angiography now clearly confirmed a fistula to the bowel. A stent graft, 9 mm in diameter and 59 mm long, was rapidly advanced and deployed across the fistula with an excellent clinical and angiographic outcomes.

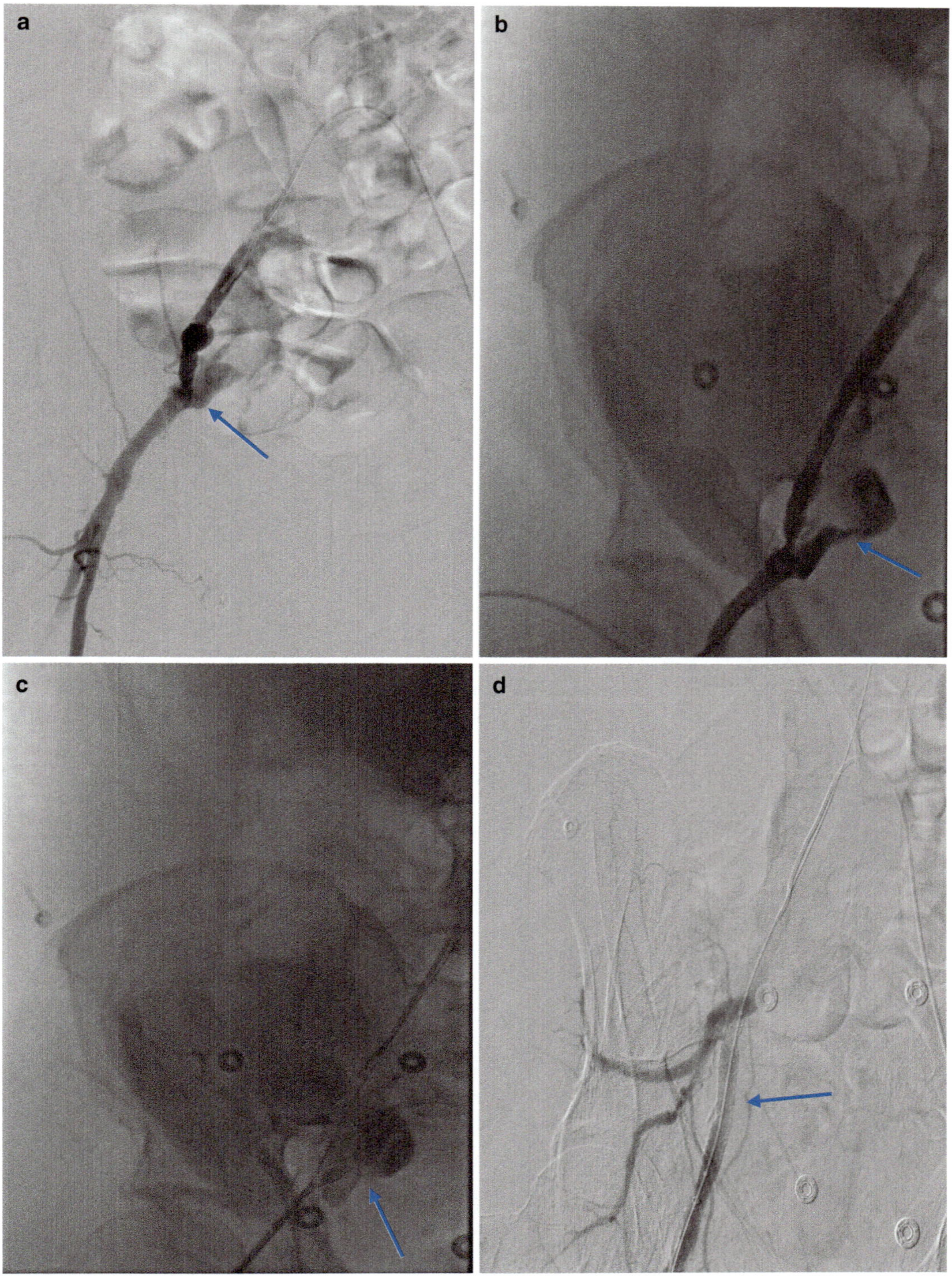

Fig. 5.20 (**a**) crossover technique and angiographic confirmation of the fistula (blue arrow). (**b** and **c**) via ipsilateral right femoral artery access, a suspected temporary coagulum was removed, and the patient's blood pressure dropped significantly; blue arrows indicate contrast inside the bowel. (**d**) control imaging after deployment of a stent graft 9 mm in diameter and 59 mm in length showing a satisfactory result (arrow)

5.7.4 Outcome

The patient did not experience any new episodes of gastrointestinal bleeding. Antibiotic treatment was continued. Control CT 1 month after the procedure showed a well-deployed stent graft and no bleeding (Fig. 5.21).

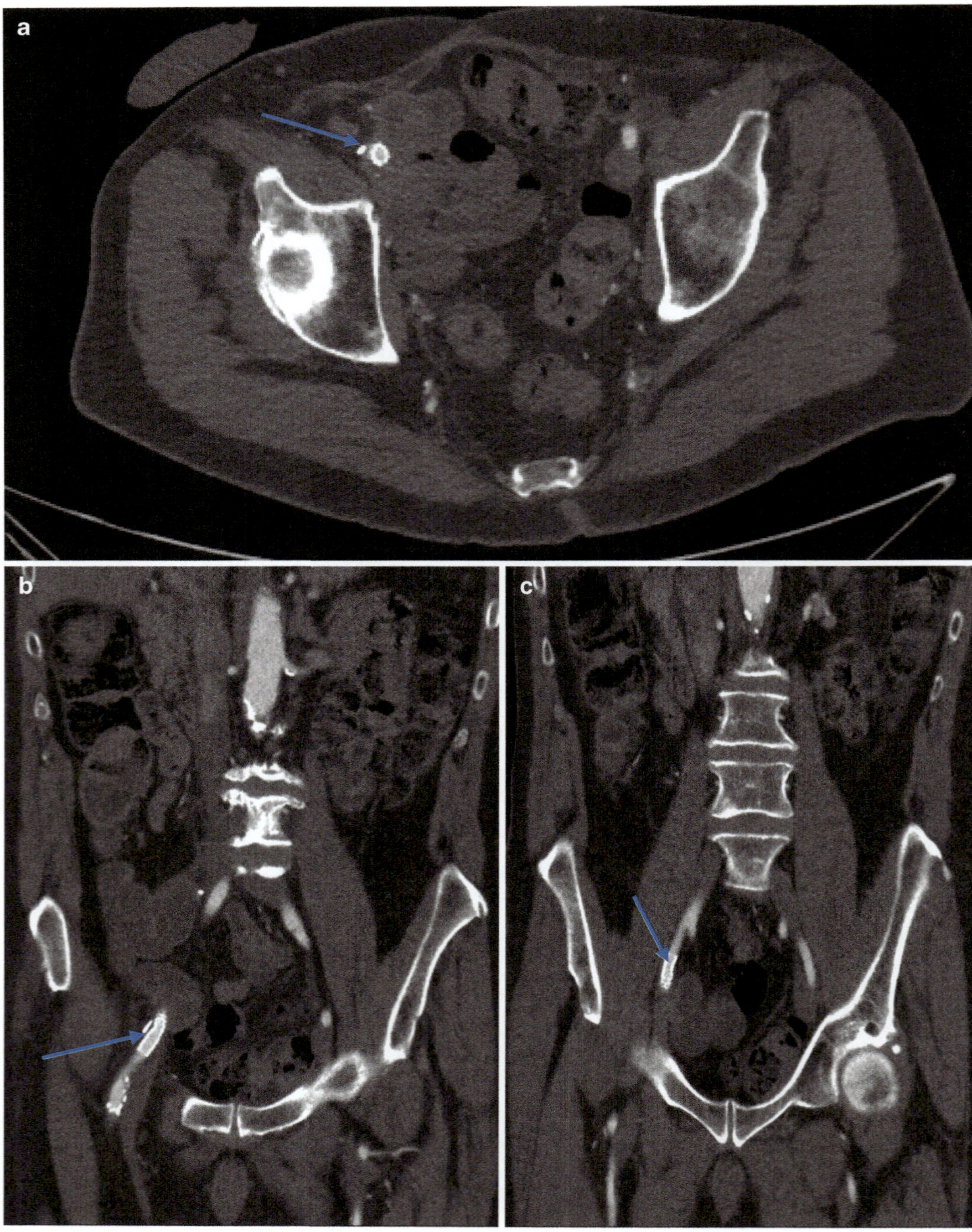

Fig. 5.21 Control CT 3 months after the intervention showing a good result; arrow indicates the stent graft

Peripheral Artery Vascular Emergency

6

Contents

S. Duvnjak, *Endovascular Treatment of Arterial Emergencies*,
https://doi.org/10.1007/978-3-030-68832-5_6

6.1 Carotid Artery

Key Points

- Arterial lesions caused by placement of a central venous line are very rare.
- A hybrid intervention with direct surgical exposure and an endovascular technique is one possible solution for challenging cases.
- The Willis polygon should be checked before occluding the vertebral artery.

6.1.1 Aetiology and Clinical Presentation

An 81-year-old patient underwent gynaecological surgery 3 months prior due to a malignancy. The patient had a central venous line placed into the right jugular vein. According to the patient record, there was no significant difficulty during central line placement. The patient was discharged from the hospital in good shape. Three months after the surgery, the patient complained of increasing hoarseness and a pulsatile mass on the right side of the neck region. The patient remained haemodynamically stable, and no bleeding events were recorded after the surgery.

6.1.2 Pre-interventional Diagnosis

Contrast-enhanced computed tomography (CT) was scheduled, and a 7 cm pseudoaneurysm arising from the right common carotid artery was discovered (Fig. 6.1).

6.1.3 Endovascular Treatment

The aortic arch had a very tortuous course, and the carotid arteries had severe calcifications. The diameter of the brachiocephalic trunk was 13 mm, and the common carotid artery had a diameter of 9 mm. We decided on surgical exposure of the right common carotid artery under general anaesthesia and deployment of anterograde an stent graft 16 mm in diameter and 82 mm in length (Fig. 6.2). The right subclavian artery and the right vertebral artery were patent. The left vertebral artery and subclavian arteries were patent,

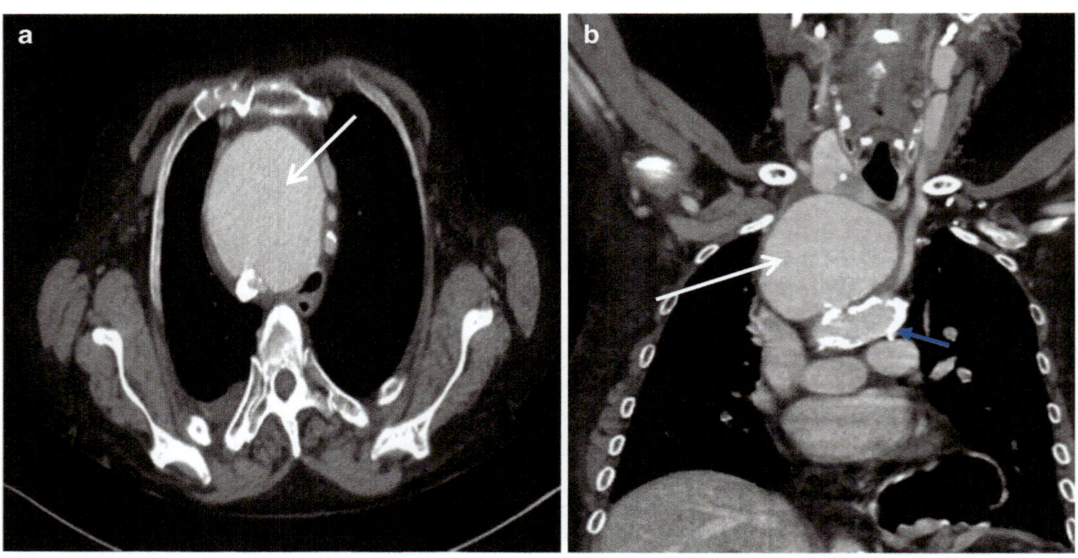

Fig. 6.1 Contrast-enhanced CT showing a 7 cm right common carotid pseudo-aneurysm (arrows): (**a**) axial image; (**b**) coronal image and (**c**) sagittal image. Note severe calcifications in the aortic arch (blue arrow)

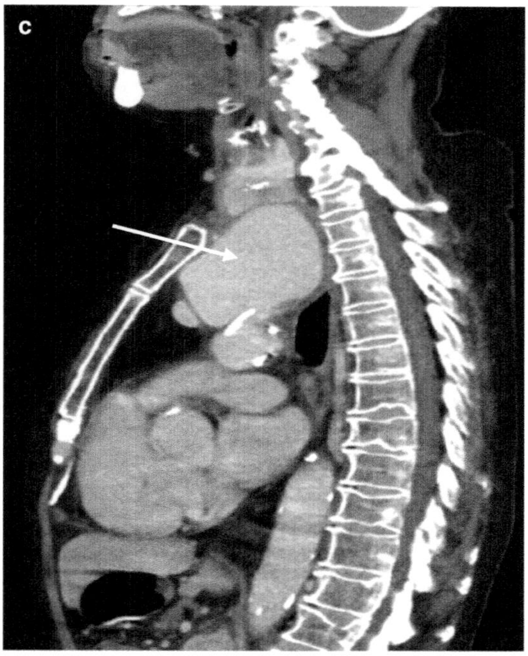

Fig. 6.1 (continued)

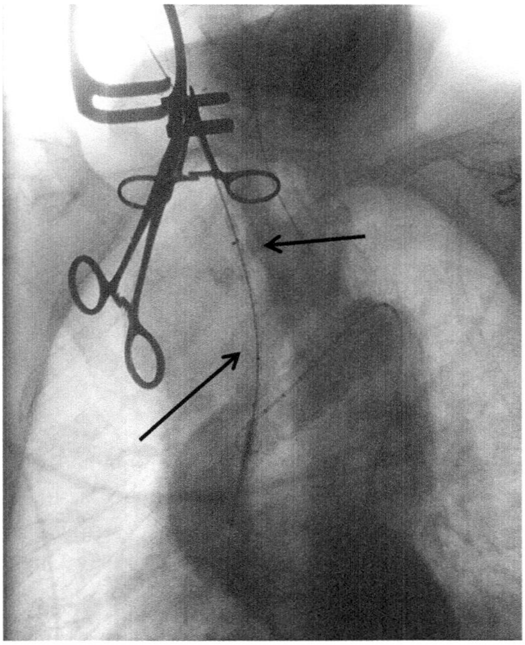

Fig. 6.2 After surgical exposure of the right common carotid artery, a stent graft was advanced over a super-stiff guidewire. Arrow indicates the stent graft before deployment

and the arteria basilaris was patent. Occlusion of the right vertebral artery could potentially result in further complications. In this case, no complications were expected after stent graft deployment across the right subclavian artery due to competent intracerebral vascularization and a competent Willis polygon. After surgical exposure and distal control angiography of the carotid artery, a super-stiff Lunderquist guidewire was advanced and placed in the ascending aorta. A bolus of 5000 IU heparin was administered. A diagnostic catheter was advanced through the right femoral artery for control angiography during graft deployment, which confirmed the complete exclusion of the pseudoaneurysm (Fig. 6.3). The arteriotomy site was stitched with 6.0 prolene suture.

6.1.4 Outcome

The patient was discharged 2 days after the operation. Three month control CT control showed a well-deployed stent graft and no contrast in the pseudoaneurysm (Fig. 6.4). The patient still experiences hoarsens but has no other complaints. The patient was on antiplatelet drugs after the operation and again began taking dual antiplatelet medication. The open surgery in the present case is a high-risk operation that requires a sternotomy, but it may be difficult to quickly perform control angiography once the sternum is open. Therefore, the endovascular option is preferred and can be performed as a "hybrid" intervention to maximize control and avoid distal embolic complications, especially when many calcifications are present in the aortic arch and manipulation with guidewires and stent grafts will inevitably cause distal embolization. The mismatch in the diameter of the carotid artery and that of the relatively stiff stent graft makes careful manipulation through the artery difficult, and follow-up evaluations are required to avoid problems including dissection, thrombosis, edge stenosis, etc.

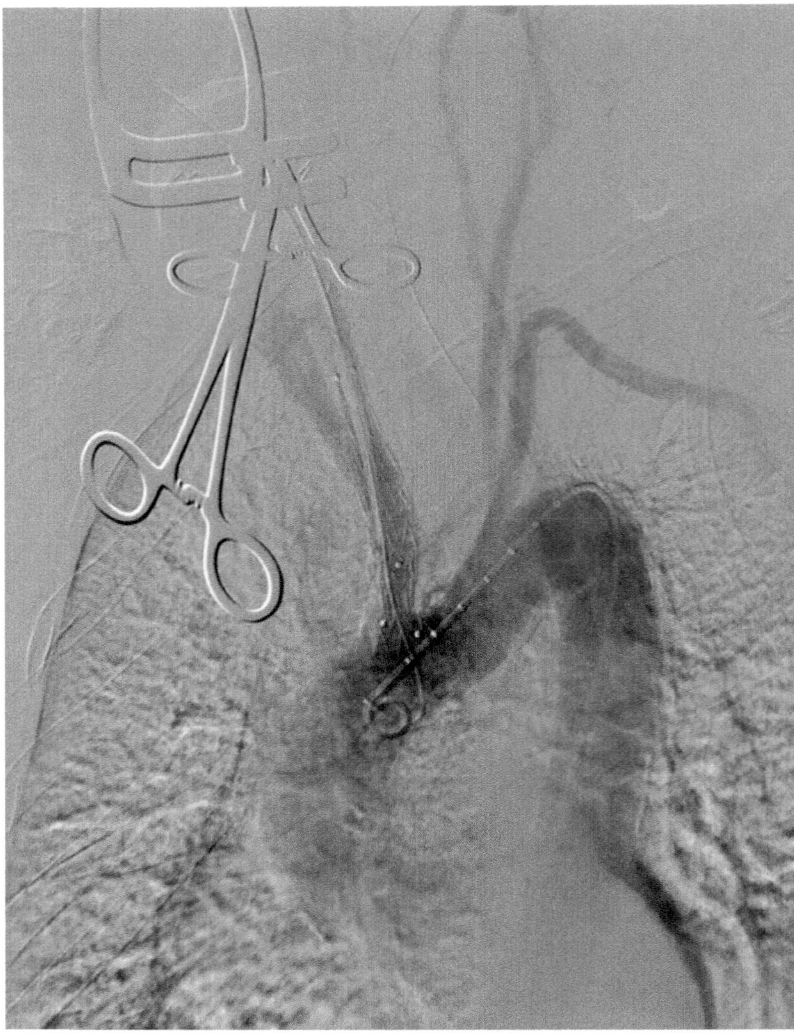

Fig. 6.3 Control angiography after stent graft deployment. Complete exclusion of the pseudoaneurysm is observed

6.2 Subclavian Artery-I

Key Points

- A traumatic pseudoaneurysm can develop slowly.
- It is important to observe the carotid artery during deployment of the graft on the right side; in some cases, the protective guidewire can slip into it.
- The intracranial circulation and Willis polygon should be checked before occluding the vertebral artery.

6.2.1 Aetiology and Clinical Presentation

A 62-year-old healthy patient complained of a pulsatile mass in the right supraclavicular fossa. The patient described that it had been gradually increasing in size over a few years. The patient had not visited the doctor before coming to our institution. During the anamnesis, the patient described trauma and right clavicular fracture that had occurred a few years ago. There were no ischaemic arm complications or other diseases present. The brachial pulse, radial pulse and blood pressure were equal on both arms.

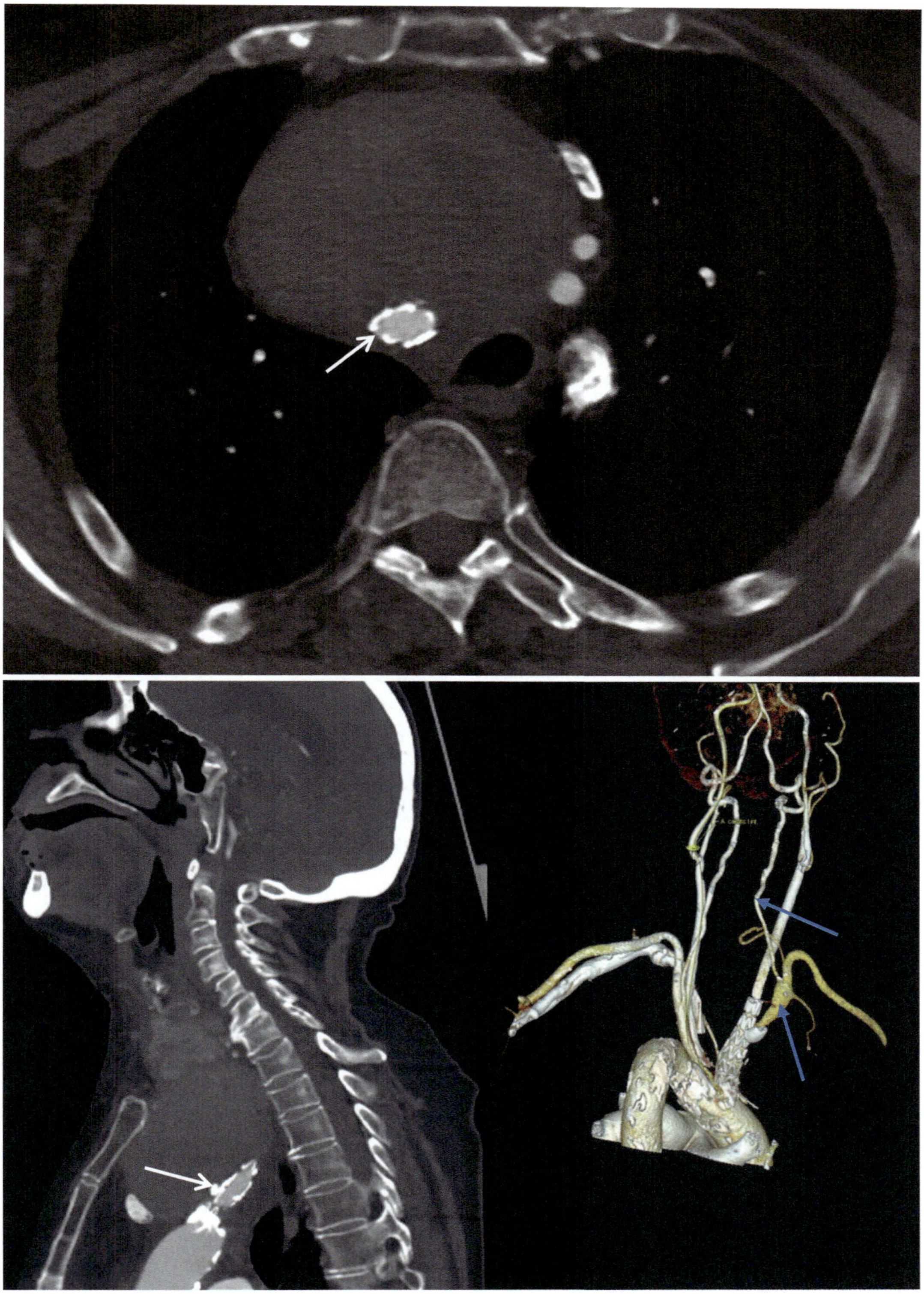

Fig. 6.4 Control CT scan showing no contrast in the pseudoaneurysm, a satisfactory result and a distally patent right carotid artery. Arrow indicates the stent graft. The right subclavian artery presents with retrograde flow through the vertebral arteries (blue arrow)

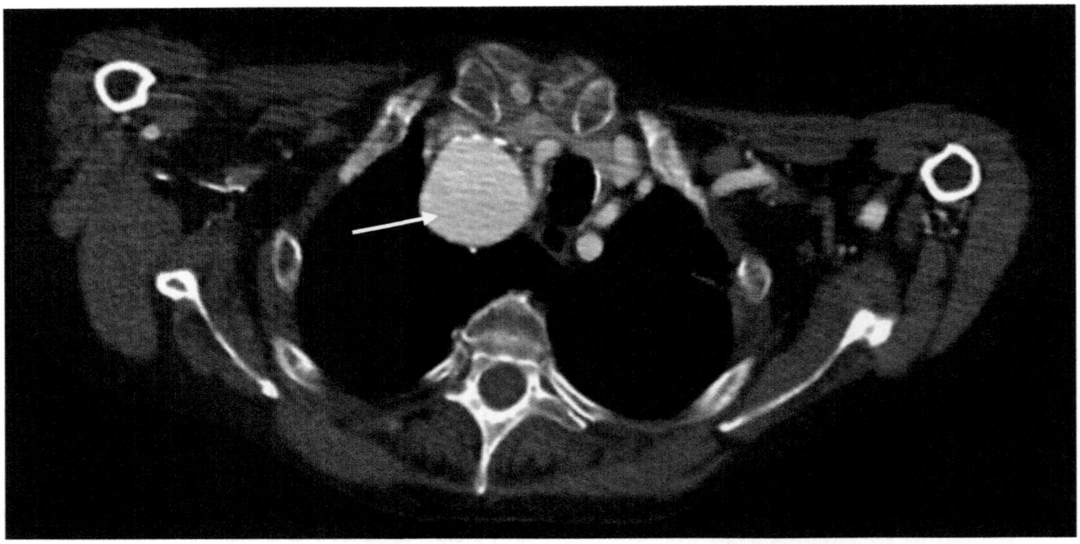

Fig. 6.5 Contrast-enhanced CT (axial reconstruction) showing a 5 cm right subclavian pseudoaneurysm (arrow)

6.2.2 Pre-interventional Diagnosis

Contrast-enhanced CT showed a 5 cm right subclavian artery pseudoaneurysm (Figs. 6.5 and 6.6). The right carotid artery was patent, and the brachiocephalic trunk lacked stenosis or aneurysm. The right vertebral artery was patent. The left vertebral artery was patent and had the same diameter as the right. Willis circulation was sufficient, and occlusion of the right vertebral artery was planned.

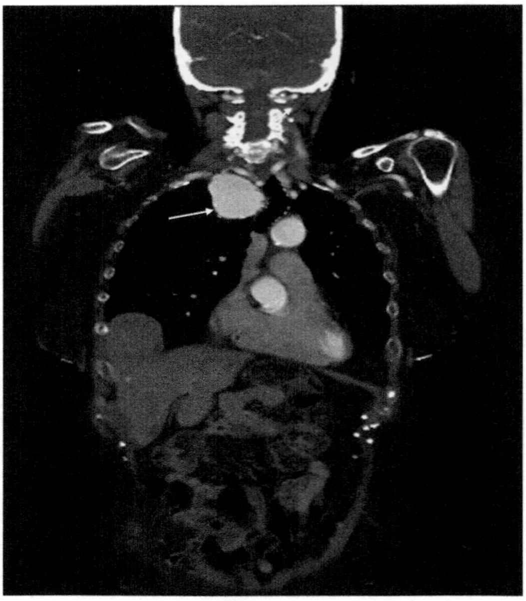

Fig. 6.6 Contrast-enhanced CT (coronal reconstruction) showing the 5 cm right subclavian pseudoaneurysm (arrow)

6.2.3 Endovascular Treatment

A diagnostic coronary catheter was inserted percutaneously through the right femoral artery and advanced over a 260 mm long stiff Terumo glide guidewire and navigated into the right subclavian artery (Fig. 6.7). A long 90 cm Destination sheath was advanced into the brachiocephalic trunk. A stent graft with a diameter of 8 mm and length of 59 mm was advanced through the long sheath into the right subclavian artery. After confirmation that it would not compromise the right common carotid artery, the stent-graft was deployed carefully (Fig. 6.8). Control imaging after graft deployment showed a good result and no endoleak.

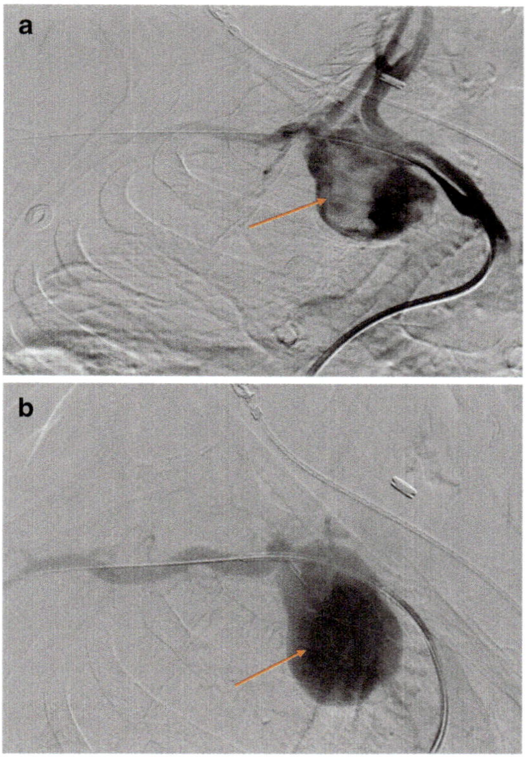

Fig. 6.7 Details from the intervention and advancement of the long 7 Fr sheath into the brachiocephalic artery. Arrows indicate the pseudoaneurysm (**a**, **b**)

6.2.4 Outcome

The patient was discharged the next day with no neurological events and a radial pulse. The patient was on dual antiplatelet therapy for 3 months, followed by continuous with 75 mg acetylsalicylic acid life-long. It is essential to analyse the importance of the Willis polygon and the patency of the other vertebral arteries before occlusion of the right vertebral artery.

6.3 Subclavian Artery-II

Key Points
- Both transfemoral and transbrachial access are needed sometimes.

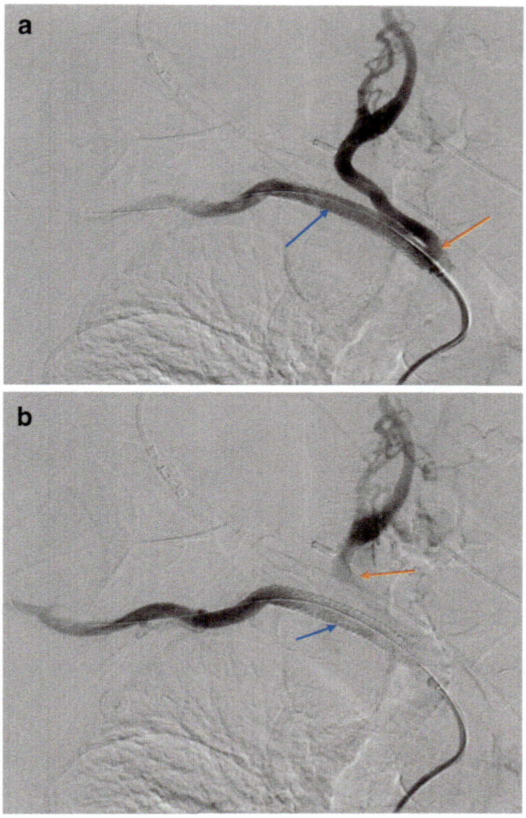

Fig. 6.8 Control angiography in the early and late phases after deployment of the balloon-expandible stent graft, showing a satisfactory result (blue arrow) (**a**, **b**). No endoleak and no compromising flow of the right carotid artery are observed (orange arrow) (**a**, **b**)

- The "through-and-through" technique can help in severe cases.
- It is important not to cover any vertebral or LIMA-LAD grafts during stent deployment.

6.3.1 Aetiology and Clinical Presentation

An 81-year-old patient underwent coronary bypass surgery (CABG) 11 years ago, including two venous bypasses to the right coronary artery and circumflex artery. The left internal mammary artery (LIMA) was used for bypass to the left

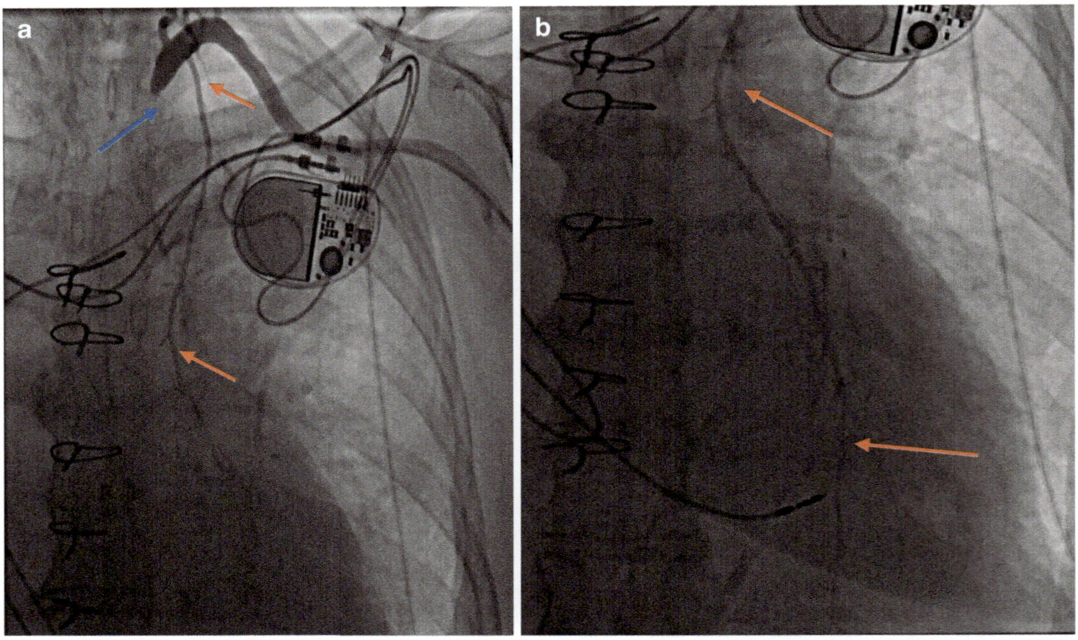

Fig. 6.9 Primary angiography showing an occluded left subclavian artery (blue arrow). Orange arrows indicate a patent LIMA-LAD graft (**a**, **b**)

anterior descending artery (LAD). Other relevant comorbidities included diabetes mellitus type 2 and hypertension. In the last month, there was increased dyspnoea and retrosternal pain, even when walking. Clinical examination confirmed that reversible ischaemia could be induced with minimal physical activity, and cardiography was scheduled.

6.3.2 Pre-interventional Diagnosis

The two venous bypasses showed no significant stenosis. The LIMA-LAD graft was patent, but the left subclavian artery was occluded (Fig. 6.9). The cardiologist colleagues attempted to recanalize the occluded subclavian artery; both thought that femoral and left brachial access would be unsuccessful.

6.3.3 Endovascular Treatment

All insertions were made percutaneously through the femoral and left brachial arteries. The first attempt was to recanalize the occluded artery via transfemoral access, but the guidewire passed into the subintimal space. Then, via the left brachial artery, a 0.014 in. guidewire was inserted and recanalized the occluded artery. The guidewire was snared through the transfemoral catheter. Finally, a transfemoral catheter was advanced over the occluded segment with the "through-and-through" technique (Fig. 6.10). After that, a 0,035-in. guidewire was introduced, and pre-dilatation with a 4 mm × 40 mm angioplasty balloon was performed. A 6 Fr, 90 cm long sheath was placed, and a stent 9 mm in diameter and 23 mm long was deployed, taking care not to compromise the LIMA-LAD graft (Fig. 6.11). Control angiography showed a satisfactory result and good flow through the LIMA graft.

6.3.4 Outcome

The patient was discharged the next day without access site complications. Clinical cardiologic control was scheduled.

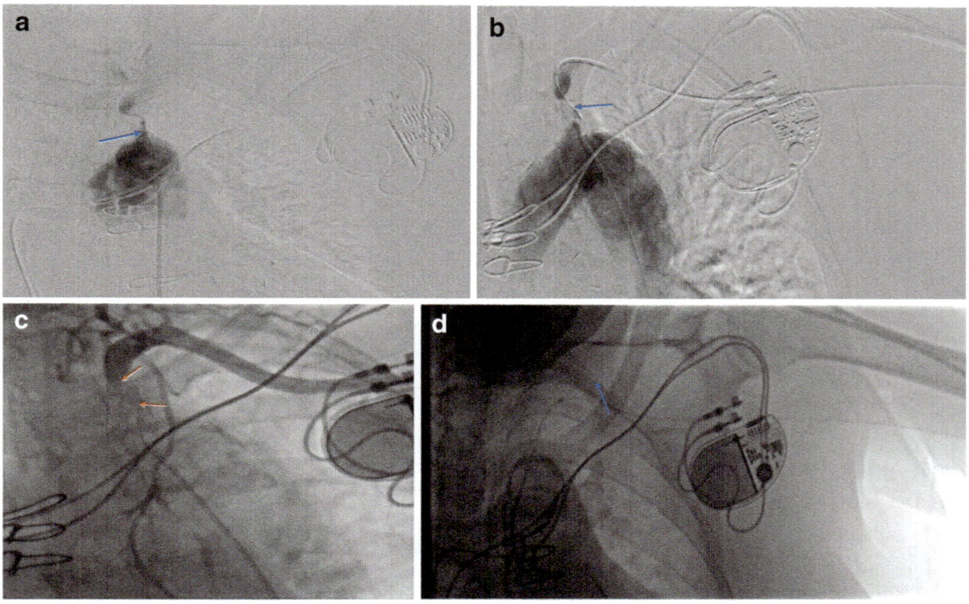

Fig. 6.10 Details from the intervention. First, recanalization of the occluded artery transfemorally was attempted. The guidewire passed into the subintimal space (arrow) (**a**). Recanalization trough the left brachial artery was achieved by navigating a 0.014-in. guidewire to the occluded segment (arrow) (**b**). The micro-guidewire was snared through the transfemoral catheter (orange arrows) (**c**). Finally, with the "through-and-through" technique, the transfemoral catheter was advanced across the occluded segment (arrow) (**d**)

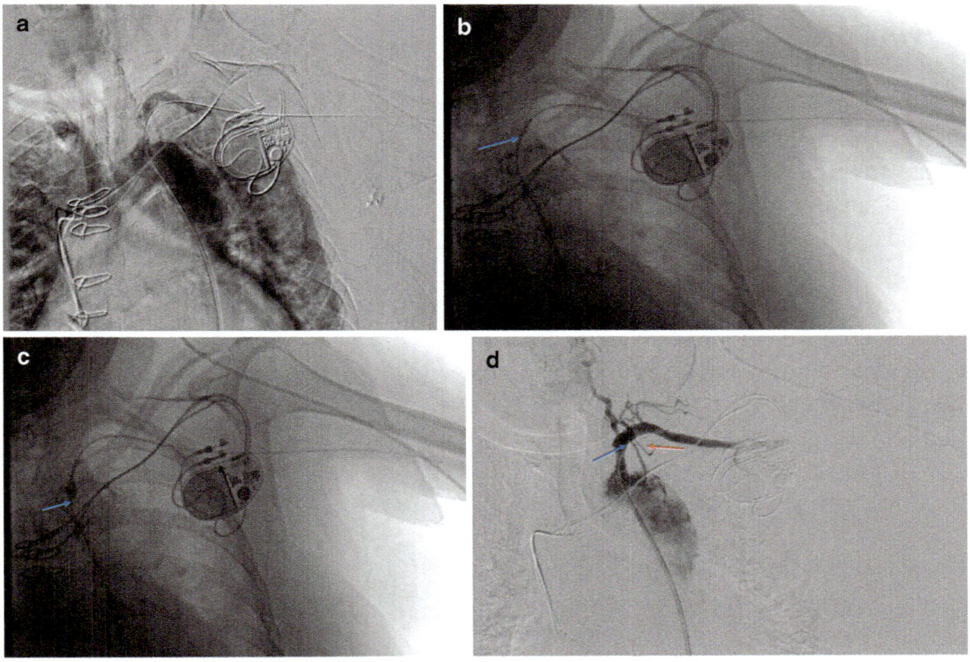

Fig. 6.11 The guidewire was exchanged with a 0.035-in. guidewire through the femoral catheter (**a**). Pre dilatation with a 4 mm balloon was performed (**b**), and a balloon-expandible stent 9 mm in diameter and 23 mm in length was deployed (blue arrows) (**c**). Orange arrow indicates the patent LIMA-LAD graft (**d**)

6.4 Femoral Artery-I

Key Points

- In elderly patients, endovascular treatment options are preferable.
- Stent graft deployment is usually straightforward.

6.4.1 Aetiology and Clinical Presentation

A 78-year-old patient was admitted to the emergency department after a fall and developing a clinically suspected left femur fracture. The patient had advanced atherosclerosis and was known to have an occluded left superficial femoral artery but no resting pain or atherosclerotic ulcers. It was not possible to measure the ABI. The left femoral region was tender and painful, and bleeding from the deep femoral artery was suspected.

6.4.2 Pre-interventional Diagnosis

Contrast-enhanced CT was ordered before orthopaedic surgery to assess the bleeding source and vascular status. CT showed a traumatic pseudoaneurysm from the deep femoral artery at the distal part of the artery (Fig. 6.12). The left superficial femoral artery was chronically occluded. There was extensive calcification of the abdominal aorta and pelvic arteries. There was a haematoma and ongoing bleeding from the pseudoaneurysm.

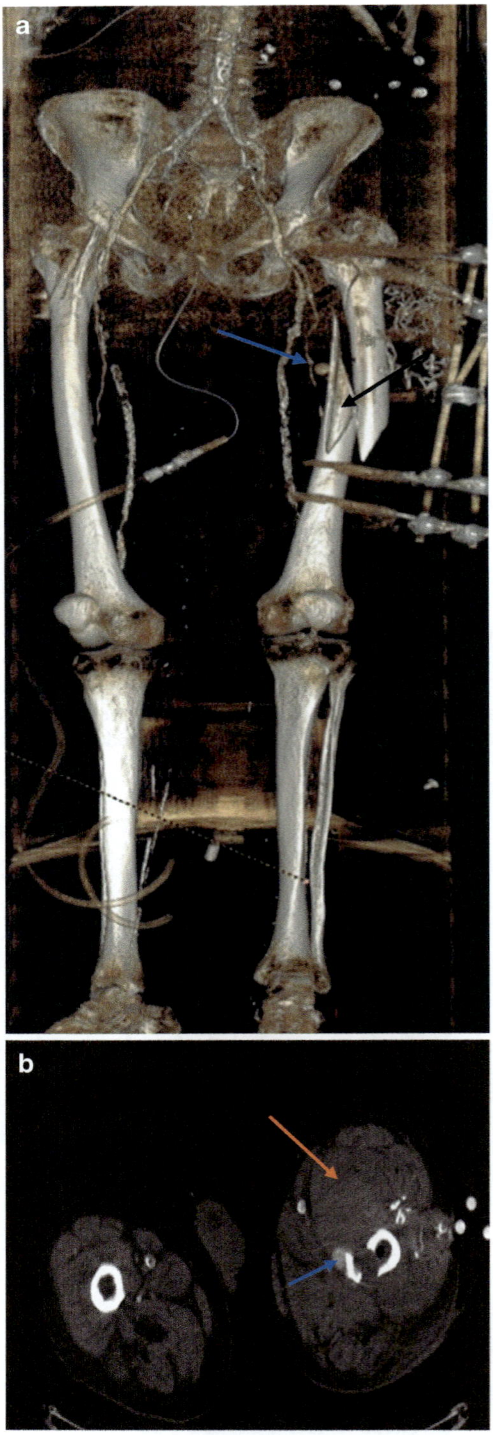

Fig. 6.12 3D and axial reconstructions (**a**) showing a deep left femoral artery pseudoaneurysm (blue arrows). Black arrow indicates a mid-shaft femoral fracture. Orange arrow indicates a haematoma in the femoral region (**b**)

6.4.3 Endovascular Treatment

The right femoral artery was percutaneously punctured. The crossover technique was used to advance a 6 Fr sheath over the aortic bifurcation into the left common femoral artery. A stiff 260 mm Terumo guidewire was advanced into the deep femoral artery. A balloon-expandable stent graft 5 mm in diameter and 38 mm in length was advanced and deployed, covering the pseudoaneurysm. No complications occurred during the intervention. Control angiography confirmed the complete exclusion of the pseudoaneurysm and lack of distal embolization (Fig. 6.13). There was

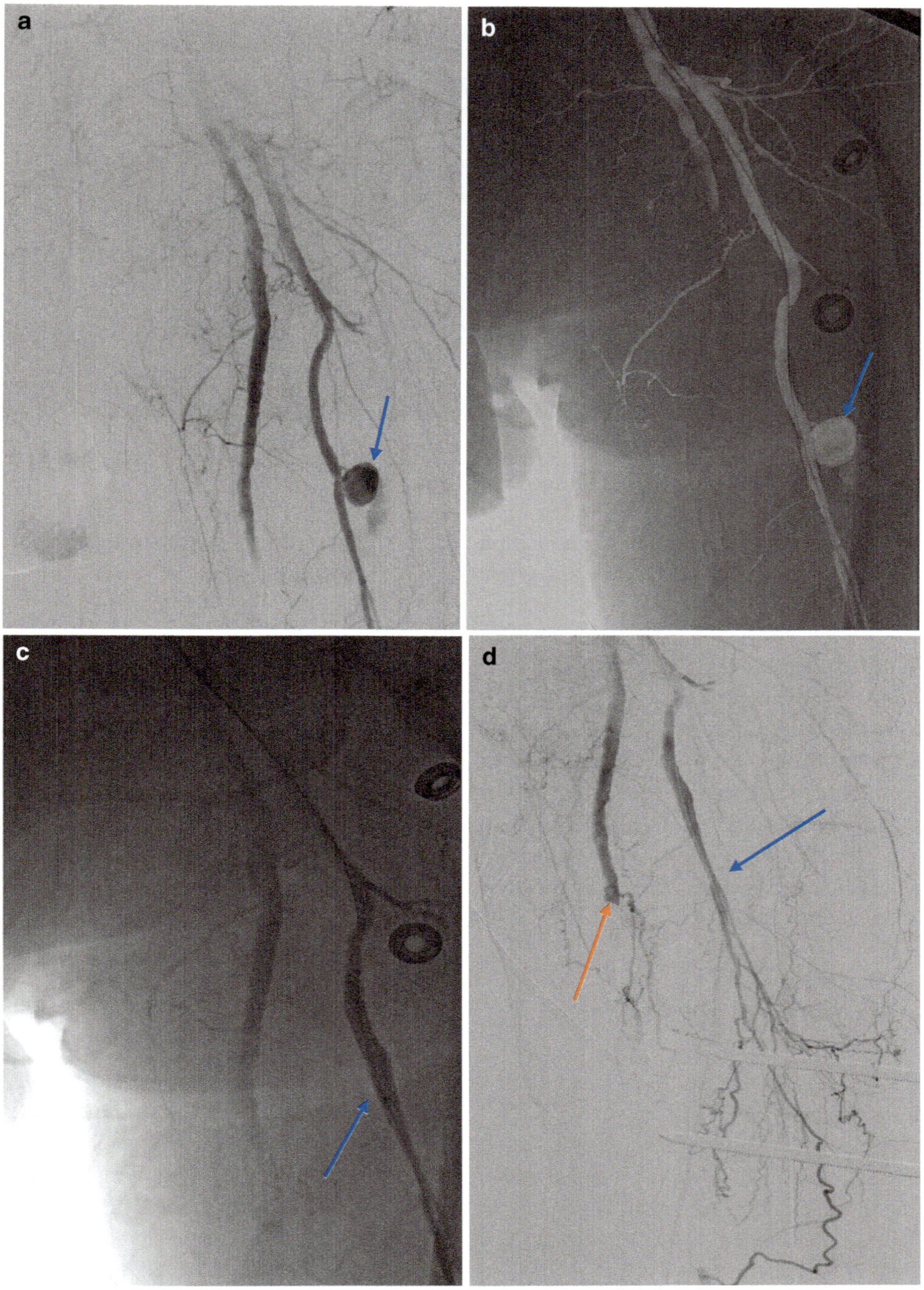

Fig. 6.13 Crossover angiography confirmed the left deep femoral artery pseudoaneurysm-(blue arrows) (**a**, **b**). Deployment of a 5 mm × 38 mm balloon-expandable led to a satisfactory result- (blue arrows) (**c**, **d**). Orange arrow indicates the occluded superficial femoral artery

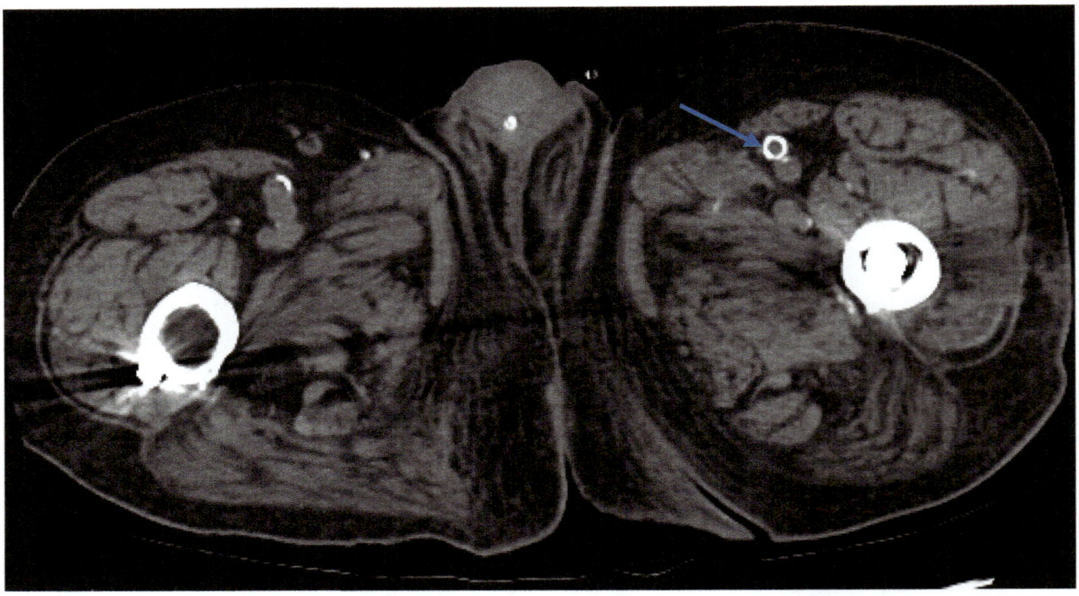

Fig. 6.14 Non–contrast-enhanced CT scan after orthopaedic femoral surgery. Resorption of the haematoma was observed, and the stent was deployed in deep femoral artery (arrow)

arterial spasm due to manipulation with multiple materials. A bolus of 5000 IU heparin was given.

6.4.4 Outcome

The patient underwent orthopaedic surgery afterwards and gradually recovered. There were no complications during the surgery and no ischaemic complications or worsening symptoms involving the left leg. A control non–contrast-enhanced CT scan 3 months later showed resorption of the haematoma (Fig. 6.14).

6.5 Femoral Artery-II

Key Points

- In elderly, multimorbid patients, we sometimes need to "think outside the box" and combine treatment options.
- Ultrasound-guided direct thrombin injection is a useful technique.
- Limb EVAR can be performed in cases of a dilated femoral artery.

6.5.1 Aetiology and Clinical Presentation

An 87-year-old patient presented with cardiac insufficiency and an ejection fraction of 15%. Right crural leg amputation was performed due to a right popliteal aneurysm and distal embolization. The patient was living alone and receiving help from the community. The patient was admitted to the emergency department after the size of the left femoral region and pain began increasing. The patient explained that the left leg started to increase in size after a fall from the bed. The patient did not seek immediate help after the event. There was no critical ischaemia in the left leg.

6.5.2 Pre-interventional Diagnosis

Contrast-enhanced CT angiography showed a large pseudoaneurysm of the left superficial femoral artery (Fig. 6.15). Generally, the femoral artery was dilated and calcified. The popliteal artery had stenosis and calcifications. The tibial arteries were patent but with multifocal stenosis and calcifications.

6.5.3 Endovascular Treatment

The left femoral artery was percutaneously punctured anterogradely, and a Proglide preclosure suture was deployed. A stiff 180 mm-long guidewire was advanced into the femoral artery down to the popliteal artery, taking care not to dislodge some plaques. A self-expandable stent graft 12 mm in diameter and 120 mm in length was advanced and deployed, starting from the proximal popliteal segment. After that, two self-expandable stents 13.5 m in diameter and 80 mm in length were used proximally to cover the pseudoaneurysm (Fig. 6.16). Control angiography confirmed the well-deployed stent grafts but remnant flow into the pseudoaneurysm due to insufficient stent graft oversizing. Ultrasound-guided percutaneous puncture directly into the pseudoaneurysm was performed, and 1 mL of 1000 IU human thrombin was administered into the pseudoaneurysm. The intervention produced no complications. There was no more pulsatile flow through the pseudoaneurysm. A bolus of 5000 IU heparin was given.

6.5.4 Outcome

The patient did not develop any ischaemic complications in the left leg, and no worsening was noted. Control Doppler ultrasound showed no flow through the pseudoaneurysm (Fig. 6.17). The patient was discharged from the hospital 3 days after the intervention.

6.6 Popliteal Artery

Key Points

- Familiarity with some thrombectomy devices is important.
- The absolute and relative contraindications for thrombolysis should be checked.
- Compartment syndrome should be considered.
- Urine output measurement is essential for acute limb ischaemia patients after revascularization.

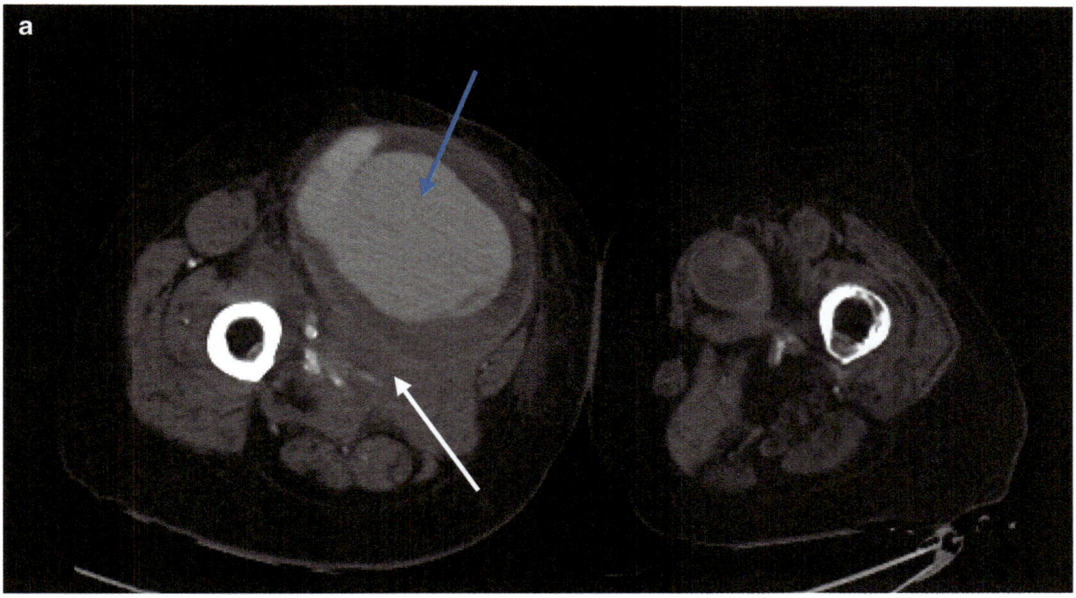

Fig. 6.15 CT angiography showing an 8 cm femoral artery pseudoaneurysm-(blue arrows) and haematoma around the pseudoaneurysm- (white arrows) (**a**, **b**). The proximal femoral and superficial arteries measured 13–14 mm on average and 10 mm distally (**c**)

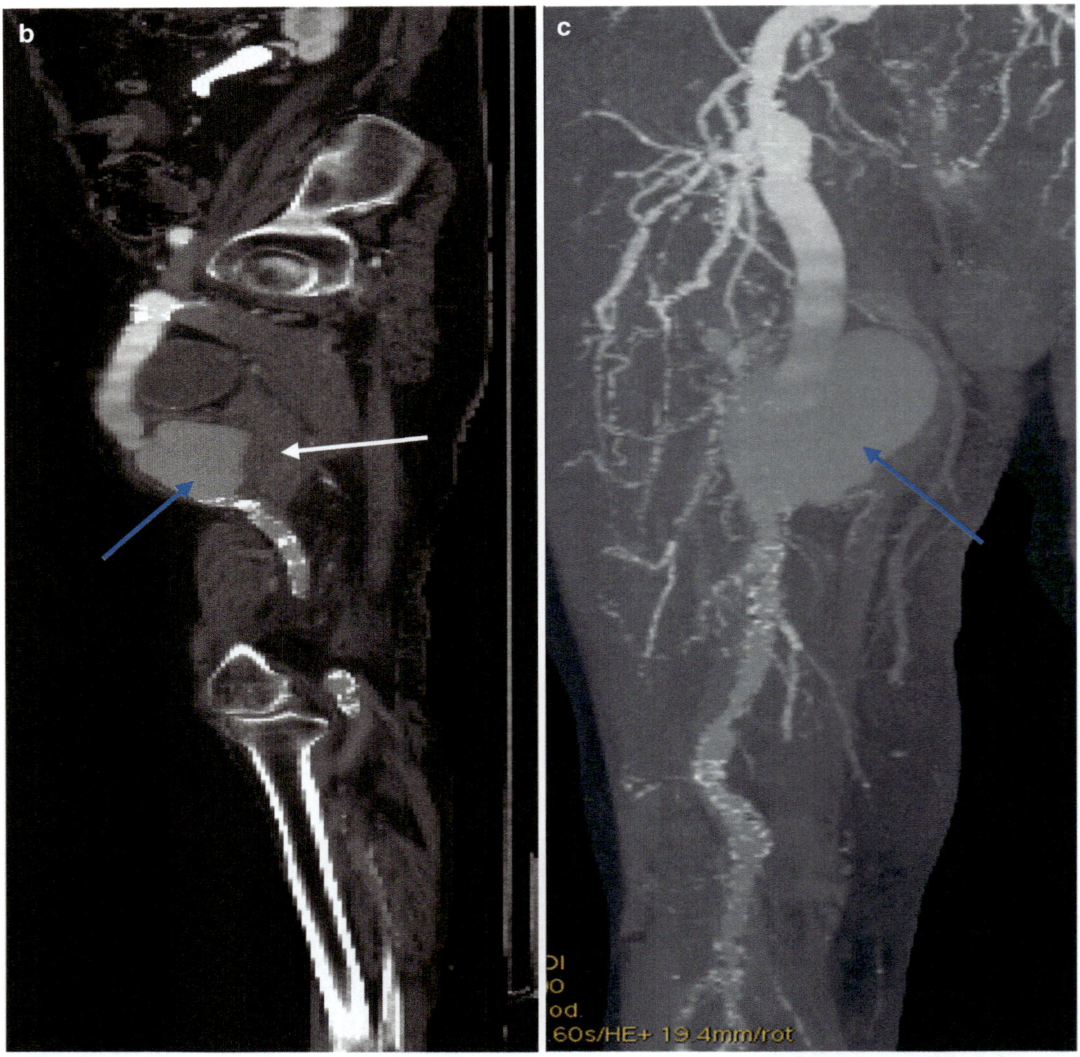

Fig. 6.15 (continued)

6.6.1 Aetiology and Clinical Presentation

A 67-year-old patient with intermittent claudication was treated with angioplasty and stent deployment in a superficial femoral artery 1 year prior. The patient was admitted with acute onset of left leg pain and changes in left foot sensitivity. There was a pulse in the left femoral artery but not in the distal portion. There was no audible Doppler arterial signal at the ankle level. The patient had been taking acetylsalicylic acid and statins.

6.6.2 Pre-interventional Diagnosis

Acute contrast-enhanced CT scanning was performed and showed a thrombosed left superficial femoral stent and occlusion of the popliteal artery (Fig. 6.18). The patient had a threatened viable left limb, and after a heparin bolus injection,

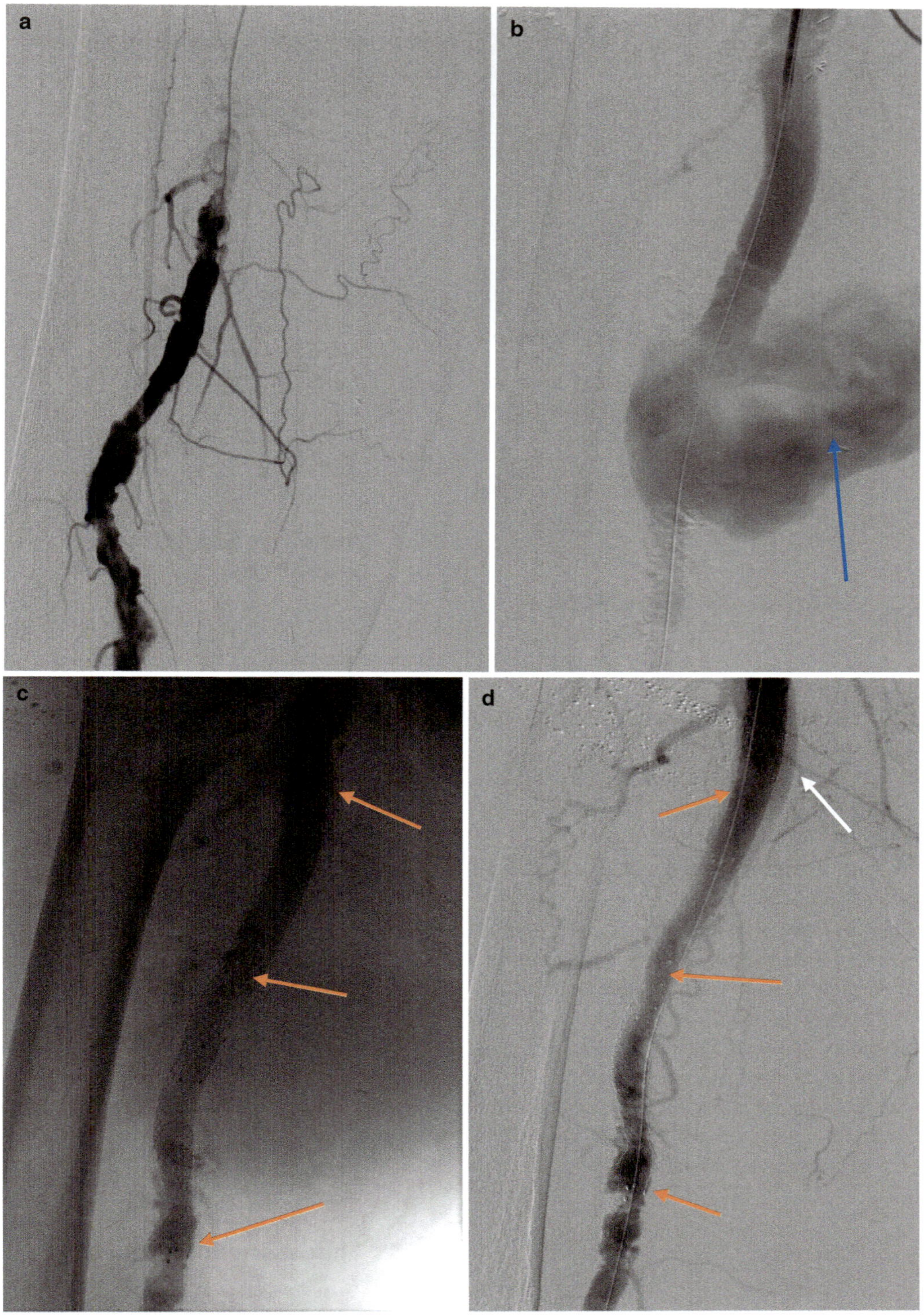

Fig. 6.16 First, a 12 mm-diameter and 120 mm-long stent graft was deployed distally (**a**, **b**). After that, two stent grafts measuring 13.5 mm in diameter and 80 mm in length were placed proximally (**c**, **d**). Finally, ultrasound-guided direct pseudoaneurysm puncture and thrombin injection were performed. Blue arrow indicates the pseudoaneurysm. Orange arrows indicate the stent grafts, and the white arrow in panel D shows remnant flow around the stent graft proximally due to the widely dilated femoral arteries

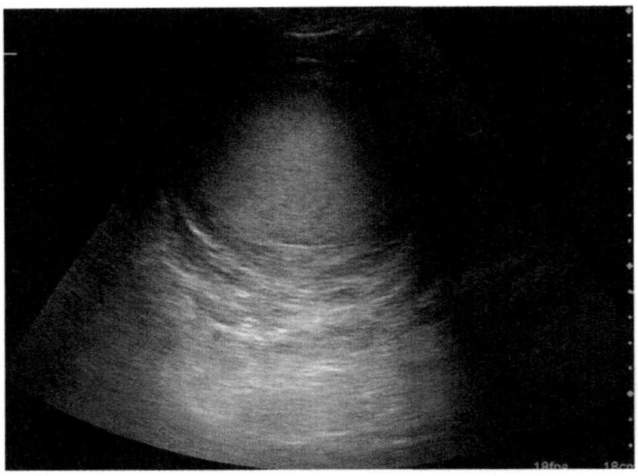

Fig. 6.17 Control Doppler ultrasound showing no flow through the completely thrombosed pseudoaneurysm following the thrombin injection

thrombolysis was scheduled. Poor filling had led to the occlusive changes of the crural vessels.

6.6.3 Endovascular Intervention

The right femoral artery was percutaneously punctured, and crossover recanalization of the occluded superficial artery was performed very quickly. A thrombolysis catheter was advanced over the wire, and local thrombolysis with 0.5 mg/h tissue plasminogen activator was performed (Fig. 6.19).

The next day, control angiography revealed an excellent result and almost complete thrombus resolution. There was tight in-stent stenosis that was treated with deployment of a new stent 6 mm in diameter (Fig. 6.20). The in-stent stenosis was probably the reason for the thrombosis. Control angiography showed distal embolization and occlusion of the popliteal artery again.

An Angiojet thrombectomy device was used for acute thrombectomy and thrombus aspiration (Fig. 6.21) with an excellent outcome.

6.6.4 Outcome

The patient regained sensitivity of the left foot, and the Doppler signal was audible. Motor function was not impaired. The patient did not experience bleeding complications during the thrombolysis.

6.7 Crural Arteries

Key Points

- Simple peripheral angioplasty can be complicated with distal embolization.
- Distal vessel patency should always be checked.
- Familiarization with some thrombectomy devices is recommended.

6.7.1 Aetiology and Clinical Presentation

A 55-year-old patient with known intermittent claudication complained of shortening of the claudication distance to approximately 100 m on the right side. The patient had been active and had reduced quality of life. The ankle-brachial index (ABI) was 55%. There was no femoral pulse on the right side. No other diseases were present. The patient was a smoker and had hyperlipidaemia treated with 75 mg acetylsalicylic acid and 40 mg atorvastatin.

6.7.2 Pre-interventional Diagnosis

Contrast-enhanced magnetic resonance angiography (MRI) was performed. MRI showed occlusion of the right external iliac artery and anterior tibial artery (Fig. 6.22). The other arteries were patent.

6.7.3 Endovascular Treatment

The right femoral artery was percutaneously punctured. The occluded external iliac artery was recanalized, and two balloon-expandable stents 6 and 7 mm in diameter and 59 mm in length were deployed. Control angiography showed a satisfactory result (Fig. 6.23).

The patient complained the same day about pain in the right leg and an absent femoral pulse again. CT angiography showed a thrombosed external iliac artery and stent (Fig. 6.24). The patient received therapeutic doses of heparin and was scheduled for re-intervention the next day. There was no motor function impairment of the right leg. The right femoral artery

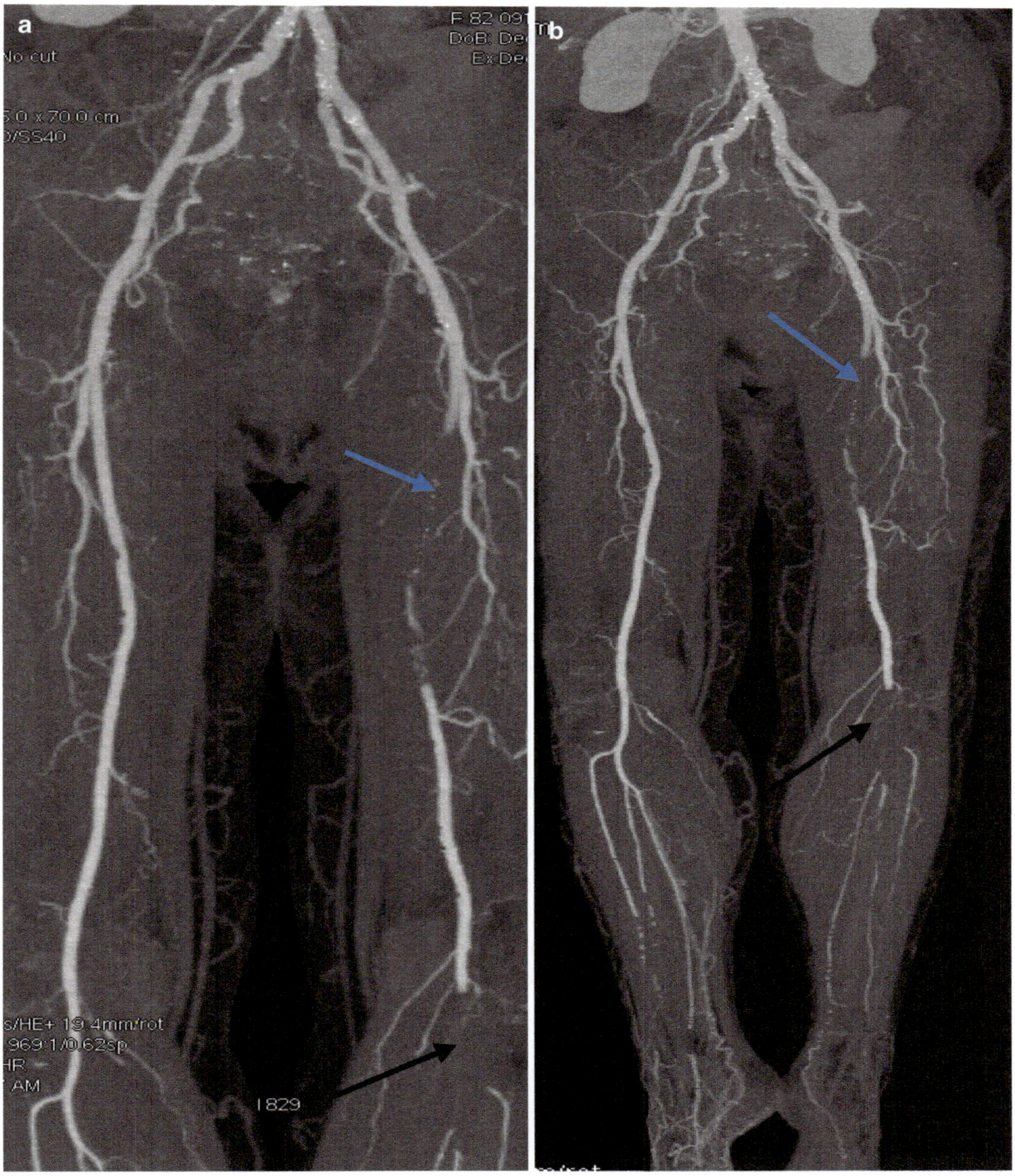

Fig. 6.18 CT angiography showing the thrombosed stent in the left femoral and superficial artery-(blue arrows). The left popliteal artery was occluded (black arrow), and poor filing of the crural arteries was evident

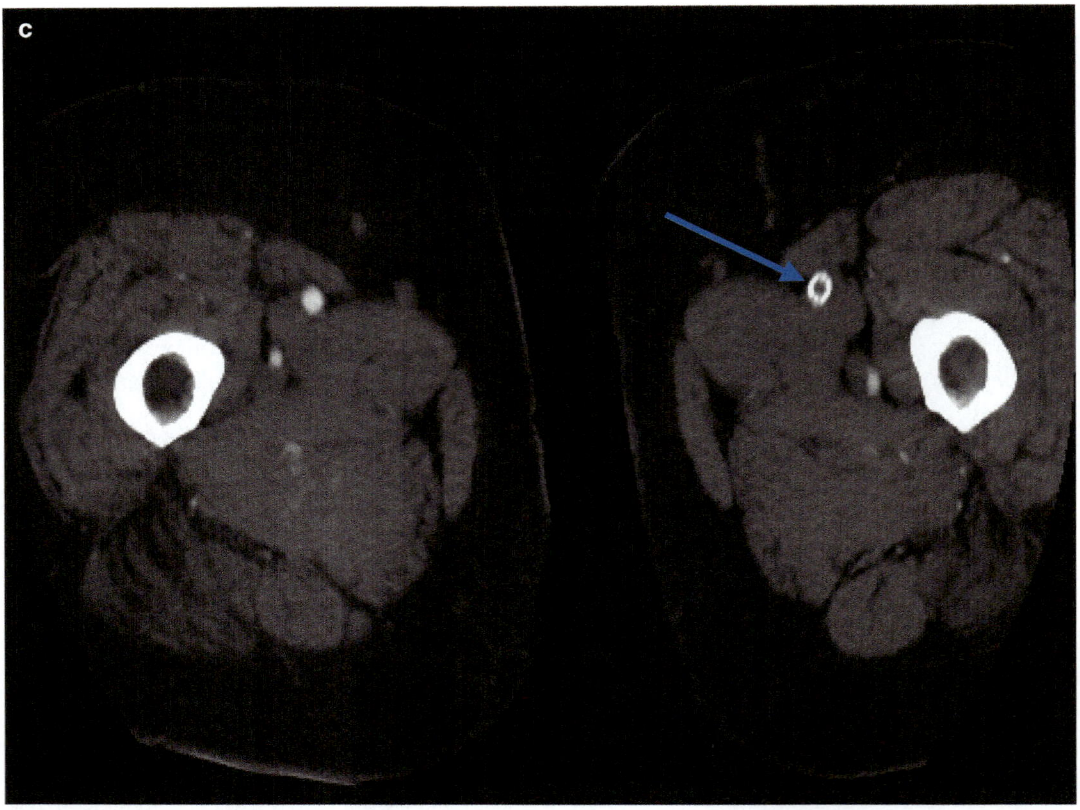

Fig. 6.18 (continued)

was punctured. The occluded stent was recanalized, and an additional stent was deployed proximally, extending into the common iliac artery. After that, two new balloon-expandable stents were used, and control angiography showed satisfactory results (Fig. 6.25). Control angiography of the popliteal and tibial arteries revealed distal embolization and occlusion of the tibioperoneal trunk that had been open before (Fig. 6.26). The left femoral artery was percutaneously punctured. The crossover technique was performed over the guidewire to advance a Penumbra aspiration thrombectomy system into the tibioperoneal trunk. After confirmation that the tip of the aspiration catheter was inside the thrombus and there was no retrograde flow, aspiration was started. It lasted approximately 2 min, and the entire thrombus was successfully removed. Control angiography after the thrombectomy showed a patent tibioperoneal trunk and posterior tibial and peroneal arteries (Fig. 6.27).

6.7.4 Outcome

The patient did not experience any complications. The posterior tibial artery pulse was present, and the ABI increased to 80%. There was no compartment syndrome of the tibial muscles. The patient was discharged from the hospital 2 days after the intervention.

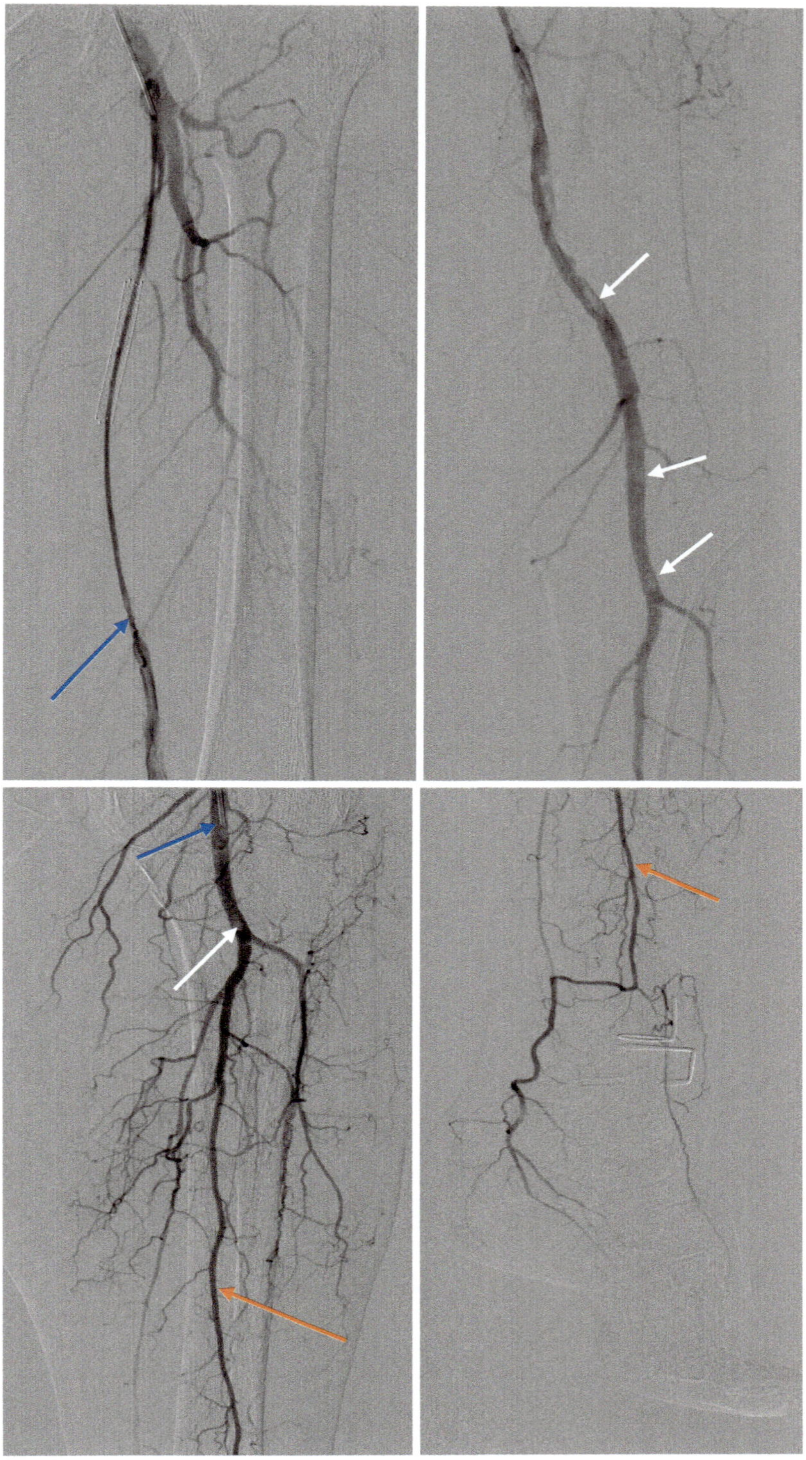

Fig. 6.19 A guidewire very easily crossed the thrombus, and a thrombolysis catheter was advanced (blue arrow). Local thrombolysis was initiated. There was some remnant thrombus in the patent popliteal artery (white arrow). The peroneal artery was the only patent crural artery (orange arrow)

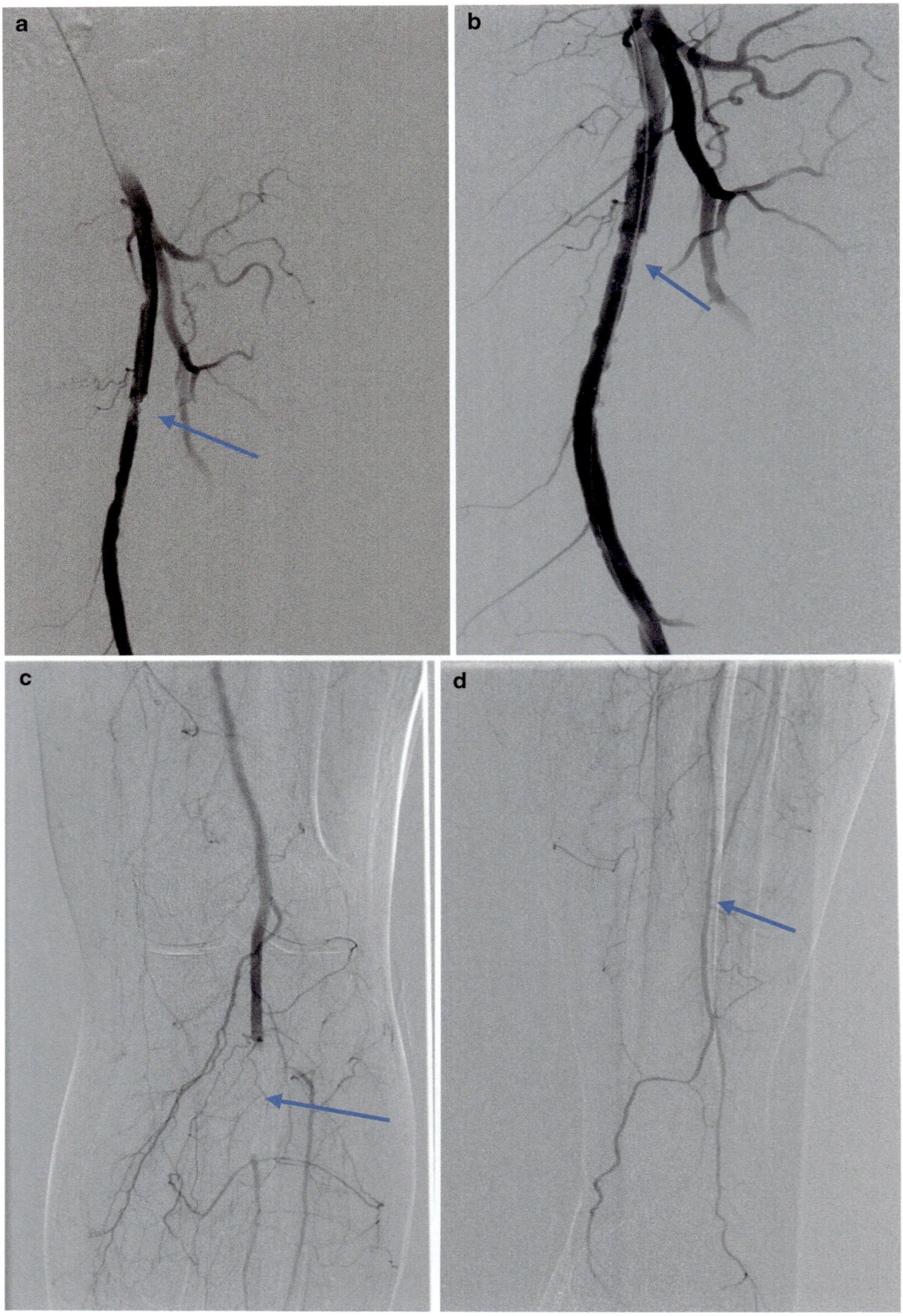

Fig. 6.20 (**a**) In-stent stenosis (arrow). (**b**) Deployment of a new stent showing a good result (arrow). (**c**) Distal embolization and popliteal artery occlusion (arrow). (**d**) Patent peroneal artery-(arrow)

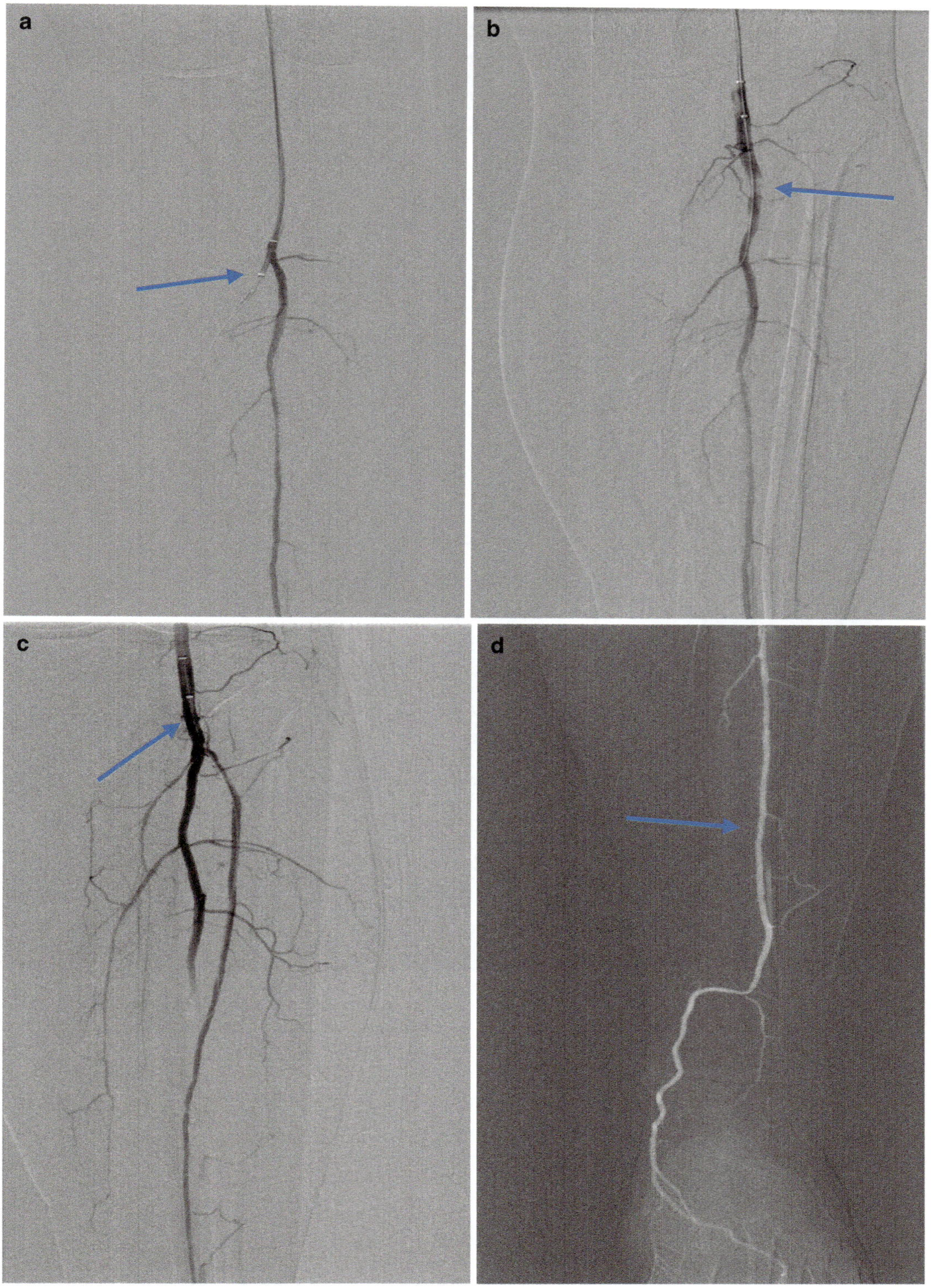

Fig. 6.21 Acute thrombectomy of the left popliteal artery. (**a**) Angiojet catheter advanced into the popliteal artery (arrow). (**b**) residual thrombus-(arrow). (**c**) control angiography after the repeat thrombectomy. (**d**) patent peroneal artery showing no distal embolization

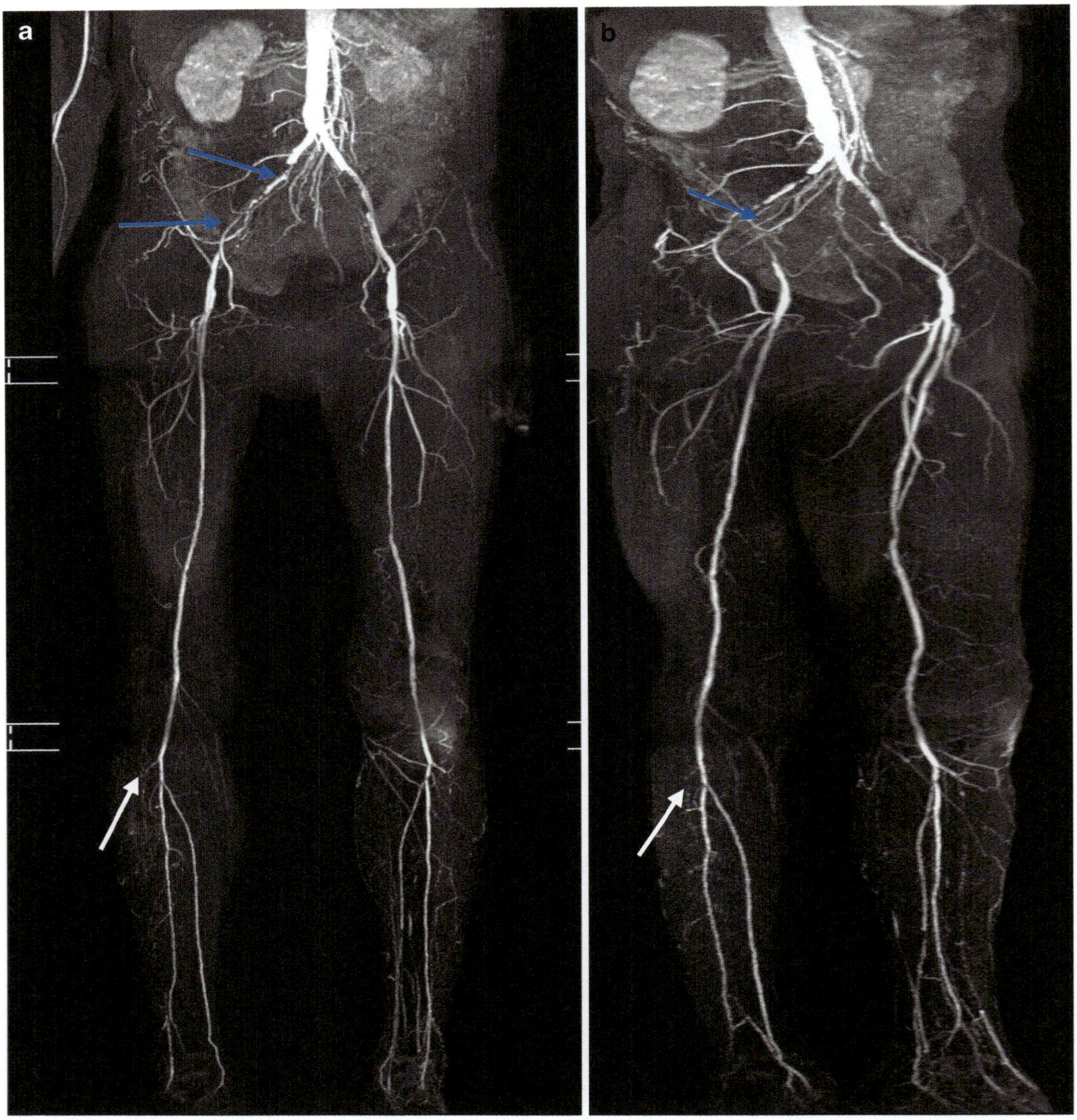

Fig. 6.22 Contrast-enhanced MR angiography showing occlusion of the right external iliac artery (blue arrows). The femoral, popliteal and truncus tibiofibular arteries on the right side are patent. The anterior tibial artery on the right side is occluded (white arrows). The posterior tibial and peroneal arteries are patent

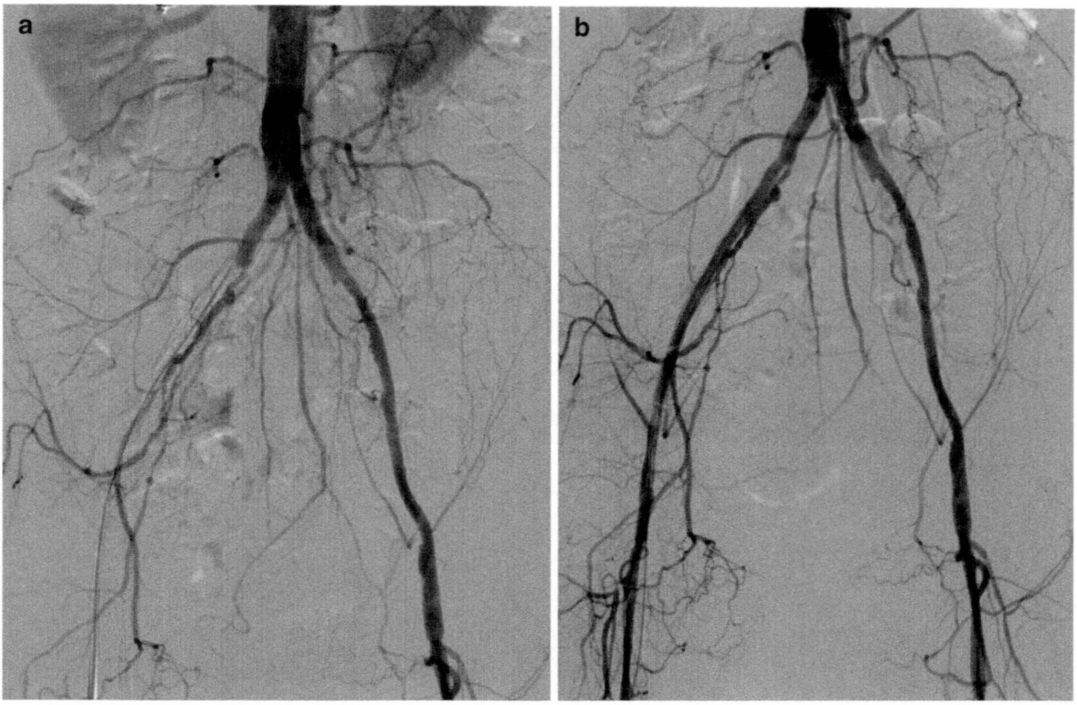

Fig. 6.23 (**a**) Recanalization of the occluded artery. (**b**) Control angiography after deployment of the 7 and 6 mm-diameter, 59 mm-long balloon-expandible stents

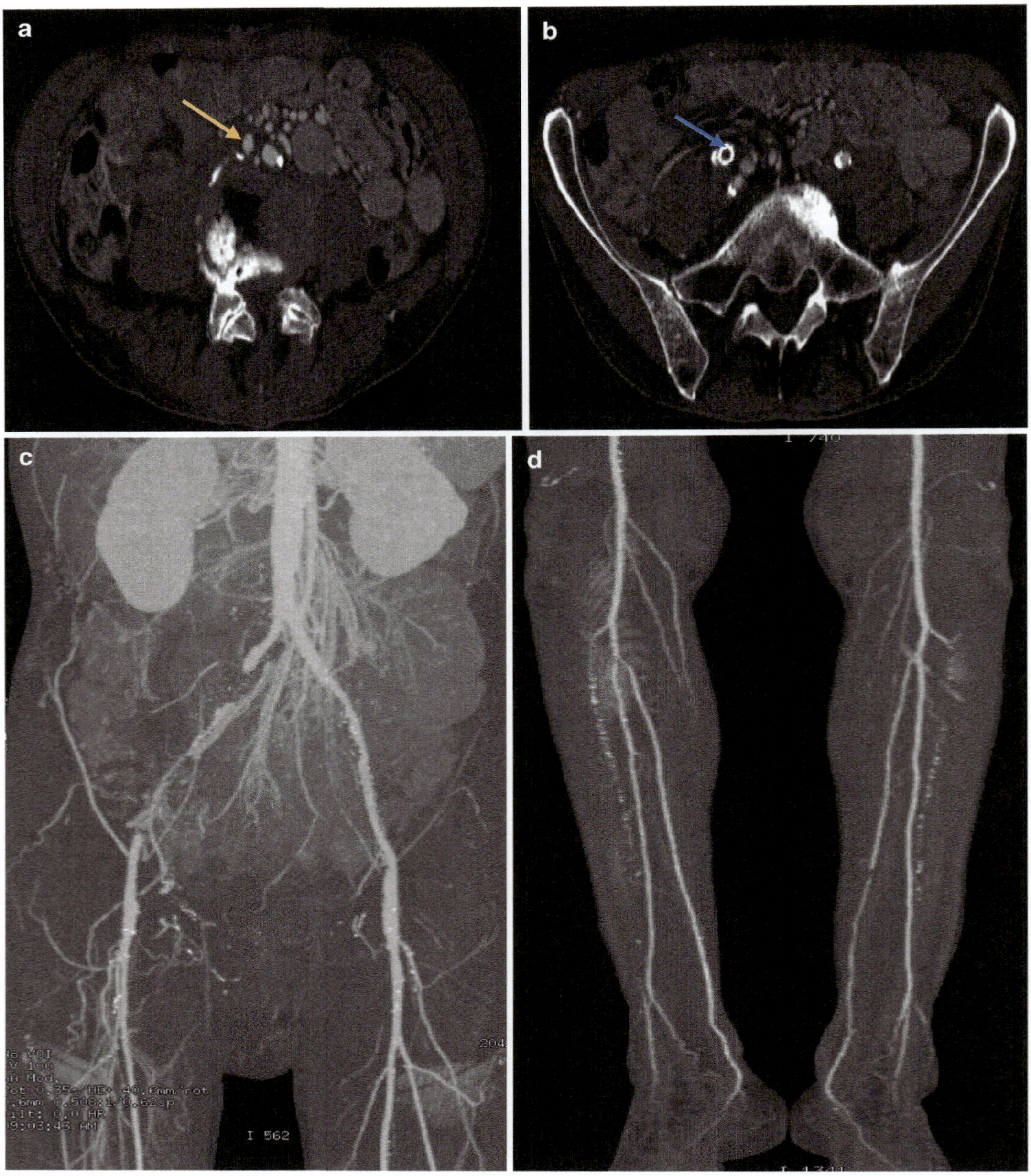

Fig. 6.24 Control CT showing a thrombosed stent and right external iliac artery (blue arrow). Yellow arrow indicates a patent right common iliac artery with approximately 50% stenosis. There was no distal peripheral embolization on CT angiography

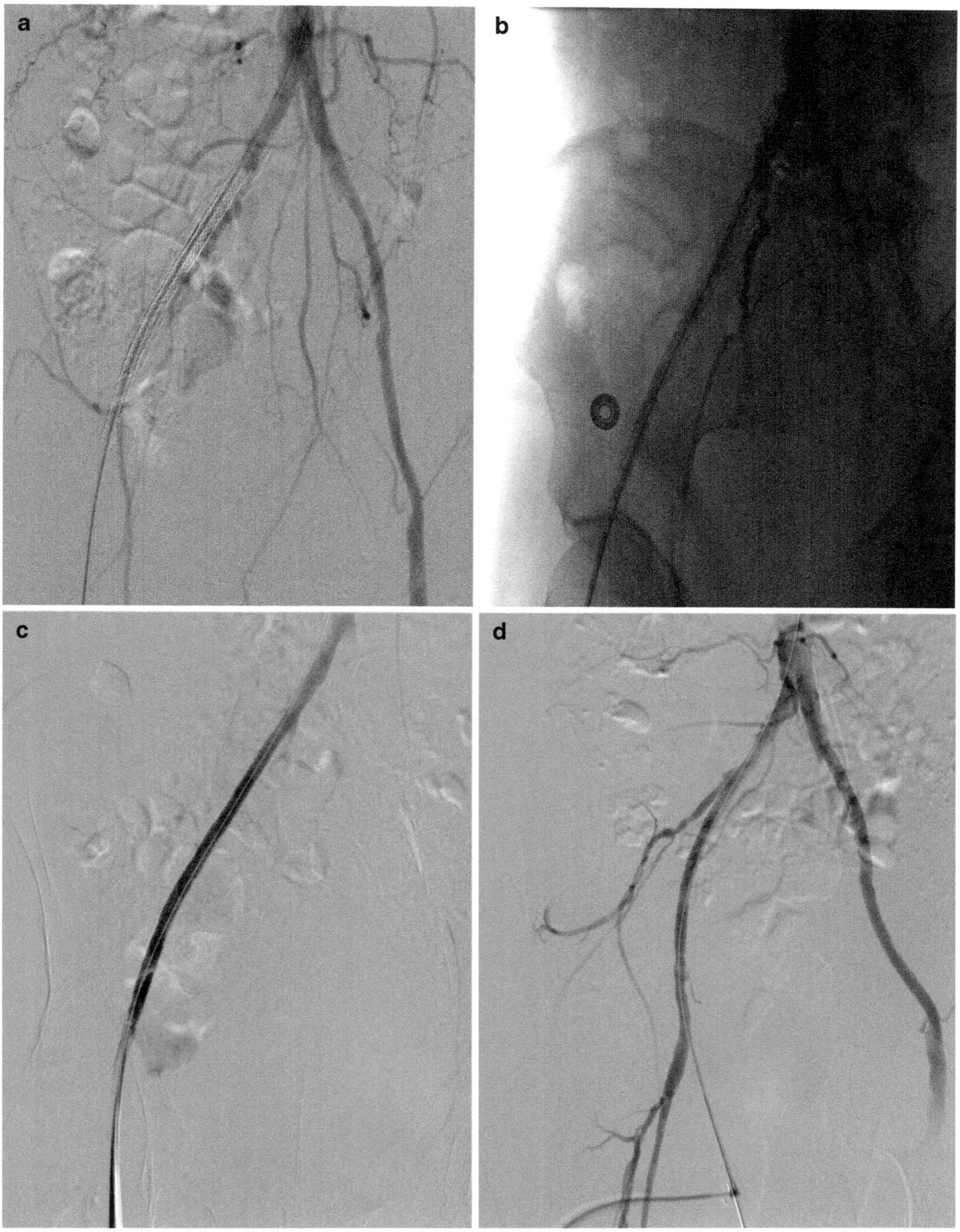

Fig. 6.25 A new percutaneous intervention with recanalization of the thrombosed stent. Control angiography after deployment of the new stent showed a good result and no residual stenosis or thrombus

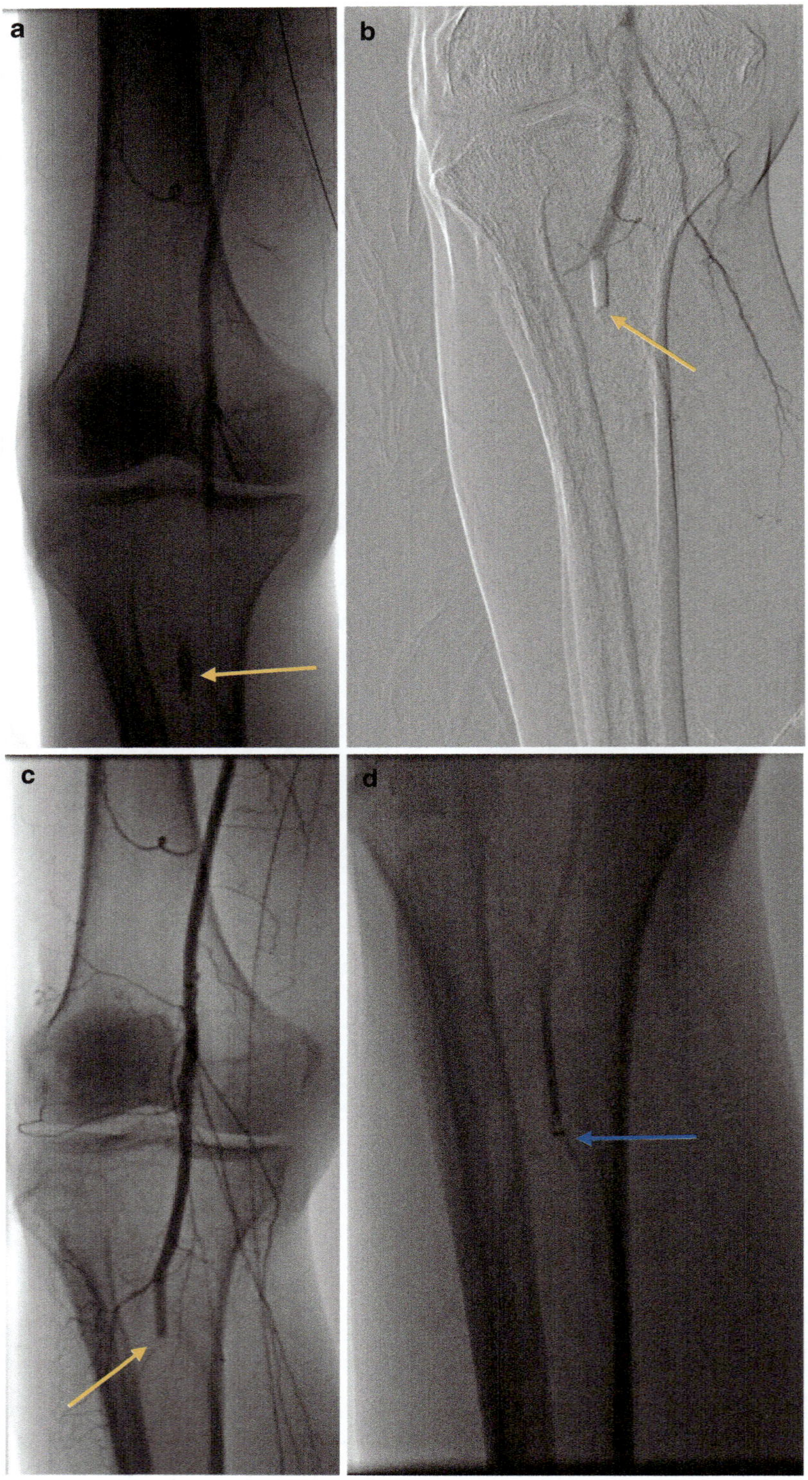

Fig. 6.26 Control angiography showed distal embolization and occlusion of the tibioperoneal trunk (yellow arrows). The aspiration thrombectomy catheter was advanced via the crossover technique and placed inside the thrombus. Blue arrow indicates the tip of the 6 Fr aspiration catheter

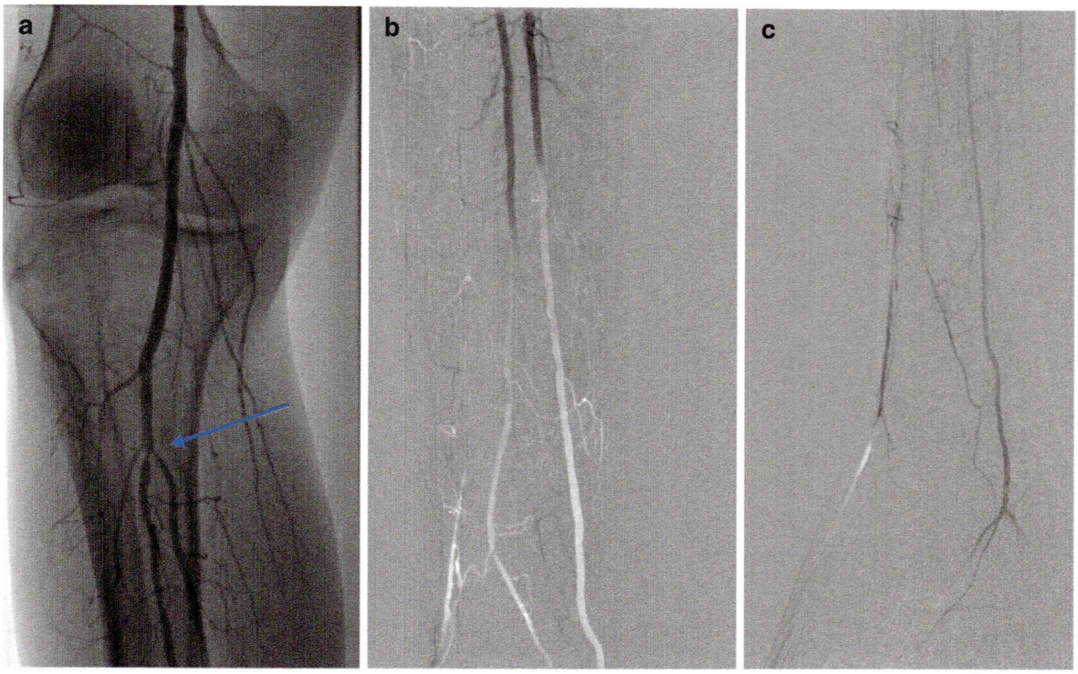

Fig. 6.27 Control angiography after aspiration thrombectomy showing a satisfactory result and complete thrombus removal. Blue arrow indicates a patent tibioperoneal trunk with some spasm. Both the posterior tibial and peroneal arteries were patent and without distal thrombi

GPSR Compliance

The European Union's (EU) General Product Safety Regulation (GPSR) is a set of rules that requires consumer products to be safe and our obligations to ensure this.

If you have any concerns about our products, you can contact us on ProductSafety@springernature.com

In case Publisher is established outside the EU, the EU authorized representative is:

Springer Nature Customer Service Center GmbH
Europaplatz 3
69115 Heidelberg, Germany

Batch number: 09224018

Printed by Printforce, the Netherlands